THE SC  N

T

Founded by C. K. Ogden

The International Library of Psychology

GENERAL PSYCHOLOGY
In 38 Volumes

THE SCIENCES OF MAN IN THE MAKING

An Orientation Book

EDWIN A KIRKPATRICK

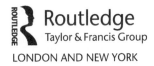

LONDON AND NEW YORK

First published in 1932 by
Routledge, Trench, Trubner & Co., Ltd.

2 Park Square, Milton Park, Abingdon, Oxfordshire OX14 4RN
711 Third Avenue, New York, NY 10017

First issued in paperback 2014

Routledge is an imprint of the Taylor and Francis Group, an informa business

British Library Cataloguing in Publication Data
A CIP catalogue record for this book
is available from the British Library

The Sciences of Man in the Making
ISBN 0415-21029-1
General Psychology: 38 Volumes
ISBN 0415-21129-8
The International Library of Psychology: 204 Volumes
ISBN 0415-19132-7

ISBN 13: 978-1-138-88248-5 (pbk)
ISBN 13: 978-0-415-21029-4 (hbk)

PREFACE

FROM a mountain-top the significant features of an extensive region may be seen better than when one is exploring a single forest or plain. Excursions into various parts, however, give a clearer understanding of what has been viewed from the mountain top. To present a complete geography of man's nature and activities in a single volume is impossible. To give abstracts only, would be uninteresting and useless. The author makes no claim to universal knowledge, but assumes to act merely as a guide in revealing some of the general truths regarding man and his place in nature, and in illustrating the methods of research employed in the various sciences of man. Without the use of extended description, exact definition, or technical terms, he hopes to give a fairly clear concept of each of these sciences, the investigations by which they are being developed, and their relationship to each other.

In most of the chapters the aim is to give in an untechnical way, some of the interesting and useful truths that have been revealed by man's study of himself individually and collectively ; while in the first chapter and in the selected researches following each of the chapters, the intention is to give an idea of scientific methods and the ways in which they are being used to study human nature and behaviour.

For several decades the author has been gleaning in many fields for his personal satisfaction in getting a broad basis for understanding human conduct. When recently he decided to organize the results of this reading into a book of the type just described, he first wrote what seemed to him most significant in the various fields ; then studied the recent literature to make sure that his presentation was in accord with the truths accepted by scientists of today ; and later spent considerable time in selecting examples of research to illustrate the scientific methods being used in each field. It was difficult to find studies that were typical, non-technical, and brief enough to be used in a book of this kind. In psychology the abundance of material made selection particularly hard ; while in such subjects as economics and sociology, objective studies, though not so numerous, were frequently long and technical.

It is the author's desire that the book be useful to intelligent men and women in, and outside of institutions of learning. Having been prepared by one man this book has the advantage of greater unity of treatment than is possible in books written by several specialists. It is hoped that the chapters on the relations of science to ethics and religion will assist in orienting the readers who are questioning whether conflict is inevitable.

The references given at the close of each chapter have been carefully selected from recent literature giving facts rather than theories.

The author is under deep obligation to scientists and publishers who have so kindly given permission to quote from articles and books, and to his wife, whose literary judgment and library training have been constantly helpful.

E. A. K.

December 1931.

CONTENTS

CHAPTER I

NATURE AND METHODS OF SCIENCE

CHAPTER II

MAN AS AN INHABITANT OF THE EARTH

CHAPTER III

VARIETIES OF HUMAN SPECIES AND THEIR MODES OF LIVING, OR ANTHROPOLOGY AND ETHNOLOGY

CHAPTER IV

HOW LIFE IS PRESERVED, OR PHYSIOLOGY AND HYGIENE

CHAPTER V

IMPROVING THE HUMAN SPECIES, OR EUGENICS AND EUTHENICS

CHAPTER VI

AVOIDING WASTE, OR ECONOMICS

CONTENTS

Chapter VIII
HOW MAN BEHAVES, OR GENERAL PSYCHOLOGY

Chapter IX
PERSONALITY DIFFERENCES, OR INDIVIDUAL PSYCHOLOGY
I.—PERSONALITY

II.—MENTAL HYGIENE

CHAPTER X

BEHAVIOUR IN RELATION TO OTHERS, OR
SOCIAL PSYCHOLOGY

CONTENTS

THE SCIENCES OF MAN IN THE MAKING

Chapter I

NATURE AND METHODS OF SCIENCE

VARIETIES OF KNOWLEDGE

IF you drop the penny you hold into the water it will sink, but if you drop a chip in, it will float. If you keep that cat under water he will drown, but if you keep this fish out of water he will die. Almost any child of school age knows these facts, but is such knowledge scientific ?

The first essential of scientific knowledge is that it shall be classified in such a way that an assertion may be made of all members of a group instead of one or two. When a child can think in general terms that all objects made of metal will sink in water, and all wooden objects will float, his knowledge is becoming scientific in an elementary way. In proportion as such knowledge becomes accurate, does its scientific character increase. All objects heavier than water sink, while those lighter than water float, is more accurate as well as more general than the preceding assertion.

The statement is not accurate, however, unless we add that in order that objects heavier than water shall sink, their shape must be such that the amount of water displaced weighs less than the object. If this were not the case steel ships would not float.

A moment's thought will show that the above general statements imply measurements of size and weight. This is one of the essentials of accurate scientific knowledge. The primitive mode of thinking which classifies as heavy or light, old or young, living or dead, intelligent or stupid, good or bad, etc., is being changed into quantitative statements, such as—the object is lighter or heavier than an equal bulk of water at the same temperature ; or still more definitely, its specific gravity is ·97 or 1·31. In age the person or animal is so many tenths as old in years as the average age attained by members of the species in the same environment ; or the bony structure of the wrist is 89 per cent. of the size of that of the average adult, or contains 91 per cent. as much mineral matter. This animal is dead in the sense that the vital organs, heart and lungs, are 100 per cent. non-functioning ; but 98 per cent. of the cells of which the body is composed are still alive. This man is good because he did right 99 times in a hundred when there were chances to be dishonest in a certain way, whereas the average for his companions is 71.

From these examples we see that the more scientifically accurate knowledge becomes, the more must its truths be expressed in mathematical terms. Mathematics uses the most accurate of language symbols, hence mathematical terms are generally employed to express truth with exactness. The statement that all men are born with two legs and all horses with four, is practically correct and reasonably scientific, yet not absolutely accurate since a fractional per cent. are born with a different number. The per cents. having an unusual number of ribs, vertebræ or teeth are considerably greater. To be accurate, classes must be so definite in the characteristics implied that the assertions of what is true of members of the class must hold for all but a negligibly small number of individuals, or there must be a numerical statement of the per cent. of cases in which any given statement holds true ; e.g. All full-blooded negroes are musical, or of a thousand full-blooded negroes between six and sixteen years of age tested, only one was tone deaf in the sense of being unable to distinguish between notes c and d.

No sharp line can be drawn between scientific and unscientific knowledge, but it is clear that the percentage of truths in our text-books which can be expressed in mathematical terms is much higher in physics and chemistry, than in botany or zoology, and very much higher than in economics or history, while those that can be so expressed in literature and other arts are few or unimportant.

Knowledge may, however, be of great value when it is not possible to express it with a definiteness which would justify its being called scientific. The knowledge of harmony gained by an experienced painter or musician may be of far greater value for artistic purposes than the more scientific formulations of physicists and psychologists as to what wave-lengths of light or sound correspond to the various colours and pitches perceived by means of the eye and the ear. In general, knowledge that is of practical and artistic value is likely to be gained regarding all sorts of things and situations before any knowledge worthy of the name scientific has been formulated. Not until scientific knowledge of common objects and situations has become extensive and definite does it correct, supplement and largely displace the less accurate knowledge gained by incidental experience in industry and art. Only within the last century has scientific knowledge come to play a large part in manufacturing, mining and agriculture ; and still more recently in the promotion of social welfare and the reproduction of things artistic.

Science is concerned not only with accurate definitions and classifications but with sequences. It assumes that objects and events are related to each other in such a way that when the combinations are the same the same results will follow as in previous cases. It is the problem of science to determine what things are of the same type, and all the conditions involved in the sequences of events. The solution of its problems is chiefly a matter of the accurate use of methods of checking the similarity and identity of objects, conditions and events by observation and experiment.

SCIENTIFIC KNOWLEDGE NOT ABSOLUTE AND UNCHANGEABLE

Science makes no attempt to gain absolute knowledge but only to discover relations between experiences. If no serious mistake has been made in the facts classified and their relations to each other, the supposed truths of science are never entirely contradicted, but the facts are always subject to more accurate determination, making possible more exact classifications or numerical statements, and simpler formulation. Every new discovery prepares the way for such further advances.

Incidental to this normal progress in knowledge, there are changes produced by examining new facts and by new theories as to general relations which may seem simpler and more satisfactory to the human mind. Extensive observation in the early history of the West and South made it certain that people living in the lowlands were afflicted with malaria more than those inhabiting the uplands. This knowledge was sufficiently general to be classed as rudimentarily scientific. The theory that the disease was caused by the moist " malarial air " seemed to fit the facts, and was in accord with other beliefs as to the part played by air in the production of diseases. Later investigations have proved that germs are the cause of many diseases, and that they are usually passed from one animal or person to another, not by means of the air but by contact. It has been demonstrated that the germs of malaria are carried from one person to another by mosquitoes. This seems quite contradictory to the original " scientific " truth. Yet the original generalization that malaria is more prevalent in the wet lowlands (unchanged by man) is as true as ever. The relation of these facts, however, is now seen differently, and explained by another and largely contradictory theory. It is not the moist air, but the little pools where mosquitoes breed, that is the significant connection of the disease with the lowlands. The disease is transmitted, not by breathing malarial air, but by the bite of a mosquito which has previously bitten a diseased individual.

The theory, now so generally accepted, that malaria and many other diseases are produced by microbes, may conceivably be replaced sometime by the view that in many cases the germs are not the cause of the disease, but the results or accompaniments of it. The scientific truth would then be differently formulated, yet the essential truth of the usual close relation between many diseases and germs, would not be contradicted.

Whenever anyone asserts that a truth of the relation of certain kinds of facts to other facts is absolutely and unchangeably true, he is making a rash statement never justified by the canons of science. All that a scientist can consistently say is, that in the light of known facts and general truths, a given statement is scientifically justified. With more accurate observations and measurements and with the study of hitherto unobserved facts, the truth is likely to need restatement. Science simply uses the best-known methods of studying causes, conditions and results, and of formulating truths and verifying them by further observation and experiment.

In a deductive and logical science like mathematics, certain definitions are given and assumptions made, and from these truths may be formulated that never change, *e.g.* " the whole is equal to the sum of its parts " and " things equal to the same thing are equal to each other." These will always be true when space, time and number are conceived in the same way ; but in the objective world with which science deals, these truths hold only to a limited extent. The sum of the bricks of which a house is composed is not the same as the pile of bricks from which it is made ; nor is a house the same as another composed of an equal number of bricks.

Given certain assumptions, mathematical and philosophical truths may be logically educed ; but the way in which things behave can never be discovered by such means. Water and many other substances contract when cooled, and logically should continue to grow smaller with increased cold, but observation and measurement show that after a certain temperature is reached, water stops contracting and expands as its temperature falls, and then changes into the form of solid ice. We cannot tell by mere logical thinking how objects will act under new conditions, but they must be observed in order to find out. Not only this, but any truth formulated is based upon observations made, and care must be exercised in formulating what will be true in future experiences. Under certain conditions water remains a fluid, and one noting the fact without considering the conditions would naturally and logically say that water *always* remains a fluid ; but when conditions are taken into account it is discovered that water may become either solid or gaseous according to temperature conditions.   This indicates the limits of inductive science. It must be based upon a sufficient number of known facts, but is always subject to change when new or more accurately measured facts are acquired.   The fundamental assumption of science is that we can judge of the unexamined and of future events, only by extensive study of similar things under similar conditions.   Any object such as iron will always have the same essential characteristics that have been observed under ordinary conditions of temperature, etc., but what characteristics it will show when the temperature is absolute zero or at a million degrees of heat, cannot be known with certainty in advance of studying it at these temperatures.

Predictions as to the behaviour of plants, animals or human beings under conditions never observed are even less probable. Experiments on guinea-pigs and rats may make predictions as to the effects of chemicals or disease germs upon them quite certain, and may justify the theory that the effects will be of the same nature upon all animals, including man ; but the latter proposition can be considered as established scientific truth only when a number of tests with various animals, including man, have verified it.   The greater the variety of facts, rather than the numbers of the same kind, confirms a theory.

Apparently well-established theories sometimes give place to others which prove to be in accord with a larger variety of facts.   By studying old phenomena more carefully or by examining new, reasons for changing old theories are often found.   Of two theories confirmed by facts, the simplest one is usually accepted as the best.   The careful scientist is therefore cautious about making assertions about what will be found in unexplored fields, yet he is always constructing theories that he regards as likely to be verified by future studies.   There are all gradations between probable hypotheses and theories, and those so well established that change is improbable.

While there is no sharp line of division between knowledge that is scientific and general truths based on experiences gained in securing the means of livelihood and comfort, yet most scientific knowledge is the result of curiosity regarding the world in which we live. Anyone who observes the stars, weather, plants, animals and people, notes similarities that serve as a basis of classification, and formulates general truths as to what may be expected of members of each class, is developing scientific knowledge. Those who make progress are likely to be raising questions as to what may be true, and then observing to see if what they thought probably true is verified. In other words, they form crude theories and then observe—not just anything—but whatever bears upon the truth of their hypotheses. If this is done in order to produce a better kind of axe or canoe, a better method of raising corn or of hardening steel, the knowledge gained is of the practical type. Such knowledge is usually limited in range and application.

In the pursuit of pure science, the essential characteristics of all cutting tools, of all floating crafts, of all animal and plant life, are studied and the classifications made in accordance with similarities, regardless of any practical purposes to be achieved. Truths as to the relationship of one set of facts to other classes are sought, regardless of whether there is any known use for such knowledge. The botanist is just as interested in studying and classifying weeds as useful grains, vegetables and fruits ; and as much concerned with conditions affecting the growth of " pussley " as of peas. Such studies are known as pure science, as distinguished from applied science.

Pure science is regarded as superior to applied science by some because it is the product of the desire to know and understand regardless of any immediate practical end to be gained. Others regard it as superior because its truths are broader and less likely to be changed by further research, and because fundamental truths are sure sooner or later to be permanently useful in gaining all sorts of desirable ends. All knowledge of plants and the conditions under which they thrive are useful in agriculture, helping in the effort to grow better crops and in the eradication of weeds. Nothing seemed more useless than a knowledge of X-rays when they were first discovered. Now such knowledge is indispensable, not only in medical practice but in many industries where there is need to know the internal structure of things. The knowledge of electricity gained in part through the curiosity of Franklin has been extended until it is now used in every home and factory, and in every phase of our modern life.

Pure science is usually surer than the narrow and immediately useful truths of applied science because of a very fundamental human characteristic. What one sees and accepts as true is determined to a very great extent by what one expects and desires. Where the truth sought has immediate bearing on any subject in which there is any emotional interest, the facts noted and their interpretation so affect the mind that often the whole truth is not obtained. At the present time it is almost impossible to get scientific knowledge of the effects of prohibition, because every one supplying data, and nearly every investigator has his facts selected, coloured and interpreted by his prejudices.

The wish that anything may be true, powerfully influences the mind toward finding it true. A researcher in pure science is usually far less influenced by prejudices and wishes than is the investigator who is aware of the practical results of his findings. Even the pure scientist is, however, likely to be prejudiced in favour of a theory that he himself has proposed or espoused. His reputation depends upon its being verified, hence in his selection of facts and interpretation of results, he is unconsciously prejudiced. This tendency to error has, however, a natural corrective. Other scientists may make their reputation by finding defects in old theories and in proving new ones. It has now become a recognized principle that evidence of the truth of a theory presented by one man cannot be accepted as reliable, even as to facts given in its support, until others have made the same observations and experiments with the same results. This is especially required when the facts reported seem not in harmony with well-established theories.

It is clear that there is a place for both pure and applied sciences. Each adds to the body of satisfying and useful knowledge, and each supplements and corrects the deficiencies of the other. The growing tendency for scientists to be employed to carry on research into problems concerned with efficiency in agriculture, mining, manufacturing, commerce and social work, is fortunately paralleled by purely scientific research in Universities and by scientific foundations. The investigator who is seeking to apply scientific truth must always spend a great deal of time in testing how various truths work out in practical situations. Laboratory tests on the effects of a given fertilizer on corn, must be supplemented by field experiments in different soils before its real value can be determined.

RELIABILITY OF KNOWLEDGE AND SCIENTIFIC METHODS

Scientific knowledge is superior in certainty and accuracy to knowledge incidentally gained in the everyday affairs of life, for several reasons : (1) The acquiring of such knowledge is the guiding purpose of the scientist rather than incidental to attainment of some other end. Such specialization naturally gives more complete and accurate knowledge of objects and phenomena. (2) The searcher after truth in any field does not wait for opportunities to study the things about which he wishes to know : he goes where the air is clearest to observe stars, and at a time and place most favourable for seeing the ones of greatest interest ; he collects specimens of rocks or plants, and studies resemblances and differences ; he systematically follows the life-history of members of a species of plants or animals ; he goes where there are many sufferers from yellow fever, pellagra, or other diseases, etc. Thus he puts himself in the way of acquiring systematic and accurate knowledge. (3) He arranges conditions so that there will be only one similarity, difference or change at a time to be studied. This arranging so that all the other factors involved shall remain the same while the effects of change in one factor are observed is the essential element in what is called experimental research. By dropping two objects of the same material and shape, but of a different size, from the same height at the same time, the truth, never observed in thousands of years of incidental human experience with falling objects, was discovered, that small objects fall at the same rate as large ones. This limiting of observation to one thing at a time by arranging that everything else shall remain constant is the most important part of experimental research.

How quickly and surely truth is obtained in this way depends greatly upon the acuteness of the investigator. There must always be some analysis to show the various possible factors and the choice of the ones most likely to be significant for experimentation. Where experience or previous research is lacking as a guide, it is largely a matter of chance. Edison, in developing electric lights, experimented with 40,000 substances, and for a time obtained his best lighting effects from carbonized bamboo. In another instance, 2000 liquids were used by him to find what would dissolve a certain substance, and in this way two solvents, formerly unknown, were discovered.

Theoretically, all the science of chemistry might be developed by a sufficient number of chance combinations of elements ; but there are so many of these possible combinations that an eternity would be required to discover the principal truths of chemistry by this method. Chance does sometimes lead to immediately important discoveries, but only when there is an acute observer present. Most discoverers of scientific truth have not only the patience to experiment and determine the effects of changing one factor after another while others are kept constant, but, guided by their knowledge of the whole phenomena, they select the most probable factors for study. Usually the results previously obtained in the scientific study of similar objects or phenomena are very helpful. For this reason scientific research is most efficient when specialized —a chemist in chemistry, a biologist in botany and zoology, a psychologist in psychology. When an eminent physicist like Sir Oliver Lodge attempts to experiment in psychology his conclusions have little weight among psychologists.

Sometimes, however, special knowledge within his own field misleads a scientist, as when investigators into the cause of pellagra wasted much time in seeking a germ, whereas, by observing the food habits of different groups of people, it was finally discovered that deficiencies in vitamins in the foods most used was the cause. Some previous experiments in animal feeding helped in this discovery, but not as much as belief in the germ theory of disease retarded its establishment. More experiments were necessary to prove that germs were not concerned than to establish the relationship of foods to the disease.

(4) Research can be accurate only by the help of measuring and counting, and the use of instruments of precision ; and these are prominent features of all modern science. Instead of depending upon accuracy of sense judgments, measurements in millimetres, degrees of heat, amperes, etc., are used to determine whether conditions are constant and how much change in result follows each change of one factor after another.

(5) Where conditions are complex and it is not possible to hold any of them entirely constant, as is usually the case in studying living things—especially man—statistics are extensively used to discover the results of marked increase or decrease in one or another of the many factors involved. How to use statistics thus is a science in itself. As generally used by politicians to show the effects of a high tariff on economic welfare, they have no value.

In measuring for scientific purposes there are developed many exact standard units of measurements that can be employed only by means of instruments (telescopes, microscopes, thermometers, micrometers, etc.) which may show differences a million times as small as can be detected by the unaided senses.

By the *use* of *instruments* instead of natural sense acuteness, by immediate *record* of *all* observations made instead of remembering those that are supposed to be significant, and by *mathematical calculations* instead of personal judgment, does scientific knowledge become more reliable and exact than ordinary knowledge. By merely keeping records and calculating the results, knowledge of weather has become much more scientific than when people, depending upon incidental observation and memory, believed that changes of moon were associated with storms, and that climate was different fifty years ago, or that thick corn husks mean a cold winter to come.

One untrained in the essentials of scientific truth-seeking is sure to have his conclusions controlled largely by personal desires. Interest once aroused in a particular fact, and the suggestion that it is typical of others, naturally leads the individual to notice and remember other facts of the same type. In this way beliefs as to weather, signs of good luck or misfortune, the characteristics of races, the value of precautions or remedies, etc., are formed and perpetuated generation after generation. Such errors can be avoided only by noting, recording and perhaps measuring *all* the facts that can possibly have a bearing on the phenomena in question, and by mathematical calculations determining how often and under what conditions the supposed truth is verified. This means that scientists must be impersonal in searching for truth. They are not necessarily cold in their emotional nature, but their desire to learn the truth must dominate over all other desires. The attitude of the artist—" Give me beauty or I die " ; of the saint, " Though He slay me, yet will I trust Him ", is paralleled by the scientist, " Let me learn the truth whatever effort is required."

SCIENTIFIC KNOWLEDGE OF HUMAN BEINGS

In all ages people have been the most important part of an individual's environment, especially in more or less helpless infancy and childhood. Knowledge of the probable behaviour of companions is well developed at an early age, and is as prominent in savages as in the most civilized groups. Early in the history of the human race some of the fundamentals of psychology, politics, and ethics were organized into systems before much had been done in the physical sciences. The truths discovered, largely by subjective means, were of considerable validity and in some respects have been but slightly improved upon by modern research. Aristotle's ethics still ranks high as a formulation of what constitutes good conduct. The success attained was due, not to the use of reliable and exact methods of science, but to the profound ability of a few great men to observe, classify, and relate the essential elements of human nature and behaviour. Their success depended upon the fundamental resemblance of all human beings and the typical character of the men who, through profound study of their own nature and observation of others, learned many things which are true of all humanity.

The difficulties of correcting, supplementing and rendering exact this body of knowledge by the use of objective scientific methods, are far greater than in the study of non-human objects and phenomena. Inorganic objects are simpler in their structure than organic, and vary far less with previous history and environment than living organisms. It is also possible to experiment on inanimate objects and discover their nature and the factors affecting them. For these reasons physical and chemical sciences developed long before those concerned with living things, and have within a comparatively short time attained a high degree of reliability and accuracy.

The study of plants has developed less rapidly and knowledge of them has not yet attained the accuracy of that gained in the physical sciences. Not only are plants complex in their organization, but every one has a history which makes it different from other similar plants, and it is responding in a more or less special way to many factors. There is also the great difficulty that experiments on living things are not reversible, as is the case with inorganic physical objects ; e.g. a plant or animal radically changed by some factor, such as heat, cannot be restored to its former state by taking the heat away, as can be done with a piece of metal. The more indirect method of experimenting with a great number of plants similar in nature and history must be resorted to, such as subjecting a certain number to the absence or presence of varying light, temperature, fertilizer, etc., and noting their average variation from those whose living conditions are not changed. By such means the characteristics of each species of plants have been accurately determined, and crops of a given size and quality may now be raised with much greater certainty and conformity to standard, than when agriculture was carried on without the help of scientific knowledge.

Animals are more complex in structure than plants, and hence the factors affecting their growth are less easily determined. When not only their structure and growth are considered, but also their behaviour, so active and varied as compared with that of plants, which for the most part remain in one place, the difficulties are greatly increased. They do not wait for man to change environing influences, but are continually moving about and varying the influence of temperature, light, and other physical forces, and using up energy and developing certain parts of the body in so doing. In spite of these complications, however, science has built up a considerable body of scientific knowledge useful in rearing and training animals.

In the study of man's body the difficulties are considerably increased by the fact that little freedom of experimentation is permitted. This is partly overcome in three ways. (1) By studying the resemblances between men and animals and judging what results of experiments upon certain animals are probably also true of man ; (2) by observing the effects of accidents and diseases ; (3) by studying the physical development of groups of people living under various conditions.

Since scientists have been freely permitted to dissect human bodies and to perform autopsies, and have had the aid of experiments on animals and non-dangerous experiments upon living human beings, the science of physiology has made great advances and has come to serve as a reliable guide in matters of health.

When man's actions are the subject of study the difficulties are even greater than in studying the behaviour of animals.

What one man does depends upon what others do, and the actions of all are influenced not only by their own nature and experience, but by what their parents and ancestors back through countless generations have done. It is impossible to experiment with the past of individuals or of their ancestors, and it is hard to get a group of human beings who are so much alike that we can be sure of the influence of the factors to which some of them are subjected, being the real and sole cause of differences observed. In spite of all this, however, much that is scientific has been learned of human behaviour, some of it helpful in practical affairs.

Progress in the study of the conduct of human beings was lacking in accuracy as long as attention was focused upon the conscious states of the individual acting, instead of upon the actions performed, and the influence of physiological and environmental conditions. These later objective studies gave more exact knowledge of details of mental activity than was attained by the early masters such as Aristotle ; but they added little to exact knowledge of mind and behaviour in their broader aspects. Within the last half-century, with increasing use of experiments with objective conditions and responses that can be measured, there has developed much accurate detailed knowledge and some of a general type which gives psychology an assured place among the sciences.

Attempts to study the geographical, economic, social and ethical life of man in relation to his environment, and the actions and interactions of individuals and groups to each other, have as yet yielded little knowledge that is scientifically accurate. The reasons for this are to be found not only in the complexity of the factors involved and the difficulty of keeping all but one factor the same while its influence is measured, but there are more serious impediments. Men usually think that the particular group of people to which they belong are superior in their nature, their customs and their beliefs, and more worthy than those of other groups. Only recently have the most ardent scientists attempted to study groups of human beings with the same scientific detachment as they study a field of corn or a colony of ants or a flock of migrating birds.

With a marked growth in this scientific attitude toward facts of human life, and with means of gathering and measuring them and learning their significance by exact statistical methods, the sciences of anthropology, economics, sociology and ethics, are gradually emerging from the clouds of superstition, tradition and prejudice. There is no reason why knowledge in these fields may not become more exact and reliable as scientific research continues and methods improve. In the nature of the case the progress will be slower than in other sciences, and the accuracy now found in physics may never characterize all of this knowledge ; but the problems of the human sciences do not differ from those of physics in kind, but only in complexity. The methods which have brought success in one, will ultimately bring success in the other.

SUBJECTIVE FACTS AND SCIENCE

A man suffering from the toothache is directly aware of the pain and may report that it is lessening or increasing. This is a subjective fact which can be observed only by the subject of the experience. Any number of other persons may hear his words or groans and may see him put his hand to his jaw, or may experiment and note that he jumps and exclaims when a certain tooth is touched. By any one or all of these facts open to general observation they may be convinced that their friend has a subjective feeling similar to something they themselves have experienced.

All phenomena that may be observed by several people are objective. They may be verified and truths formulated in accordance with scientific methods. The subjective fact of pain itself, since it can be observed directly by one person only, is not subject to such direct verification. The fact of pain and the degree of pain, if any, can never be directly determined except on the testimony of the person suffering. By studying the objective accompaniments found in many persons who claim to have toothache, truths may be formulated which will help in deciding the truth of a patient's statement, but no immediate observation or measurements of such facts are possible to a scientific investigator.

The work of a scientific investigator in dealing with subjective facts is chiefly in making constant the objective conditions under which subjective observations are made, and noting variations in reports of subjective experiences as one or another of the objective conditions are changed to a measured extent. He may also observe and measure physiological changes, *e.g.* in blood pressure, that occur as certain subjective states are reported. By such means greater accuracy of subjective description and estimates of changes in degree are secured and their correspondence to objective facts ascertained. When many persons have been tested generalizations may be made as to the usual objective accompaniments of pain. The individual who gives different reports from others, or the same reports without the usual bodily accompaniments is probably mistaken or falsifying, but it is almost impossible to *prove* that such is the case. The claim of an individual seeking to collect insurance money on the grounds of pains experienced are difficult to disprove, as are also the mental satisfactions reported as resulting from certain religious practices. It follows from the above that scientific methods, although not directly applicable to subjective facts, may be used in getting more accurate data and in testing the probability of individual observations and reports.

In everyday life we assume that the people around us are experiencing feelings and acting purposefully because this is usually true of ourselves. This assumption is near enough to the truth to serve fairly well in dealing with our fellow-men. We can adjust our actions to those of others better by inferring their emotions and purposes than by mere observation of their objective behaviour. If a rolling stone approaches us we observe its direction of motion and get out of its path ; but if a person moves toward us we infer from objective signs whether his *purpose* is to greet us or attack us, and act accordingly. We can thus adjust quickly and fittingly to actions of companions on the basis of inferred subjective

B

states better than by observing and acting on objective facts only.

The same is true in dealing with all animals of the higher type. We deal with them as if they were animated by purposes, and not as we do with non-living objects and machines. The actions of men and animals may be mechanically determined, but under ordinary circumstances we can adjust to them more successfully by supposing them to be animated by purpose than by any knowledge we have or can gain of their usual organic mechanisms. Man always has made and probably always will thus make use of inferred knowledge of subjective states in reacting to his fellow-men.

Among many tribes of people not only are fellow-men and animals considered as animated by subjective purposes, but to a greater or less degree all things in nature are so considered. The growth of common sense and scientific knowledge among such people was greatly retarded by this subjective view of the world. Instead of observing objects, conditions and results more carefully, the phenomena of nature was regarded as partly or wholly determined by the subjective states of spirits in, or associated with them. Superstitions and religions are, in part at least, the development of a subjective view of the world.

Objects resembling those known to produce certain results, or things associated with such objects, are uncritically supposed to be effective in bringing the results because of such resemblance or contiguity.

SELECTED RESEARCHES

"THE ELEMENTS AND SAFEGUARDS OF SCIENTIFIC THINKING." By Professor ELLIOT R. DOWNING, Univ. of Chicago. From *Scientific Monthly*, March 1928. *Quoted by Permission.*

The teacher who endeavours to direct pupils in acquiring skill in scientific thinking must have a clear-cut notion of the elements that constitute such thinking ; he must be on the alert to detect and correct the errors that pupils are most likely to make in the process. The elements of scientific thinking are essentially the same as for any reflective thinking. It is by increasing the awareness of the safeguards that must be thrown around the successive steps in the thought process that science has made its thinking constantly more cautious.

The following outline will present these elements and safeguards :

Elements of Scientific Thinking	Safeguards
Purposeful observation . .	*a.* must be accurate ;
	b. must be extensive ;
	c. must be done under a variety of conditions.
Analysis—Synthesis . .	*d.* The essential elements in a problematic situation must be picked out.
	e. Dissimilarities as well as similarities must be regarded. Danger of analogy.
	f. Exceptions are to be given special attention. Selective interpretation.
Selective recall . . .	*g.* A wide range of experience is necessary.
Hypotheses	*h.* All possible ones must be considered. (Fertility of suggestion.)
Verification by inference and experiment . . .	*i.* Inferences must be tested experimentally.
	j. Only one variable is permitted.

Elements of Scientific Thinking	*Safeguards*
Reasoning by :	
1. Method of agreement.	k. Data must be cogently arranged.
2. Method of difference.	l. Judgment must be passed on the adequacy of the data.
3. Method of residues.	
4. Method of concomitant variation.	m. Judgment must be passed on the pertinency of data.
5. Joint method of agreement and difference.	
Judgment	n. must be unprejudiced ;
	o. must be impersonal ;
	p. must be suspended if data are inadequate.

Aloisio Galvani (1737–1798), a physician and professor at Bologna, was preparing frogs' legs for his wife. She was ill with some stomach trouble and this delicacy had been prescribed for her. He had skinned a number of the frogs' legs and had laid them on the table when he was called out of the room. A student of his was experimenting with a frictional electric machine on the same table. His wife happened to touch a scalpel to the nerve of a frog's leg when a spark jumped from the electric machine to the scalpel and the leg twitched violently. She related this to Galvani. He recognized in this a problem, not merely a curious fact. He tried to get additional facts. He hung frogs' legs on iron wires, on an iron trellis in his garden while a thunder-storm was in progress. The legs twitched violently. He laid frogs' legs on metal plates indoors, and touched the nerve with one end of a wire, the other end of which was in contact with the metal plate. Again he observed the twitching of the legs. When, however, he laid the legs on a glass plate and used a glass rod to connect the plate and the nerve, there was no twitching. In these experiments he was trying to define his problem, which finally shaped itself into the question, whence came the electricity into these frogs' legs ? He later decided, erroneously, that it was generated in the nerves. In spite of a wrong solution he had seen and defined a problem. . . .

It is very desirable to inculcate pupils with ideals of scientific accuracy. . . .

De Saussure thought he saw the microscopic animalcules reproduce by fission and so reported the fact. But Ellis, an Englishman, denied this, claiming that the young came out of the body of the parent. He said he was able to see the children inside the parent and even the grandchildren inside the children. Spallanzani put a drop of broth swarming with infusoria on a glass slide ; near it he put a drop of pure water. He connected the two drops by a tiny bridge by drawing the broth out with a fine brush until it connected with the drop of water. Under the lens he watched this bridge until he saw one animalcule swim over into the drop of water. He then wiped the bridge away and sucked the drop of water with its one animalcule up into a fine glass tube. He watched this one animal continuously, saw it divide and the two offspring redivide. This he did again and again until he was sure that De Saussure was right. . . .

Observations need to be made under a variety of conditions. Newton desired, if possible, to make a telescope free from chromatic aberration ; that is one in which the image would not be surrounded by a halo of colour. He knew that light passing through a lens is broken up into its component colours just as it is in passing through a prism. He thought that it might be possible by a combination of lenses to overcome this defect. To test the possibility of this, he put a glass prism in a prismatic vessel filled with a sugar of lead solution. The apex of the glass prism pointed in the opposite direction from the apex of the prismatic vessel. His idea was that one prism might undo the dispersive effect of the other. He found, however, that the light after passing through both prisms still showed colour bands, and concluded that the achromatic lens was impossible. If he had varied the condition, however, using a variety of solutions, he would have discovered that some solutions would correct the dispersive effect of the glass prism much more than others might, then have hoped to find one that would correct the trouble entirely. Due to this failure of his to vary the conditions under which he worked and due to the great weight of his authority, the discovery of the method of making the achromatic telescope lens was delayed for more than a century. . . .

. . . Wolf relates that in a certain hospital in Dublin many deaths occurred among the patients located on the first floor of the hospital, while few died in the second floor ward. It was concluded that for some unknown reason the first floor was very unhealthful. One essential element in the situation had been overlooked, however. The hospital porter was in the habit of sending all patients upstairs who could walk up, while those who were too sick to climb the stairs were put in the ward on the first floor. . . .

It is exceedingly important that in all experiments to test the inferences from an hypothesis, or for that matter in any experiments, all factors be kept constant except the one variable whose effect is being tested. Some of Pasteur's opponents, unconvinced that the bacteria were the cause of anthrax, drew blood from a sheep that had died of the disease and injected some of this into rabbits. These rabbits died promptly, although no anthrax bacteria were to be found in their bodies, showing, to their way of thinking, that the bacteria had nothing to do with the death of the sheep. But they had waited so long before introducing the sheep's blood into the rabbits, that putrefaction changes had developed poisons that killed the rabbits before the anthrax germs had a chance to multiply. A whole set of new variables had arisen that vitiated the results of their experiments. . . .

. . . In 1846, Dr. Marcy of Boston removed a tumour while the patient was under ether. In 1847, Dr. J. Y. Simpson used ether and chloroform to relieve suffering in childbirth, and persisted in spite of tremendous opposition, based on the biblical curse pronounced on Eve.   One would think that so great a scientist as Dr. Simpson, with his background of experience, would be open-minded on a scientific problem.   Yet he opposed Lister's method of antiseptic surgery, biased against Lister apparently because Lister had devised a method of tying blood-vessels, in operations, with gut, which replaced Simpson's method of closing the vessels with needle-like instruments.   Simpson could not free himself from personal animosities and judge solely on objective evidence.

SUGGESTED READINGS

Biographies like those of Pasteur, by Vallery-Radot, are helpful in giving beginners a good idea of scientific work. A number of such biographies are given in an interesting way by De Kruif, Paul, in *Hunger Fighters*, 1928.

Methods in the social sciences are discussed by :

LUNDBERG, GEORGE A., *Social Research*, 1929.

ODUM, H. W., and JOCHER, KATHERINE, *An Introduction to Social Research*, 1929.

Chapter II

MAN AS AN INHABITANT OF THE EARTH

MAN'S IMPORTANCE

THE human race is only one of the millions of species of animals that the earth has brought forth ; many of which were in existence long before man appeared. For countless millenniums after his appearance his numbers were few as compared with those of other species, but during the last two centuries human population has increased manyfold in Europe and America, and there are now portions of these countries more densely populated by man than it ever was by any other of the larger animals. However, his total of less than two billion individuals can be duplicated in numbers by the lower forms of life found in any small pond, or in a few rods of soil.

Numbers are an indication of only one kind of importance of a species as an earth inhabitant. Every species of plant and animal, in maintaining its own life, affects in some way the life of every other species, and thus increases or decreases the total life on the earth. Until comparatively recent times the new species, man, maintained existence without attaining prominence among his fellow-creatures. He fed upon natural plants and some animals were his prey. He lived in favoured spots, or wandered from place to place in securing food and other comforts. but did little to disturb the balance of plant and animal life, or to modify the earth. Probably the earth was more changed and made more productive through the earlier ages by the lowly earth-worm than by man.

The progress made by man during the last few millenia, and especially during the last few centuries, has, however, been in the direction of power and dominance as an earth-dweller. He has decreased and even exterminated many species of plants and animals, increased others, transformed many by domestication, and has long been changing species by selective breeding into forms more useful or more beautiful to him. He is now employing the forces of wind, water, sun, fire and chemistry to aid in feeding and sheltering himself, and in extending his rule over the earth and its inhabitants. He holds in his hands the destiny of every other species, except, perhaps, some of the microbes and insects which have such tremendous capacity for reproduction that his victory over them, although ultimately probable, is not yet in sight.

These facts justify the claim that of all the earth's inhabitants, man is the most powerful and therefore the most significant subject of scientific research. There are reasons for believing that during the time of his great advance in power and position, his essential structure and nature has remained practically unchanged. It is, therefore, well worth while to inquire by what qualities and means he has attained his present supremacy.

PHYSICAL ENDOWMENT

Like all other living things, man is a self-preserving, self-repairing, self-reproducing organism. In anatomic structure and modes of functioning, every species differs, but in those of the mammalian type to which man belongs, the similarities are marked. In essentials of physiological functions, man is nearly the same as the higher four-legged species. His four limbs are more specialized than those of any other quadruped ; one pair for supporting and transporting the body, and the other for ready manipulation of things. He has not the strength of the tiger, the swiftness of the deer, nor the power of claws and teeth possessed by lions and tigers ; but in skill of hand he has no rival. His senses are in themselves much the same as those of other mammals, but in variety and range of vision, in facilities for directing and focusing the eye, he is superior to all others, though he is surpassed by many in the ability to use the sense of smell.

None of the higher mammals are less protected than man by outer covering against cold and wounds. On the other hand, the internal mechanism of muscles and nerves for controlling the parts of the body are more varied and closely associated than is the case with any other animal. This superiority is shown in the brain, which serves as a switch-board for connecting all parts of the body with each other, and for responding to the stimulation of the surrounding world. With such a bodily structure, man has a versatility and a unity of action which more than balances his lack of strength or of formidableness in weapons of attack and defence.

As a chemical-physical mechanism man depends upon food and air for the energy which he uses in keeping his bodily organism functioning, and for muscular activity of all sorts. As a transformer of food energy into heat and into work of various kinds, he is not greatly different from other animals, and not much more efficient than the best steam- or gas-engines of today.

MENTAL NATURE

In view of the important position man has gained among earth's inhabitants without marked superiority in physio-logical structure, we must conclude that this dominating position is due to the greater versatility, adaptability and efficiency of the central office or switchboard within his skull. The functioning of the human brain in adjusting and directing bodily organs in the accomplishment of ends favourable to the continued existence and prominence of man, is what is implied by the term mental nature of man. This nature may be studied (1) by observing man's objective behaviour only ; by (2) studying his subjective states only ; (3) by concentrating on the physical and chemical nature of brain functioning ; or by (4) using facts from all these fields.

When we observe the behaviour of an individual man in natural surroundings in competing for food and safety with squirrels, deer, bears, etc., the mental superiority of the man does not seem great. If the man wins, it is usually because he has the aid of other men present, or because he makes use of knowledge, weapons, traps or other means previously prepared by someone else. Evidently he has a kind of intelligence which enables him to co-operate with his fellow-men and use their skill and experience in gaining his own individual ends. It is because of this use of what the race has learned that man, especially in recent times, has become the most powerful of all earth's creatures.

It is not easy to demonstrate in detail the differences in the intelligence of man as compared with that of other species. He is known, however, to have by far the largest and most complex brain of any animal of his size. Experimental studies of men and animals show striking similarities in learning to adapt themselves to situations. In general, animals can do some things better than man without apparently having to learn to do them (walk, swim, etc.) ; but man learns a much greater variety of things and learns many things more rapidly.

The most marked difference is in the extent to which man learns to guide himself by elements in the situation not present at the moment. A dog learns quickly to go to an opening where a certain light is shown and get food ; but if the light is shown and then turned off for several minutes before he is allowed to go to the food receptacle, he is likely to be confused as to its location. In other words, dogs and other animals direct their behaviour chiefly by present stimuli, while, as is well known, man is guided largely by absent stimuli.

This elementary difference is greatly increased by language, which man has invented. By visual and verbal signs he is able to suggest things not present that guide the conduct of himself and others more than things sensed at the moment. Consequently each man may direct his actions not only by his own experiences, but he can also make use of the experience and knowledge of other men. This greatly increases two possibilities : (a) effective co-operation in using means for attaining an understood end, and (b) accumulation of knowledge of means of successfully meeting situations like those that have been met by companions and ancestors. An animal draws upon his native endowment and upon the knowledge and wisdom gained from his own rather limited experience, while man uses the tools others have discovered and made, and draws upon the illimitable store of knowledge others have accumulated.   An individual man thus equipped does not have to be greatly superior to an animal in intelligence in order to dominate him.

With an intelligence such as man possesses certain physical handicaps have even proved to be of advantage to him.   He is quite inferior to many animals in means of attack, defence, and in protection from the cold, and in order to survive he began to supplement these deficiencies by artificial weapons and coverings.   This started his development in a direction different from that of any other creature.   Animals in a new environment change not only their behaviour but also their physiological structure ; while man changes the things in his environment so as to make them more satisfactory to himself. As a result, animals produce few and incidental changes in their environment, while man transforms the surface of the earth, its stones, trees, plants, animals and rivers, extensively and consciously in order to give himself all the satisfactions found in the most favoured regions, and with a minimum of effort.

This line of development which man has followed because of comparatively slight differences in type and degree of intelligence between himself and the animals, has been furthered by what at first seems like another handicap, *i.e.* the extreme and continued helplessness of the young of the human species.   Instead of depending upon his native endowment, as is the case with the horse or the pig, the young of man is started on a course of learning under the tuition of persons who have learned many things by their own experience and have drawn upon material resources and the knowledge and wisdom acquired by their ancestors.   The period during which the child must and may learn is a long one ; while in animal development this period is short and the aid given by adults is limited to a small portion of their own experience.

Another result of the prolonged period of infancy among men is that the family unit, which among animals continues to exist for a few weeks or a year or two, lasts for a dozen or more years, if not for life. This not only fosters continued learning, but renders inevitable continued co-operation between members of the family group. This in turn prepares the way for more extensive co-operation of families and groups of families. By co-operating in securing a common end, what is impossible to one individual or group is easily accomplished by using the combined strength and special skill and knowledge of each. It is through such co-operation that man has so rapidly gained control over all objects, creatures, and forces of nature during the last century.

BIOLOGY AND THE SCIENCES OF MAN

As the biological sciences have developed, there has been a very natural tendency to take the position that as man is an animal very much like the other of the higher animals, the various fields of knowledge embraced in the sciences of man are mere enlargements and specializations of the field of biological science. Up to a certain point this view is in accordance with many fundamental truths. Physiologically man *is* an animal, and most of what is true of animals, especially the mammals, is true of human beings with slight variations in detail. Mentally the higher animals show many of the activities and interests of human beings. Socially there are also resemblances between the family and group life of animals and of human beings. Some animal groups form customs (*e.g.* an Eskimo dog team) and maintain class distinctions of dominance and submission, or of equality. Leaders exercise rudimentary control over the pack. Many animals show some economic activity in providing food and shelter. The young animals of some species receive a little schooling in conformity to herd law.

In general, animal behaviour is determined by physiological structure, by physical environment and by the reactions of other animals. Man is influenced by all these, but still more by the culture of the group to which he belongs. These cultures are not determined entirely by experience in reacting to the environment; but beliefs in supernatural powers, cultural traits based on animistic, superstitious, magical and religious beliefs, and æsthetic, social, and intellectual interests, all of which play a large part in the life of man. When scientific knowledge becomes dominant man is influenced by many phases of the environment that have no effect upon animal or primitive human behaviour. His reactions are not controlled by the here and now only, but because of transportation and communication facilities distant stimuli are powerful; and because of language, especially written, the past and the future control behaviour even more than the present. For these reasons cultural traits are of more significance in most of the sciences concerned with man than climatic and biological factors, although the latter exert a constant influence that cannot be disregarded.

Man's development in every line, in its beginnings, resembles that of animals, but it takes such a different direction and becomes so dependent upon new and different conditions, that the truths of biology do not carry us very far into the complexities of human psychology, sociology, economics, political economy and ethics. Man, while remaining akin to animals physically and mentally, and subject to the same physical environment, is continually changing that environment, putting it to new uses, continually adding to knowledge and experience, and always modifying behaviour by what has been, and by what it is desired shall be.

The phenomena with which the sciences of man deal are as different from those of biology as the leaves, blossoms and fruits of a tree are from the roots upon which their life depend; also they are as closely related. The roots of all civilization are biological, but the sciences concerned with the various activities of civilized man cannot be extensively and correctly developed from a study of biological phenomena only. Just as trees are modified, not only by the soil conditions, but also by outside elements and nearby growths above the ground, so are human activities modified by man's inventions and by his customary organized activities. This involves the consideration of many factors not distinctly biological. The phenomena of human living is not, therefore, merely biological living, but also an immensely varied complex of activities more or less remotely related to biological processes and conditions, and directed by the products of past living and purposes for the future.

MAN AND CULTURE

The preceding discussion shows us that man is the only creature in which the past experience of the species in any given environment has a dominating influence upon behaviour. All the material constructions of man and all knowledge of ways of doing things which are passed on from one generation to another, constitute what in the social sciences is called culture. The term as thus used is evidently much broader than in its ordinary signification of the finer and less necessary elements of civilized living. It includes, as Folsom points out : (1) Material constructions such as tools, roads, houses, etc. ; (2) Elements of social structure such as relationships, governments, etc. ; (3) Sentiments or attitudes as to clothes, conduct, rituals, etc. ; (4) Skills in dancing, archery, music, art ; (5) Symbolic elements such as languages ; (6) Beliefs and knowledge of all sorts.

Each generation is born with natural endowments fitting it for a certain mode of living, but the special behaviour by means of which life is maintained and enjoyed, is, in man, determined chiefly by the culture of the group to which he belongs rather than by his native endowment and the natural physical environment. It is because man is a culture-forming creature and a ready acquirer of the culture by which he is surrounded, that the biological sciences alone are inadequate to interpret and explain man's nature and his social development.

MAN'S ORIGIN

Man, like other species, probably evolved from some lower form of life. In his structure, quality of blood, and in complexity of behaviour, he resembles the ape more than any other animal. The resemblance is close enough to justify the belief that man and the ape descended from a common ancestor.

The universal tendency of similar individuals to mate, and of like to produce like, perpetuates separate species of animals. The observations of one person, therefore, and the records of centuries of history, make it appear that every species of plant and animal remains fundamentally the same generation after generation ; but actually during the æons of earth's development there have been innumerable and profound changes and transformations in species. How these changes have been brought about has long excited theoretical speculation and, more recently, careful observation and experimentation.

There is positive evidence that all species are modified by changed geographical and other conditions. Every species produces an excess of young, many of which die before reaching maturity. It is not wholly a matter of chance which ones die. When environment changes, individuals having different traits survive. By experimental breeding of organisms for many generations in water of a temperature above their optimum temperature, those surviving after many generations were vigorous in water at a temperature which would have killed their ancestors. Others bred in colder water thrived in temperatures so low as to have destroyed their ancestors. By means of such procedure, two distinct varieties have been produced, one highly resistant to cold and the other to heat. At first such changes were supposed to be the result of individual adaptation transmitted to descendants. Another explanation, however, is now more generally accepted as the chief cause of species modification. The individuals which can least endure a given change, such as increased or decreased heat, die, and only those most resistant survive and produce descendants. The two varieties are resistant, one to heat and the other to cold, chiefly because they are descended from ancestors having that native capacity, rather than because of their acquiring it by practice in adapting to the change.

This theory of environmental change and natural selection is not, however, sufficient to fully account for the origin of distinctly different species. Individuals that are descended from the same ancestors, living in a constant environment, differ slightly from each other ; and since each descendant has two slightly different parents, it has a chance of getting slightly different traits from the others of the same parentage. To produce a new species, however, there must be a union of individuals differing from each other in a much greater degree than is found when both belong to the same variety of the species. If parents are chosen from widely different varieties of the same species, the descendants will differ from each other in a marked degree, yet not enough to give rise to a new species.

If an attempt is made to interbreed distinct species, there may be few or no descendants. When there are any, they are usually incapable of producing young. To produce individuals differing so greatly from each other as to originate a new species is not readily accomplished by means available to man. Nature has undoubtedly produced countless new species from pre-existing forms of life. This has probably been accomplished through the combined effects of differences in the two parents, and of changes in environment that have taken place during the history of the earth. Researches such as that of Muller, quoted at the end of this chapter, may be of great assistance in solving the problem of the origin of new species. Further archæological studies are likely to give clearer evidence of man's origin, essential nature, and ancestral relationship.

C

SELECTED RESEARCHES

"THE METHOD OF EVOLUTION." By Professor H. J. MULLER, Univ. of Texas. From *Scientific Monthly*, December 1929. *Quoted by Permission*.

All modern genetic work converges to show that the heritable differences between parent and offspring, between brother and sister, in fact between any organisms which can be crossed, have their basis in differences in minute self-reproducing bodies called the genes, located in the nucleus of every cell. The genes themselves are too small to be separately visible, but hundreds or thousands of them are linked together into strings, and these strings of genes, together probably with some accessory material, are large enough to be seen through the microscope by the cytologist; they constitute the sausage-shaped bodies called chromosomes. We know that, ordinarily, each individual gene in a string is different from every other gene in the same string, and has its own distinctive rôle to play in the incomparably complicated economy of the cell.

. . . Nevertheless, if one individual differs from another individual in regard to just one of the genes that do take part, it will be seen that the given characteristic in the two individuals will be different, and so, conversely, a difference between two individuals in regard to a certain characteristic, let us say eye colour, may be due to a difference between just two given genes in them rather than other genes. We may then call these for short the genes " for brown " and " for blue " eyes respectively, while remembering that really, in both individuals, many other genes are present also which are helping to produce the exact eye colorations seen, but that these other genes happen to be alike in the two individuals in question, and therefore are not causing this particular difference, between this brown eye and this blue eye.

When two germ-cells that differ in respect to a certain gene, *e.g.* the egg having the gene for brown and the sperm that for blue eyes, fertilize each other, neither gene is lost, but the resulting individual possesses both genes in every one of his cells, even though his eyes may show preponderantly the brown colour, brown being said to be the dominant gene and blue the recessive. Half the germ-cells formed by an individual of such mixed composition (" heterozygous," we call him) will carry the brown gene and not the blue one, the rest carry the blue gene and not the brown, and so there is as good a chance for any one of his children to inherit the blue gene as the brown one. Moreover, it is found that neither the blue gene nor the brown one, when inherited by the next generation, shows any weakening or other trace of its former sojourn with a gene of opposite character. It persists through the generations uncontaminated by its associate-genes. . . .

Most of modern genetics has been occupied with tracing down the above " facts " (if this term may now be used, subject to the qualifications previously expressed). They relate essentially to the method of transmission, to later generations, of gene-differences that are already found to exist between individuals. They show the universality of these differences, their comparative permanence and their recombining capabilities. But they leave untouched what now becomes the major question—how do such differences originate in the first place ? What is the origin of variation ? . . .

Each gene-difference arises suddenly and full-fledged, though we may not be aware of it at once. . . .

The new gene, once it has arisen, is ordinarily as stable as the old. The change is definite and fixed, evidently of a chemical nature. Once it has occurred, we have a new mutant gene which will eventually either spread throughout the population or be killed off, according to whether the individuals which carry it reproduce more offspring or fewer. . . .

. . . In addition to this work, efforts have been by no means lacking, on the part of numerous investigators, to find the cause, or a cause, of visible mutations, by trying all sorts of mal-treatments in the attempt to produce changes. In the course of this work, animals and plants have been drugged, poisoned, intoxicated, etherized, illuminated, kept in darkness, half-smothered, painted inside and out, whirled round and round, shaken violently, vaccinated, mutilated, educated and treated with everything except affection, from generation to generation. But their genes seemed to remain oblivious, and they could not be distracted into making an obvious mistake in the reproduction of daughter genes just like themselves. The new genes were exact duplicates of the old ones, showing no demonstrable mutations, or at most such a scattering few as might have occurred anyhow.

Either the technique used for finding the mutations was inadequate or the treatments had little or no effect upon the composition of the genes, or both, and I am inclined to think the latter is correct. And yet mutations certainly do happen, even though rarely. In the examination of over twenty million fruit-flies, not specially maltreated, over four hundred visible mutations have been found. These mutations must have causes. What then can the causes be ? What subtle conditions are they ? . . .

The genes are not only protected by a cell membrane but by

a nuclear membrane inside of that, and possibly again by a chromosomal envelope of some kind ; they may be well shielded, therefore, from the reach of any poisonous substances or unusual products of metabolism. They cannot, however, escape the interplay of the helter-skelter molecular, atomic and electronic motions that are continually taking place both within and around them, on the part of the substances of which they and their neighbour molecules are naturally composed. . . .

. . . Among the agents of an ultramicroscopically random character, that can strike willy-nilly through living things, causing drastic atomic changes here and passing everything by unaltered there—not a ten-thousandth of a millimetre away, there stands pre-eminently the X- or Y-ray and its accomplice, the speeding electron. There is nothing in protoplasm which can effectually stop the passage of X-rays or the related waves of shorter wavelength—gamma and cosmic rays. For the most part, in a cell, the rays will pass through ; but at isolated, unpredictable spots, depending upon unknown " chance " details of energy-configurations, a definite portion, a " quantum " of the rays will be held up, and part of the energy thus absorbed will issue forth in a hurtling electron, shot out of the atom that stood in the way of the radiation. The atom will be changed thereby, and hence the molecule in which it lies may undergo a change in its chemical composition. But for every atom thus directly changed there are thousands of other atoms changed indirectly. . . . If a gene is a molecule, then, with properties depending upon its chemical composition, it can be shot and altered by the electrons resulting from the absorption of X-rays or rays of shorter wavelength. The only question would be, can enough mutations be caused in this way to be detectable by our present methods, with doses of rays small enough not to kill or sterilize the treated organism ? . . .

With these points in mind, the author undertook in the fall of 1926 a series of experiments designed to test the question at issue. The fruit-fly, Drosophila, was used, since it so easily and rapidly bred in large numbers and since it rendered possible the employment of special genetic technique for the finding of mutations, that had been elaborated in the course of my previous work on linkage and mutation in this organism. . . .

In these experiments the adult flies—in some cases males, in other cases females—were placed in gelatin capsules and subjected to doses of X-rays so strong as to produce partial sterility, though the other functions of the flies are not noticeably disturbed by a dose several times stronger than used here. The treated flies were then bred to untreated mates, and at the same time numerous control matings of the same genetic type were carried on for comparison, consisting of untreated males crossed by untreated females. Thousands of cultures were used in this and subsequent experiments, in order, if possible, to settle the matter beyond any doubt.

All types of mutations large and small, ugly and beautiful, burst upon the gaze. Flies with bulging eyes or with flat or dented eyes ; flies with white, purple, yellow or brown eyes or with flat or dented eyes ; flies with curly hair, with ruffled hair, with parted hair, with fine and with coarse hair, and bald flies ; flies with swollen antennæ, or extra antennæ, or legs in place of antennæ ; flies with broad wings, with narrow wings, with upturned wings, with downturned wings, with outstretched wings, with truncated wings, with split wings, with spotted wings, with bloated wings and with virtually no wings at all. Big flies and little ones, dark ones and light ones, active and sluggish ones, fertile and sterile ones, long-lived and short-lived ones. Flies that preferred to stay on the ground, flies that did not care about the light, flies with a mixture of sex characters, flies that were especially sensitive to warm weather. They were a motley throng. What had been done ? The roots of life—the genes—had indeed been struck, and had yielded.

It must not be supposed that all the above types appeared congregated together in one family. The vast majority of the offspring that hatched still appeared quite normal, and it was only by raking through our thousands of cultures that all these types were found. But what a difference from the normal frequency of mutation, which is so painfully low ! By checking up with the small numbers of mutants found in the numerous untreated or control cultures, which were bred in parallel, it was found that the heaviest treatment had increased the frequency of mutation about 150 times—that is, an increase of 15,000 per cent. . . .

" *Note.*—Although it cannot be doubted that natural radiation must be responsible for *some* mutations in untreated Drosophila, the question as to whether some other factor or factors cause the *large majority* of these ' natural ' mutations has, since date of the above writing, been decisively answered in the affirmative by experiments and calculations carried out by L. Mott-Smith of the Rice Institute and the present writer.

H. J. MULLER (Feb. 20, 1930).

" STABILITY." By Professor T. WINGATE TODD, Western Reserve University. From *Scientific Monthly*, December 1924. *Quoted by Permission.*

During recent years it has fallen to my lot to study rather intensively the variability in pattern of man's bodily features and, in order to have some standard of comparison by which this variability may be judged, I have found it instructive to use as a contrast the variability in pattern of the bodily features of other forms of life which are at least similar in design. . . .

The example which I propose to take as a test is drawn from the very core of man's physical being, namely, the character of the vertebral column, a feature which every one would admit is ancient and fundamental. In the chest and loins of a man's body there are, as a rule, seventeen separate bones or vertebræ. But if we enumerate the bones in a large number of human beings, we find some people who have, not seventeen, but sixteen or perhaps eighteen vertebræ in this region. This variability in itself is rather striking, for we have reason to believe that the earliest mammals to make their appearance on the earth had nineteen, whereas certain mammals of today have more than nineteen, but others have less. . . .

VARIABILITY IN NUMBER OF THORACICO-LUMBAR VERTEBRÆ

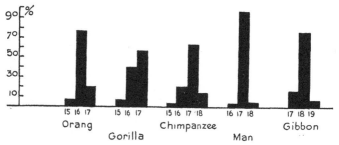

To render clearer the variability in number of thoracico-lumbar vertebræ found in man, I append a chart showing in black columns the percentage of individuals possessing, respectively, sixteen, seventeen and eighteen. The series upon which these observations were made totals about 850 skeletons ; there is no doubt, therefore, of its essential accuracy. The percentage of individuals possessing eighteen vertebræ in chest and loins is very small, and the percentage with sixteen is negligible. Now for comparison I have included black columns analysing the similar bones in existing anthropoid apes. The difference between all these anthropoid figures and that representing man is sufficiently distinct. The characteristic of man is his stability of pattern contrasted with the instability of pattern in the anthropoids. . . .

" A MILLION YEARS OF EVOLUTION IN TOOLS." By MILDRED FAIRCHILD and Dr. HORNELL HART, Brynmawr College. From *Scientific Monthly*, January 1929. *Quoted by Permission.*

In the attempt to measure past changes in human culture the longest and most complete series of data available consists in the tools with which man has cut and shaped his materials.

This series extends in unbroken line over immense stretches of time. . . .

If a quantitative statement of progress in cutting tools is to be made, the first problem is to arrive at the nearest feasible approximation to an objective scale of points by which to rate such tools. Analysis indicates that at least five variables enter into the efficiency of man's cutting tools : (1) Keenness and durability of the cutting edge ; (2) differentiation and specialization ; (3) effectiveness of mechanisms employed to apply the blade to the materials to be cut ; (4) utilization of auxiliary power ; and (5) mastery displayed in the technique of manufacture. . . .

TABLE I

RATINGS OF THE EFFICIENCY OF CUTTING TOOLS AT VARIOUS CULTURE EPOCHS FROM EOLITHIC TIMES TO THE MACHINE AGE

Period.	Date.	Keenness.	Specialization.	Mechanisms.	Power.	Technique in Manufacture.	Total Rating.
1	2	3	4	5	6	7	8
Machine Age .	A.D. 1915	20	20	20	20	20	100
Iron	500 B.C.	16	15	7	8	14	60
Bronze .	2000 B.C.	12	13	6	5	13	49
Copper .	4000 B.C.	9	12	4	2	12	39
Neolithic	6000 B.C.	7	10	4	2	11	34
Mesolithic	8000 B.C.	5	8	4	2	9	28
Magdalenian .	16,000 B.C.	4	7	2	2	8	23
Solutrian	40,000 B.C.	4	6	2	2	7	21
Aurignacian .	75,000 B.C.	3	6	2	2	5	18
Mousterian	200,000 B.C.	3	2	2	1	4	12
Acheulean	400,000 B.C.	3	2	1	0	3	9
Chellean	600,000 B.C.	2	2	1	0	1	6
Cromerian	850,000 B.C.	2	1	1	0	1	5
Foxhallian	1,150,000 B.C.	2	1	0	0	1	4
Sub-Red Crag	1,300,000 B.C.	2	1	0	0	1	4

The above figures given by the authors are, of course, estimates rather than actual measurements.

SUGGESTED READINGS

Material in this field is so various, ranging from Palæontology and Geography, through Biology and Anthropology, and Psychology to Sociology and Religion, that it is almost impossible to cite single works which adequately describe the distinctive characteristics of the human species. Two books only will be named :

CONKLIN, E. G., " Has Human Evolution come to an End ? " *Princeton Lectures,* Vol. I, No. 1, 1921.

RITTER, W. E., and BAILEY, E. W., *The Natural History of our Conduct,* 1927.

CHAPTER III

VARIETIES OF THE HUMAN SPECIES AND THEIR MODES OF LIVING, OR ANTHROPOLOGY AND ETHNOLOGY

RACIAL DIFFERENCES AND RESEMBLANCES

SUPERFICIALLY people of various regions are quite unlike, yet we find no such extremes as in domestic animals, *e.g.* the draught-horse and the Shetland pony, the lap-dog and the Great Dane. No race of men consistently averages above 5 ft. 10 in. in height, and in only a few small tribes is the average below 5 ft. Hair varies in human beings in colour, texture and quantity, but there are no fundamental differences in the bony skeleton, though some races have more individuals with round heads than others. The comparative size and shape of the vital organs, the location and connections of the main nerves and the principal blood-vessels, are practically the same in all races. Physicians and surgeons make no more variations in treating Negroes, Whites or Indians than they do in treating an office worker and an outdoor labourer of the white race.

This marvellous similarity of all human beings in anatomy and physiology is probably due in part to the fact that man has remained in the same geographical region less consistently than other animals; but chiefly because instead of changing himself physiologically when in new physical surroundings, he changes those surroundings to more perfectly match his essential nature. Such changes are especially necessary as he goes into regions of extremes in temperature.

Superficial thinkers imagine the future man as losing nearly all his muscular power because of the development of the automobile and other substitutes for muscular exertion. Such speculations show not only lack of a knowledge of heredity, but failure to allow for the general tendency of man to preserve his fundamental characteristics. As he uses his muscles less in work, so much more does he employ them in play. In acting so as to live and be comfortable and healthy, he inevitably, consciously and unconsciously, preserves the typical human form and functions of parts. However much civilization may change conditions of living, man will remain much the same physically and mentally. He is not original enough to make himself into a different creature from the man nature made, but can only refine and specialize himself in various ways.

The early classification of man into five races on the basis of colour is partly justified by more careful study of the characteristics of different peoples. The distinction between the White or Caucasian race and the Negro or Negroid race, is pretty definitely drawn when traits other than colour are considered. The Caucasians have wavy hair, considerable body hair, narrow nose and generally tall stature ; while the Negroids have woolly hair, smooth body, broad nose, with stature variable and colour of skin generally darker than the Hindu, who is the darkest Caucasian.

In general, the Negroid races inhabit the warmer, moister regions ; the Mongolian, the drier and less warm regions ; while the White race usually occupies the colder sections having greater seasonal changes. The two most important factors in climate are latitude and elevation. So far as is known, the oldest civilizations were on the mesas extending across Southern Europe and Asia. The variations in seasons, length of day and night, and moisture are less in these regions than in the forest and grass regions farther from the Equator.

The Mongoloid race is nearer to the Caucasian than to the Negroid type, having straight hair, little body hair, medium width nose, and light brown skin. The American Indian or Red Man is now included in the Mongoloid race, as are also the Malays.

The Melanesian and Australian are considered Negroid, although they have some resemblances to the Caucasians.

The Polynesian, Ainu, and other smaller groups, are of doubtful classification.

Width of head does not distinguish the chief races from each other, but it does help to classify Nordic and Mediterranean varieties of the Caucasians ; also to distinguish Red Men from the more typical Mongolian variety. The Caucasians are most consistently a tall race, and are the only race having a blue-eyed and very white-skinned variety.

There are no marked physiological differences in the races in rate of breathing, pulse rate or bodily temperature. Some evidences of difference in basal metabolism has been found seemingly independent of food and exercise habits, but it is not certain that it is an inherited trait. The same may be said of differences in glandular activity.

How far races may differ in intelligence remains to be established. The attempt to settle this by weighing brains, gives variable results, dependent more upon size and individuality than upon race. When judged by cultural inventions and success in transforming environment, the White race has actually achieved more than the Negroid or Mongoloid, but we have no means of knowing how much of the difference is due to climatic influences, glandular activity, or cultural trends and contacts.

Intelligence tests give higher ratings to white than to coloured people in the United States. The differences are less when persons of presumably the same social status are compared, but do not entirely disappear. Either because of real differences in type of intellectual activity or for other reasons, negroes rank higher when the tests involve real objects, than when they deal with abstract symbols.

Comparisons of various national and racial groups in the United States are of doubtful interpretation, not only because of differences in language, education and occupation, but because some groups have a larger proportion of inferior individuals than do other of the immigrant groups.

Every group has some individuals of unusual size, strength, agility, intelligence, etc., and others that are markedly inferior. The chief differences among national and occupational groups is that some have a larger number of individuals who are average or superior in some tested ability than others. To say that a person is a southern negro or a white common labourer does not necessarily classify him as to intelligence. He may be the one in ten of his race or group who is superior to the average citizen.

As already pointed out, instead of adapting their bodies, men in a new environment proceed to change that environment so as to make it serve them. The articles constructed and the new modes of acting are cumulative, and as a consequence the cultural differences between the inhabitants of various regions become infinitely greater than the anatomical and physiological ones.

A museum visitor in passing from room to room observing the material constructions of Egyptians, Romans, Greeks, Africans, Chinese, and Indians, cannot fail to be impressed with the fact that each is of a different type. The traveller who visits in out-of-the-way regions, is still more impressed with differences in customs relating to food, marriage, religion, morals and government. He is often quite unable to properly interpret some of the behaviour. Their foods may nauseate him, their acts of politeness seem to him insults, and their religious rituals crude or horrible. A psychiatrist who attempted to deal with the *mental* disorders of an individual belonging to a strange cultural group would be hopelessly perplexed, while the physician could successfully use the means of cure with which he was already familiar.

Every group of people living for some time in the same environment develops special customs of dealing with plants, animals and persons. A few examples from Lowie will show their extreme diversity. In some places women do all the milking, but a Zulu will not allow women to go near the cattle, lest the productivity of the cows be decreased. It is a sin for an Eskimo to eat venison *with* seal meat, because it is believed that this would excite the wrath of the sea-goddess and bring some punishment upon the tribe. A Masai husband and wife must never eat together. Customs as to parts of body that are covered differ greatly. A nude South American woman blushed violently when a plug which she usually wore was removed from her nose. In some places men have many wives, and in others women have many husbands. Some tribes insist on chastity before marriage, and others afterwards. The Gommera order the killing of any man who reveals the bull-roarer to a woman, and a man in love with a woman of a forbidden clan commits suicide. In New Guinea it is a man's duty to support his sister's children rather than his own. A Crow Indian must not speak to his mother-in-law. Among the Plains Indians, to begin hunting buffalo before the signal to do so was one of the most serious of crimes. To catch and eat lice is a pleasant social pastime among some Eskimos.

At first glance it might appear that such great varieties of human culture indicate that mentally human beings differ much more than they do physically. A more careful study of peoples of all varieties of cultures, however, reveals fundamental similarities. All have the same needs and desires and show a certain amount of intelligence in satisfying them, and in adjusting their conduct to others. Scientists are becoming very cautious about comparing the intelligence of the different races and the value of the cultures each has developed in its own surroundings.

ANTHROPOLOGY USING SCIENTIFIC METHODS

In any science there is need for an analytical and critical examination of a great collection of facts in order to find the most promising ways of classifying them for a more exact study. This phase of scientific development so prominent in botany and zoology a hundred years ago, now receives only a minor proportion of attention. This is partly because this preliminary work has been done, but more because facts upon which classification depend are less helpful in understanding plant and animal life than was expected. We learn little of practical or scientific value by merely determining the characteristics which distinguish the rose family from the lily family, or the order Mammalia from the order Reptilia.   More is gained by looking upon all organisms as being composed of living cells having similar characteristics, and being influenced in much the same way by environment. The factors exercising general control over life are found to be of more significance than the forms of the typical specimens of each species.

Anthropologists were previously much occupied with such classifications, but have come to realize the greater advantages of studying the factors concerned in producing differences in physiological traits and cultures. For a time they were misled by the theory that all groups of men must pass through the same cultural stages, such as the " stone age ", the " iron age ", the " agricultural age " or the " mechanical age ".   In a very general way such terms have a value in characterizing cultures, but many errors have grown out of the belief in their universality and in the order in which they become prominent.   Still more misleading is this theory when applied to special behaviour types. Not until Westermarck published his monumental study of marriage, was the idea that every group of human beings must pass through the same stages of promiscuity, community of wives, polygamy and monogamy, abandoned. Much effort was also partly wasted in searching for primitive forms of religion, language, etc., from which all others were supposed to have developed. The way to truth has been cleared by the rather general abandonment of the theory of universality in origins and stages of culture.

There has recently been much improvement in methods of verifying and recording observations. Psychologists have shown that unless special precautions are taken, observations of people are less likely to be accurate than those made upon natural phenomena. In describing people, reports are likely to be made, not of objective acts, but of subjectively selected and interpreted traits. Much of the extensive data given by untrained observers after a limited contact with the peoples described is a poor basis upon which to found scientific knowledge. Notwithstanding this unreliability and inexactness of the anthropological facts earlier gathered by Spencer, yet when treated statistically some of them are significant ; for instance, the frequent combination of pottery manufacture with the use of maize as a food, and of polygamy with pastoral life. Careful surveys have also shown that many specimens and varieties of pottery are found in certain centres, and in decreasing quantity and variety in places more distant from this centre. It is often correctly concluded from such studies that the area of greatest variety and abundance of this cultural object is a centre from which it was diffused to the surrounding regions, and that the most widely diffused variety was the type first originated. The same reasoning has been used in the study of culture customs. These assumptions, supported by Wissler and others, have been shown by Dixon to have many limitations.

The facts regarding culture traits of a people cannot be interpreted and evaluated separately, but must be considered in relation to all other traits. The culture of a people is a complex more or less perfectly balanced. This means, as Malinowski has shown, that the whole cultural system of a people must be studied in order to understand the significance of any one trait. Facts are valuable, not so much because of their resemblance to those found in other culture systems, as because of their relation to other facts in the same system. Such a custom as that of killing aged and helpless parents may, under certain conditions of tribal life, be found to mean, not hard-hearted cruelty but real kindness ; or what seems to a Westerner like community of property, may actually be a system of reciprocity in service and obligations analogous to our Christmas giving.

Terms used in describing cultures cannot easily be differentiated ; but in general, a cultural trait is relatively elementary, while " pattern " implies a quality found in several traits, and " complex ", a group of traits.

FACTORS INVOLVED IN CULTURE DEVELOPMENT

The most important factors to be considered are (1) the climate and physical conditions of the locality inhabited; (2) the plant environment; (3) the animal inhabitants; (4) human nature and the culture already acquired.

(1) *Physical Surroundings and Culture.* The direct effects of temperature, moisture, sunshine, air composition and pressure, length of day, etc., upon the physiological functionings of man are considerable, and are still more marked upon culture. Where all these physical factors remain nearly the same, there is comparatively little stimulus to physical and mental activity, and hence to culture development. When changes are marked, culture develops not merely because of efforts to make life more comfortable, but because of the greater mental stimulus. In the drier tropical regions, where the contrast between bright sunshine and brilliant starlight are the most prominent daily changes, knowledge of astronomy and myths associated with the stars are likely to be features of the cultures of the people inhabiting those regions. In places where seasonal changes are great, man must develop cultural types of behaviour adjustments in order to live and be comfortable, but also he is mentally stimulated to form mythical or more or less scientific knowledge of these changes and their causes. Variations in day and night and winter and summer temperatures, and the phenomena of storms, lead not only to protective acts but to various observations and fancies, many of which become prominent forms of culture. The action of winds, the light and cloud effects on water, are not without their influence in stimulating the imagination to form explanatory myths.

It is clear that some kinds of culture could not possibly originate with, or even be diffused among a people whose physical environment does not favour them. Ways of dealing with ice and snow could not originate among dwellers in the tropics; nor could myths of mountains and seas be formed by plains people. The effects of chemical and physical environment on bodily vigour and culture have been strongly emphasized and traced in some detail by Huntington. It is probable that the relative vigour and intelligence of people inhabiting certain regions are greatly affected not only by climate, but by the amount of iodine in water, and the vitamins contained in the foods most used. The effectiveness of these and other influences decreases as man becomes able to modify his environment.

Material objects prevalent in a given region often determine the particular form the culture of the people shall take. Where stones are plentiful they are often used in forming tools, utensils and ornaments. In other places shells serve the same purposes. Where copper is easily accessible it is likely to be made into utensils, weapons and ornaments, while in other places iron is employed for similar purposes. The Eskimo with few suitable stones, no copper, only an occasional bit of meteoric iron, and a very limited amount of wood, makes much use of bones, teeth, sinews and skins. When he obtains the rarer materials he uses them in his own cultural way, as when he sets a flake of iron in a bone for use as a knife. The presence of coloured clay is an important factor in developing the art of pottery-making and in decorating objects, including the human body.

(2) *Plants and Cultures.* Plants have played a large part in the development of culture in all ages and in most regions. When there is an important food plant in abundance all the year round, especially if little needs to be done to it before eating, the development of cultural traits in connection with it is not marked. Yet there will be knowledge of where it is plentiful, when it is ripe, various customs as to how it shall be transported and eaten, what individuals or groups may use it and under what circumstances, and these may constitute a definite culture complex.

When the food material must undergo considerable treatment before being eaten, or must be stored for future use, the cultural traits are more extensive and complex. This is especially true if it becomes an article of trade among individuals or between groups. Among all peoples, plants are used to a greater or less extent for clothing and shelter,

D

and in every region the forms used and the methods of preparation are distinctive.

The environment is changed by the agricultural operations of clearing away non-useful plants and planting those desired. Such action, with the inevitable choice of specimens to be planted, results in what is called the domestication of plants. Even comparatively backward races have sometimes made profound changes in plant species. The principal grain foods—rice, rye, wheat, oats, barley, and corn—are all grasses which have been changed from the original wild species by domestication.

Of these man-changed food grasses, none have been so completely modified and specialized as maize, or Indian corn. There is no wild species that can easily and surely be identified as the parent of the domestic varieties. Most of these changes were produced by Indians in various sections of the Americas before the coming of white men. They developed varieties of corn able to survive in places marked by extremes of temperature, length of summer, and kind of soil. Corn differing from two to ten feet in height, and with ears from three to thirteen inches long, varieties suitable for eating when green, for grinding into meal when dry, and for popping, were produced. Some of these mature in half the time required for others. Customs of seed selection, depth and spacing for planting, means of fertilizing, cultivating, gathering and storing, were distinct culture complexes for each tribe, and for each variety of corn. The south-western Indians planted their corn deep in the sandy soil where the variety used would find its way to the surface through nearly a foot of sand. Not only were the characteristics of the species corn and the industrial habits of the people changed in the process of domestication, but intellectual and religious life was modified and moulded, as is shown by the corn myths (some of which are given in Longfellow's " Hiawatha "), and in dances and religious ceremonials associated with the planting and gathering of corn.

Plants such as the cocoanut palm, the breadfruit palm ; the banana, apple, cherry and other fruit trees ; the grains—

corn in America, rice in Asia, wheat and barley in Europe ; fibre plants, such as flax, cotton and hemp ; and trees supplying barks and woods, have been important factors in the development of culture traits, patterns and complexes, distinctive for each geographical area.

(3) *Animals and Culture.* In an early stage of human existence, man was merely one of many competing species of animals, some of which were naturally much more powerful than he, while others were an easy prey for him. Man learned to preserve himself by the help of stones and sticks, which he modified in various ways into effective weapons against dangerous animals, and into means for the capture of both small and large animals. Myths, legends and folk-lores deal extensively with animals and their relations to man. They have profoundly stimulated his inventive imagination, and coloured his thoughts of heavenly bodies, of spirits and gods, and of the origin of tribes of men. Some of the animals figuring in these numerous myths are supposed to be larger, more powerful or wiser than the present members of the species ; while others are not like any animals found on the earth at the present time. We know that myths and lores regarding the characteristics of certain animals which have impressed man, *e.g.* the fox, have persisted for thousands of years, and it may be that animals now extinct were the source of stories of dragons and other monsters found in folk-lore.

Whether the product of real experience or of imaginative invention, there can be no doubt that the presence of animals in man's environment, especially the dangerous and domesticated ones, were powerful emotional and intellectual stimuli to human beings. The beauty of plant and animal life is reflected in literature and art. Animals supposed to have special characteristics of greed, slyness or shrewdness, were influential in determining the epithets applied to individual men. Clans among Indians are often named after animals, and members of a clan usually treat animals whose names they bear, with respect.

Besides these general influences of wild animals upon man, those which are sources of food, clothing and shelter are of especial importance in the culture of many tribes. All the Plains Indians had a culture dominantly of the bison type ; the Eskimo of the seal and caribou types ; those of the North Pacific region, of the salmon type ; while those of the Lake and Atlantic coast regions did not have their culture complexes so completely dominated by any one type of land or water animal. The deer, the squirrel, the beaver, the fish and some birds were prominent.

There is evidence that before the dawn of recorded history many animals were first domesticated as pets or companions ; some also were later used as means of transportation, and for providing food, covering and shelter. Evidences of such early domestication are found in drawings and in the frequent presence of the bones of men along with those of domestic animals. In this process of domestication animal species have been modified into many varieties. In dealing with them, man has been modified, not only in his behaviour toward them and the things upon which his and their welfare depend, but also in his religious thoughts and emotions.

The culture complexes which develop in connection with the same species of domesticated animal are quite diverse— the dog may be a companion, protector, helper, hunter, playmate and friend, or a scarcely endured nuisance. He may be an important source of food and clothing, or a valuable means of transportation, either as a pack-animal or as a drawer of sleds, carts or the travois. The horse is a steed, a pack-animal, a drawer of various types of vehicles, a source of food and clothing, and has frequently been used in warfare. The elephant and the camel play similar rôles with special cultural complexes for each group of people. The cow may have any of these uses, but in many places is now kept chiefly as a source of supply of milk. The sheep is a dominant animal in many regions, although used only for food and clothing. Other creatures, notably the falcon, have been the cause of special and extensive culture patterns, which dominated the thought and behaviour of certain classes. The art of every nation has been profoundly influenced by animals, especially the domesticated varieties.

(4) *Human Nature and Culture.* Physiologically man has certain needs such as food, optimum temperature, etc., and he has natural means (teeth, hands, feet, etc.) of securing what is needed. He has certain native activity tendencies, but these are much modified by his own experience and the reaction of others to what he does. Thus are social customs and cultures formed which are more dependent on man's nature than on his environment of objects, plants and animals. He is of two sexes, and both for physiological and psychological reasons this results in mating. He has a long period of infancy, and this helps to develop the family and other groups. He has capacity for communicating and co-operating with others, and thus individual activities are adjusted to those of other individuals.

The truth that all varieties of the human species are fundamentally the same although differing in details, is positively proven, as Wissler points out, by the fact that all have cultures of the following types, although no two tribes have exactly the same culture patterns. (1) All communicate with others of their group by signs, words, drawings or visual symbols ; the essential condition in all such communication being that the persons communicating are similar in nature and experiences so that a part of an experience will suggest the whole. A gesture connected with food taking, a drawing of a food object, a sound associated with food taking, or a written word, may be the means of arousing in the minds of others ideas of eating. No group of human beings has ever been found which did not have at least an oral language. (2) Every group of people has characteristic habits regarding food, shelter, means of transportation, dress, tools and weapons used, industries carried on, and ways of co-operating. (3) All have their special types of art, play, games, amusements, forms of carving, drawings, paintings, music and dances. (4) None are without special conceptions of the world in the form of myths, and of more or less classified and reasoned knowledge. (5) None are without special ritualistic activities associated with birth, sickness, death, etc., known as religious practices. (6) Everywhere are families, initiated and perpetuated by some sort of marriage, which involves various systems of courting, relationship, inheritance and responsibility. (7) Property rights in some form are observed in the life of all people, and with them are associated systems of trade and means of determining values. (8) In all groups larger than the family (an almost universal condition) there is some sort of government or form of exercising control.

Since these types of culture are found in the most diverse physical environments, and in every known stage of man's life on the earth, we may be positive that they exist because man's nature is what it is. He inevitably develops them wherever he lives. The special form which the culture takes among different peoples is, however, largely determined by the surroundings.

Human Interaction. In the early days when men were few, their influence upon each other outside the family life was probably not greater than that of the animals with which they came in contact ; but it has been increasing until now in the great cities contact with human beings is almost the sole culture stimulus obtained from living things.

Mating and family life are important factors in the life of all the higher animals. Instinctively and by habit, they act in special ways because of the presence of mates, companions and young. In man the influences of family life are more continuous and much more prolonged, because there are no definite mating seasons, and because of the extended helplessness of human young. Besides this, men, much more than animals, emphasize the natural physiological differences between the sexes by means of dress, family responsibilities, and occupations.

Special family organizations are prominent features of the culture of every tribe that has been studied. Rarely is equality found between husband and wife, never between parents and children, and usually not between older and younger children, or those of different sex. The principle of dominance or subordination in the relations of human beings to each other, is in general recognized. This dominance may be founded upon the natural helplessness of children and the sympathetic care-taking tendencies of adults, or upon the tendency of the strong to dominate, and of the weak to submit. In most parts of the world adults of both sexes dominate over children, and the man is usually the head of the family. Such family customs lead rather naturally to the establishment of more or less autocratic control by head-men, warriors and rulers over tribes and nations.

In adulthood, much of the association of persons with each other may be chiefly of a different type—that of equals with equals. If one does not take account of the reactions of other people, when surrounded by equals, he is likely to be thwarted at every turn in his efforts to get things needed or desired. Because of this fact, members of a group who remain together for some time refrain from actions which are resented by others of equal or greater strength, and increase those which call forth favourable actions from others. This inevitably leads to co-operation rather than fighting among those who belong to the same group. After a time, each knows what to expect from others and acts accordingly, whether the others are equals, stronger or weaker. There is disappointment or resentment when any individual acts contrary to such expectation. Thus does the idea of justice and right originate and become an important part of the culture of every group. These ideas of what one should do in various situations and relations are never exactly the same in different parts of the world, but in every permanent group they are connected with customs which, of all that have been tried, are regarded as most satisfactory.

In the development of these approved customs, rights and obligations are always closely related. If you control an individual's time and effort, you must feed or pay him; if you get food and care from parents, you must obey them; if you take fruit from another's tree, you must permit him to take from yours; if he loans you a boat, you must give him some of the fish you catch, etc.

The social and moral traits of a tribe can never be understood by studying their acts or customs singly, but only by studying the whole system of customs. These are always found to secure some sort of balance between rights and obligations of the various individuals and social groups. Such a balance must be recognized, because any great variation is corrected sooner or later, either by rebellion of the less favoured, or by the self-interest of the dominant ones. Even a slave-owner is limited by self-interest in what he may do to his slaves.

Origin and Spread of Cultures. The origin and spread of culture depends upon three principal factors, as Dixon shows. (1) There must be something in the environment and in the previous culture which makes the new object, symbol or custom possible. Boats could never originate from, or diffuse into, a desert region ; the word kilowatt, among a people with no knowledge of electricity ; nor an eight-hour-day law, where there are no organized industries. (2) Not only must there be facilities in the surroundings and culture patterns for originating and receiving a new culture trait or complex, but there must be members of the group intelligent enough to invent, or to lead in using what is introduced from without. (3) The trait must be useful or in some way attractive to many members of the group, else the inventor or introducer will not be able to secure its adoption. In a large proportion of cases, after its invention or adoption, a cultural trait undergoes development changes in form or in its grouping with other traits. The theory that the spread of cultures is in concentric circles often fails to conform to the facts because of the influence of the above factors upon the acceptance of culture traits brought to a group. Nor is it certain that the places where the most highly developed traits are found was the centre of origin. The evidence that a given place was the centre for the diffusion of a trait is greater, if various stages of its development are represented there. However, even then it may be possible that the latest form of the trait was brought to that place, then degenerated for lack of skill in construction, imitation, or use. This fact that culture traits may decline instead of developing into more specialized perfectly functioning types, renders conclusions as to what traits are older difficult of determination.

Tendencies of Cultures to Persist. Formerly there was much talk about the " lost arts " ; but now it is believed that the only way any cultural trait could be *completely* lost, would be in an isolated tribe which became extinct before it had contacts with other inhabitants of the earth. Languages may become " dead ", in the sense that they are no longer used, more readily than any other forms of culture ; yet rarely do they " die " without having produced some changes in languages that are still in use. Art objects of certain materials and designs cease to be made, but usually leave their mark upon those that take their place. Religions and rituals survive in spite of many changes in environment, and some of their characteristics are assimilated by surviving religions. Superstitions have not wholly lost their power even after generations of scientific teaching. Weapons, utensils, and machines change in material and form, but each new type is a development from those previously constructed. (Note the resemblance of the early railway cars and automobiles to horse-drawn vehicles.) Family, social, economic and ethical customs are especially persistent.

Every discovery, invention, and habit of an individual which is of sufficient interest to others to lead a whole group to adopt it as a cultural trait, has in it a more or less universal appeal. Such cultural traits of a group constitute the most influential portion of the environment of the new generation of the same people, and have a stimulating influence upon surrounding groups. Adults naturally continue habits once formed, and the imitativeness of children and the prestige of parents almost insure the perpetuation of customs in succeeding generations. It follows, therefore, that cultural traits once established tend to remain the same so long as the group to which they belong stays in the same physical environment and makes no new contacts with other groups.

Factors Favouring Culture Changes. Opposed to these general influences toward preservation of cultures are factors favouring change—(1) experimentation by children and young people ; (2) discoveries and inventions by talented individuals ; (3) modification in conduct by powerful leaders ; (4) changes in general or special economic conditions ; and (5) finally and chiefly, contacts with outside cultures. In an isolated group the first four factors are rarely strong enough to do more than improve upon cultural types without radically changing them. Changes in population affecting economic conditions are sometimes great enough to affect all phases of social life. In general, better economic conditions favour increase of population, except when standards of living increase more rapidly than the population. If there are two or more classes nearly equal in numbers or power so as to provide constant competition, the probabilities of change are much greater than when one class fully dominates the other. If the people migrate to a new environment or if a new kind of domestic plant or animal, weapon, utensil or religion is brought from without, there are sure to be modifications of cultural traits, and sometimes of many of the cultural complexes associated with them ; but usually the utilitarian traits are adopted earlier than the social or religious patterns associated therewith : *e.g.* the Indians' methods of planting and using corn were adopted by whites without the religious ceremonies.

During the historical period, changes in the culture of a people have been stimulated most by contacts with people of other cultures. In nearly all cases the influence of great leaders has played a conspicuous part in modifying and perfecting cultural traits already present. Such leaders may be inventors of devices or religions, but are frequently those whose personalities give them power and prestige in inducing others to adopt new traits originated by other individuals of their group, or taken over from some other group.

Development of Cultures. Every culture trait is the result of adaptation of a group of people to the exigencies of life presented by their physical, plant, animal and human environment, and conditioned by traits and complexes already existing. With so many factors involved, the chief similarity in order of development that may be expected is that the simpler forms will be produced earlier in the centres of origin, and will become more complex and more closely integrated into tribal patterns and complexes as time goes on. When a trait is introduced from without, not infrequently its most complex form is adopted, but the integration with other tribal traits is likely to remain imperfect for some time, *e.g.* guns and automobiles may be *used* by people who have no knowledge of the principles involved in their construction and operation. Chapin finds many facts in support of the theory that old customs dominate in a new situation for a time, followed by more or less random or trial changes, which after a time give way to a uniform and more satisfactory adjustment. This is best shown in the development of utilitarian and legal customs.

The construction and use of a bow presents little perceptible uniformity of development among different peoples. The materials of which the bows and arrows are constructed depend much upon the materials found in the locality ; the size, form, etc., depend upon their uses and the skill and ingenuity of their makers. The use of poisoned arrows would not ordinarily be a development from using heavier blunt or sharp arrows that kill, but might well develop in one tribe from coming in contact with another that used poisoned arrows in a blow-gun, especially if there were large animals that could not be killed by direct arrow wounds. The cross-bow, on the other hand, is an undoubted instance of development from a simpler form. Only under certain conditions, such as a need for it in warfare, and facility in the use of mechanical appliances, would it become a weapon of the type used in mediæval warfare. A spring-gun might be considered as a more complex form of the blow-gun, but it could not be invented where there was only slight knowledge of mechanics. However far advanced in mechanical knowledge and skill a people might be, the modern gun would never have appeared without knowledge of explosives and their use for other purposes. No kind of propulsive weapon or machine will survive when introduced from without, unless it either continues to be obtainable by trade, or the knowledge and skill necessary to produce it is acquired.

What is true of weapons is true of all significant culture traits. A people cannot be accurately classified as to degree of general culture development by such terms as the hunting, the pastoral, or the agricultural stage, etc. These may vary greatly in complexity, or several of the types may be combined. A mechanical stage of development is, however, necessarily a more advanced and complex development than a tool age. Characterization by some much used material, such as stone age, bronze age, iron age, is not significant in itself; but in general more varieties of knowledge and skill are likely to be associated with the construction of iron tools, than with stone or copper ones. Some tribes using no iron, however, have more varied and complex cultures than others making use of it, *e.g.* the Eskimo, without metals, has developed rather complex traits and patterns in using skins, bones and tusks of the animals of his region.

In the light of such facts as these, it is clear that the idea of a fixed order of culture development cannot be used as a safe guide in anthropological studies. It is much more profitable to study the effects of local surroundings, of group contacts and of cultures already developed.

The factors concerned in the development of material cultural objects that are chiefly utilitarian and many of the complexes associated with them, are comparatively easy to study. But many of the culture traits associated with objects of use, and shown in all sorts of customs and rituals, are not the product of material surroundings, but of the human imagination which has peopled the world with spirits, and coloured all things by mental attitudes of approval and disapproval. It is therefore necessary to give some space to forms of culture not directly objective in origin.

Subjective Attitudes and Cultures. In the healthy reactions of anthropologists against unscientific subjective and theoretical explanations of the origin of cultural traits and complexes, an important characteristic of human nature may not be given sufficient weight. Man has the capacity to observe his mental states, as well as to perceive and react to the things affecting his senses. His own feelings when manipulating things, are often more interesting to him than the things themselves or the changes he produces in them. This subjective interest seems to be very prominent in children in their earliest voluntary movements. People are of great interest to them also, because their acts bring relief from pain, and pleasant experiences of various kinds. From his own experience, the child finds that by making certain motions he may change one feeling into another more pleasing : hence these motions are made frequently to effect such changes. He naturally infers that people in performing certain acts, get the same feeling that he does. He thus gets the idea of *purpose* as the important factor in action. Much of what people do affects his comfort, so it is of advantage to him to know what they are going to do, especially when his acts and desires may be thwarted or modified by theirs. Trying to anticipate objective movements to be performed, teaches him to look for signs of purpose in others. Thus he can more effectively meet human situations than by waiting until people have performed an act before he responds to it. This tendency to think of the actions of self and other human beings in terms of purpose developed in childhood, continues in adult life and is often so strong that it is readily carried over into experiences with animals ; often also to observed changes in plants, clouds, heavenly bodies and fire ; and not infrequently to falling stones and other changing objects. Man has, therefore, always been surrounded by a subjective world projected from his own conscious states.

This subjective world has had a profound influence upon the behaviour of men individually and as groups. Good and evil spirits are conceived as animating plants and animals, and sometimes even non-material objects. This immaterial world has played a large part in man's religious practices and beliefs, his myths, his literature and art, and has influenced and sometimes almost completely dominated his practical conduct in many important phases of life. It has developed in him all sorts of taboos and rituals in relation to plants, animals, and natural phenomena, especially at critical times of planting, harvesting, going on expeditions or beginning construction, and in emergencies of birth, death, sickness and marriage. Not man's conduct alone has been modified and directed in important ways by superstitions and religious beliefs, but also his ways of thinking and of reasoning about the world, and about all things.

Magical Thinking. Fundamentally all thinking is based on the idea that things associated in time or place, or resembling each other in appearance, are, or may be, causally related. These assumptions are used uncritically in magical thinking, while in scientific thinking they are carefully tested by observation and experience. Common sense uses experience as a check, but uses it less accurately than science. In magical thinking there are usually no tests used, or they are non-conclusive because of beliefs that invisible spirits, as well as things, are concerned in happenings. Signs, protective talismans, magic words or formulas, and rituals are sometimes employed because of chance coincidences ; yet most of them originate in, or are made to seem probable by reasoning based upon some fact of contiguity or similarity in the things, or in the assumed spirit of the things. A barren woman must not be concerned with the planting of seed, lest it be unproductive ; the crop will be good if the motion made in sowing is like that of a well-grown field of grain waving in the wind, etc. Sickness may be cured by a medicine resembling some symptom of the disease ; the red planet Mars is connected with war, so is any one born under it ; the heart of a brave man, when eaten, will give courage to the one eating it, etc.

The evidence of a universal human tendency to make such inferences is found in common folk-lore everywhere, and in the early behaviour of all children. A child who imitates some feature of an act of his elders, or uses something resembling an object they have used, attains in imagination, and sometimes actually, the ends he has seen gained by them, *e.g.* a child imitating an automobile driver. Among all people objects which have belonged to some great individual, or were found where he lived, are of the greatest interest and value. It is only a short step from the treasuring of souvenirs to using them for the cure of disease, for protection against danger, or as a means of attaining success in all sorts of undertakings. Civilized people are in part restrained from taking this step because of their more complete knowledge of causes and of known relation of means to ends ; but whenever people lack this knowledge the tendency to superstitious and magical thinking asserts itself. In games of chance and in all new ventures, magical means of insuring good fortune are universally invoked in some form. Even the results of scientific research are made use of in similar ways, *e.g.* the powerful but unseen force of electricity is the basis of countless fake cures for disease, and of false logic regarding thought transference.

Religious Cultures. Religion, so universal among all peoples, is the inevitable result of attempts to adjust to the serious situations of life by some sort of appeal to unseen spirits associated with things and events. In dealing with plants, animals and forces of nature, North American Indians and most savage tribes believe that spirits must be invoked when anything is done in relation to them. For example, if an individual bear is killed, the spirit of bears as a species must be propitiated. With most primitive peoples rituals are, therefore, a prominent feature of daily life, especially in affairs of importance.

The more the knowledge of natural causes acquired through · observation and scientific study, the fewer are the occasions for the use of magic objects, rituals and prayers. Such increased knowledge has resulted in a very great decrease of religious performances among civilized peoples in the last century ; but since man will always be faced by mysteries, and subject to uncontrollable and terrible experiences, religious rites are likely to continue to be used for protection and comfort in great emergencies. Religious culture is as surely the outgrowth of man's nature as are tools, machines, social customs and political organizations.

SELECTED RESEARCHES

From "ANTHROPOLOGY." By A. L. Kroeber. 1923. London:
George G. Harrap & Co. Ltd. New York: Harcourt, Brace
& Co., Inc. *Quoted by Permission.*

After showing the probable order in which four types of ritual
culture developed among California Indians (assuming that the
one most generally found in all the tribes was the oldest), Kroeber
attempts to determine the probable age of these rituals in the
following ways :

California began to be settled about 1770. The last tribes
were not brought into contact with the white men until 1850.
As early, however, as 1540 Alarcon rowed and towed up the
lower Colorado and wrote an account of the tribes he encountered
there. Two years later, Cabrillo visited the coast and island
tribes of southern California, and wintered among them. In
1579 Drake spent some weeks on shore among the central
Californians and a member of his crew has left a brief but spirited
description of them. In all three instances these old accounts of
native customs tally with remarkable fidelity with all that has
been ascertained in regard to the recent tribes of the same
regions. That is, native culture has evidently changed very
little since the sixteenth century. The local sub-cultures already
showed substantially their present form ; which means that the
Fourth Period must have been well established three to four
centuries ago. We might then assign to this period about double
the time which has elapsed since the explorers visited California ;
say seven hundred years. This seems a conservative figure,
which would put the commencement of the Fourth Period
somewhere about A.D. 1200.

All the remainder must be reconstruction by projection. In
most parts of the world for which there are continuous records,
it is found that civilization usually changes more rapidly as
time goes on. While this is not a rigorous law, it is a prevailing
tendency. However, let us apply this principle with reserve,
and assume that the Third Period was no longer than the Fourth.
Another seven hundred years would carry back to A.D. 500.

Now, however, it seems reasonable to begin to lengthen our
periods somewhat. For the Second, a thousand years does not
appear excessive : approximately from 500 B.C. to A.D. 500.
By the same logic the First Period should be allowed from a
thousand to fifteen hundred years. It might be wisest to set
no beginning at all, since our " First " Period is only the first

of those which are determinable with present knowledge. Actually it may have been preceded by a still more primitive era on which as yet no specific evidence is available. It can, however, be suggested that by 2,000 or 1,500 B.C. the beginnings of native Californian culture as we know it had already been made. . . .

The archæologists have tried to compute the age of Ellis Landing mound in another way. When it was first examined there were near its top about fifteen shallow depressions. These appear to be the remains of the pits over which the Indians were wont to build their dwellings. A native household averages about seven inmates. One may thus estimate a population of about 100 souls. Numerous quadruped bones in the mound prove that these people hunted; net sinkers, that they fished; mortars and pestles, that they consumed acorns and other seeds. Accordingly, only part of their subsistence, and probably the minor part, was derived from molluscs. Fifty mussels a day for a man, woman and child seem a fair estimate of what their shell-fish food is likely to have aggregated. This would mean that the shells of 5,000 mussels would accumulate on the site daily. Laboratory experiments prove that 5,000 such shells, with the addition of the same percentage of ash and soil as occurs in the mound, all crushed down to the same consistency of compactness as the body of the mound exhibits, occupy a volume of a cubic foot. This being the daily increment, the growth of the mound would be in the neighbourhood of 365 feet per year. Now the deposit contains roughly a million and a quarter cubic feet. Dividing this figure by 365, one obtains about 3,500 as the presumable number of years required to accumulate the mound.

This result may not be accepted too literally. It is the result of a calculation with several factors, each of which is only tentative. Had the population been 200 instead of 100, the deposit would, with the other terms of the computation remaining the same, have built up twice as fast, and the 3,500 years would have to be cut in half. On the other hand, it has been assumed that occupation of the site was continuous through the year. Yet all that is known of the habits of the Indians makes it probable that the mound inhabitants were accustomed to go up in the hills and camp about half of the time. Allowance for this factor would double the 3,500 years. All that is maintained for the computed age is that it represents a conscientious and conservative endeavour to draw a conclusion from all available sources of knowledge, and that it seems to hit as near the truth as a calculation of this sort can.

One verification has been attempted. Sample of mound material, taken randomly from different parts, indicate that 14 per cent of its weight, or about 7,000 tons, are ashes. If the mound is 3,500 years old, the ashes were deposited at the rate of two tons a year, or about eleven pounds daily. Experiments with the woods growing in the neighbourhood have shown that they yield less than one per cent of ash. The eleven daily pounds

E

must therefore have come from 1,200 pounds of wood. On the assumption, as before, that the population averaged fifteen families, the one-fifteenth share of each household would be eighty pounds daily. This is a pretty good load of firewood for a woman to carry on her back, and with the Indians' habit of nursing their fires economically, especially along a timberless shore, eighty pounds seem a liberal allowance to satisfy all their requirements for heating and cooking. If they managed to get along on less than eighty pounds per hut, the mound age would be correspondingly greater.

This check calculation thus verifies the former estimate rather reasonably. It does not seem rash to set down three to four thousand years as the indicated age of the mound.

This double archæological conclusion tallies as closely as one could wish with the results derived from the ethnological method of estimating antiquity from the degree and putative rapidity of cultural change. Both methods carry the First traceable Period back to about 1,500 or 2,000 B.C.

"RACIAL GROUPS IN A UNIVERSITY." By Prof. EDWARD CARY HAYES, Univ. of Illinois. From *Scientific Monthly*, February 1928. *Quoted by Permission.*

In view of the discussion of racial traits by a great company of writers, from Gobineau and Vacher de Lapouge to Wiggam and Madison Grant, and in view of current fears as to the mongrelizing of our stock, it occurred to the writer to study the racial groups represented in the University of Illinois. The number of students is sufficiently large to have significance. The individuals are tested for four years in similar pursuits. They come after twelve years of similar schooling. Against such a background of cultural similarity, racial traits might be expected to stand out definitely.

The university department of hygiene which examines every student admitted was asked to record for each student the measurements from which cephalic index is computed, eye colour and hair colour, distinguishing a number of grades of each, stature, build and racial parentage, as understood by the matriculant.

After thousands of these records had accumulated, a graduate student, Mr. George M. Proctor, was asked to sort out the records of the first hundred Nordics, the first hundred Alpines, the first hundred Mediterraneans, and of all the Chinese, other foreigners, Jews and Negroes encountered. However much doubt there may be as to whether his Nordics, Alpines and Mediterraneans are actually pure-bred representatives of distinct racial stocks, there is no doubt that they are as distinctively classifiable by race as white American citizens ever are.

The investigator was directed to give primary importance to

cephalic index and secondary importance to eye colour. Hair colour and stature were recognized as less significant but treated as corroborative evidence when, for example, blond hair and high stature accompanied a dolichocephalic index and blue eyes, or when medium stature, stocky build and chestnut hair accompanied a brachycephalic index and hazel eyes. The race of their parents as given by the students, and their names were also treated as having some corroborative value.

The first result of his investigation was that relatively few of the students at this university could be definitely assigned to any racial group. Our student population is very thoroughly mixed in blood and is descended mainly from European populations, each of which is very mixed.

The second fact disclosed was that of those who could be so classified an overwhelming majority were Nordics. Mr. Proctor classified as Nordics about one-tenth of the first thousand, but after going through the records for eleven thousand students, he had found only seventy-two whom he felt confident in classifying as Alpines and only ten whom he could classify with confidence as Mediterraneans. Italian parentage and name were not proof of membership in the Mediterranean race. There is too much Lombard and Alpine blood in Italy, and too much departure from characteristic Mediterranean traits was found among those who call themselves Italians.

The Jews were a racially heterogeneous group. Thirty-four per cent of them had grey, blue or greenish eyes, two had red hair. In respect to cephalic index they were distributed pretty evenly all the way from 72·5 to 88·6, that is from those very decidedly dolichocephalic, through sub-dolichocephalic, mesocephalic, sub-brachycephalic, to very decided brachycephalic. They showed no tendency to centre about a cephalic type. Many of the Jews are indistinguishable in appearance from other Americans. Others among them " look Jewish ", that is foreign. The foreignness is often Syrian or Hittite, rather often Spanish. So far as this group of ninety-three indicates, they do not represent a racial type.

The 435 students included in the seven groups treated as classifiable had a scholastic average distinctly below that of the racially unclassifiable mass of students in the university. In this institution a student's grade is computed by counting a grade of A equal to 5, B equal to 4, C equal to 3, D equal to 2 and E equal to 1. E is failure. Each course grade is multiplied by the number of hours' credit given for the course. The sum of these products is divided by the student's total number of credit hours to give his average grade. The average of all the men in the university is found each semester by averaging the averages of a thousand men selected at random. In the nine semesters ending January 1925, the average grade of all men has ranged from 3·157 to 3·314. The average of the nine semesters has been 3·235.

The 435 students belonging to classifiable groups taken together had for their entire time of their residence at the university an average scholastic grade of 2·934. To one familiar with our grading system this is a marked inferiority.

The seven classifiable groups had the following averages :

Chinese	3·35
Jews	3·18
Nordics	3·00
Foreign students, excluding Chinese . .	3·00
Alpines	2·94
Mediterraneans	2·83
Negroes	2·55

Only the Chinese equal the average for unclassified men.

The ten individuals among the 435 classified having the highest grades were :

A Nordic	4·94
A Chinaman	4·82
A Jew	4·73
A South African	4·68
A Nordic	4·68
A Nordic	4·65
A Chinaman	4·48
A Chinaman	4·47
A Jew	4·41
A Negro	4·29

The first six in the above list have grades entitling them to election to Phi Beta Kappa or Tau Beta Pi. No others of the 435 classified are clearly eligible to such election. Three per cent of those classified as Nordic appear in the list of ten best students, 8·33 per cent of the Chinese, 2·15 per cent of the Jews, 1·57 per cent of foreigners, excluding Chinese, 1·66 per cent of the Negroes, no Alpine and no Mediterranean. In the case of the Mediterraneans, at least, the number involved is too small to have any significance.

In view of the alarms that have been sounded as to the degeneracy to be expected from hybridization, perhaps the most interesting of these facts is that the aggregate of 435 classifiable students, including thirty-six Chinese slightly superior to the average, should be so distinctly lower in scholastic standing than the unclassifiable mass. The hundred Nordics are decidedly below the average of unclassified students. So are the Jews.

The figures given are reported merely as a bit of evidence to be put with other evidence for what it may be worth.

SUGGESTED READINGS

The general field of Anthropology is perhaps best covered by the following:

DIXON, ROLAND B., *The Racial History of Man*, 1923.
GOLDENWEISER, A. A., *Early Civilization*, 1930.
KROEBER, A. L., *Anthropology*, 1923.
TOZZER, A., *Social Origins and Social Continuities*, 1925.
WALLACE, WILSON D., *An Introduction to Anthropology*, 1926.
WISSLER, CLARK, *Man and Culture*, 1923.
WISSLER, CLARK, *Social Anthropology*, 1929.

Of more special studies which may be mentioned are:

GARTH, THOMAS RUSSELL, *Race Psychology*, 1931.
MALINOWSKI, BRANISLAW, *Argonauts of the Western Pacific*, 1922.
REUTER, E. BYRON, *The American Race Problem*, 1927.
REUTER, E. BYRON, *Race Mixture*, 1931.
WISSLER, CLARK, *The American Indian*, 1922.

Those interested in the American Negro should also consult the *American Academy of Political and Social Science*, November 1928, edited by DONALD YOUNG.

The influence of environment on man and his culture is emphasized by HUNTINGTON, ELLSWORTH, *Civilization and Climate*, 3rd ed., 1924, and other writings by Huntington.

Chapter IV

HOW LIFE IS PRESERVED, OR PHYSIOLOGY AND HYGIENE

THE BODY NATURALLY CARES FOR ITSELF

Man, like other animal organisms, is an active centre for receiving, transforming and using energy, and it is by virtue of such an organization that he continues to exist and function as a unit, composed of many diverse parts. The permanence and vigour of his existence depends upon the preservation of suitable balance between processes, while varying the degrees of activity in adjusting to the environing stimuli.

One of the most important conditions for preserving this balance is that the body shall be kept at the same *temperature* all the time (98·6° F.), whatever the temperature of the surrounding air or water. Like other animals he takes in food and oxygen, and by means of elaborate co-operating mechanisms his body is automatically kept at about the right temperature whether he is resting or active, so long as the surrounding temperature does not vary too much. If this is forty degrees below that of his body, more clothing, more food and perhaps some exercise is necessary to keep him at the usual temperature, than if the surroundings are only twenty or thirty degrees below. When the outside temperature is almost the same as that of the body, especially if exercise is being taken, the temperature of the body would be raised above normal if its regulating mechanism did not act in a cooling way. This mechanism, when in a healthy condition, is remarkably prompt and effective in adjusting so as to cool the body when surrounding temperature of air or water is high, or to warm it when temperature is low. One of the advantages of a varying climate, and of hot and cold showers, is that they keep this mechanism in good working order. When it has been little used or over-exercised in acting in one way, a change to a more variable climate or to one demanding an opposite kind of adjustment, may be of advantage, if the change is not too sudden or extreme.

The adjustment needed to keep the body at normal temperature when in water at sixty degrees is much greater than when in air of the same temperature, because the water takes up the heat of the body much more rapidly than the air. For a similar reason moist air demands more adjustment than dry air. Moving air also takes away more heat than motionless air, not only because new particles of air touch the skin, but because already warmed moisture is removed.

The *pressure* of the *air* upon the body and its variations in composition and electric conditions, all of which vary with elevation and other factors, make many physiological adjustments necessary. If changes are suddenly made by deep diving, or rising suddenly from the deeps, or by going swiftly up a mountain or rising in an airplane, the mechanism may not be equal to the task of adjusting to the changed pressure and decrease of oxygen. However, in this as in the case of temperature, moderate and not too sudden changes probably keep the mechanism in good order. A change from sea-level to elevated regions, or the reverse, is often invigorating when one has remained at the same elevation for some time.*

Man's activities, like those of other animals, vary from the most vigorous exercise to a passive condition of sleep,

* Numerous experiments by biologists, and statistical studies of man in different physical environments by Huntington and others, emphasize the importance of physical conditions of temperature, moisture, air pressure, and foods, in the development, physiological health and activity of all living things. Each species of plant and animal thrives when these are of optimum degree, and slows up and perhaps dies when they become too strong or too weak. Young rats may be fed in such a way that they will remain the same weight for a long period of time. Hybernation of woodchucks may be shortened or lengthened by regulation of temperature ; of toads, by control of moisture ; and the hatching of eggs may be accelerated or delayed by variations in heat and light. Flowers may be brought to bloom or to seed at any time of year by appropriate control of kind, duration and intensity of light. A slight change in temperature or moisture at a critical time in the development of pests, such as the codling-moth, may make them very plentiful or very scarce. Lack of iodine in water

in which there is decreased activity of heart and lungs and no external movement. These changes are naturally rhythmic in character and under ordinary conditions there is at least one rather long period of sleep during each day, with periods of considerable activity followed by comparative quietude. When the exigencies of living do not demand a large amount of activity, there is likely to be some of a playful character.

Moving the limbs and body keeps not only the muscles in good working condition, but incidentally the internal organs of breathing, circulation, digestion and other apparatus concerned in heat regulation and in digestion. All parts of the body are stimulated and kept working harmoniously by exercise that is not too violent or prolonged, or too dominantly of only a few parts. Under ordinary natural conditions, exercising and resting like adjusting to temperature and pressure, are likely to take place in men as well as in other animals without much thought on their part.

Another essential to the maintenance of life and health in man is *food*, which supplies the energy required to keep the body at the same temperature and the internal organs active ; and also that required to move the body and limbs in getting food, escaping enemies, seeking comfortable surroundings and in play and work activities. Man like other animals has natural means of securing food and of digesting it. He also has appetites which in a very general way cause him to take the kind and amount of food needed at more or less regular intervals. The amount of food taken and, to a less extent, the kind taken, is naturally varied with the temperature of the surroundings and with the amount of muscular activity, as well as with the quality and quantity of food available.

A rather natural sequence in animals and men is to be externally active in getting and taking food, then to rest and

and food, or of ultra-violet rays of light, may profoundly modify the health and activity of the inhabitants of a region.

Civilized man is able to regulate indoor temperature accurately, but finds it difficult to get the same combinations of temperature, moisture, light, and electric conditions that are found in the open air. As yet the prescription of more outdoor life is surer to promote health than attempted exact regulation of indoor conditions.

perhaps sleep, while internal processes of digestion continue, and to follow this by playful activity. The more strenuous and prolonged the activity of any kind (if not excessive), the greater the amount of food taken, which in turn supplies energy for future activity. This natural adjustment is disturbed if no exercise is taken, or if too little or too much food is eaten. There is enough stored-up energy in the body to prevent serious disturbance being produced by temporary decrease or absence of food. Declining energy is quickly restored when a proper food is supplied. The effects of over-eating, *i.e.* taking in more energy-producing materials than are needed, are often more lasting and serious. There is a limit to the amount of energy that can be stored up in the body, and without the stimulus of exercise the digestive organs may not be able to take care of the larger amount of material to be disposed of by the bowels, kidneys, lungs and skin. These difficulties are often slight after one or two excessive meals, but are cumulative if there is continuous over-eating.

ONE BODILY ACTIVITY AFFECTS ANOTHER

Physiological processes are all closely related to each other. A change in one kind of activity demands a change in other activities to restore the harmonious balance upon which health depends. If the rate of breathing changes, so also does the heart-beat. If the muscles are vigorously active they are supplied with more oxygenated blood. If the brain is vigorously active it receives more blood, while after a hearty meal the digestive organs use an increased amount.

There is a normal pulse and breathing rate, varying with age and associated with a standard degree of blood-pressure. Individuals varying greatly from these standards are less likely to live long and vigorously than those near the standard. Variations from the norm in an individual usually indicate poor health. The disturbance of health is less severe if *all* the activities vary so as to keep their relative vigour the same, than if one increases, and the others decrease or remain the same. In health there are adjustive processes which keep the activities in harmony with each other, and they are thus more or less automatically regulated. This is most strikingly shown in the repairing of wounds.

A recognition of these relations plays an important part in hygiene. If circulation is poor it is not advisable to stimulate the heart to greater action directly, but improvement is often brought about by prescribing certain breathing and muscular exercises. The value of muscular exercise is not chiefly in increasing the size, hardness and flexibility of the muscles concerned, but in the effects upon respiration, circulation, digestion, and upon the activity of all sorts of glands, particularly those of the skin. Rarely can any physical disorder be permanently cured by direct treatment in accordance with older theories of medicine. Scientific health building, on the contrary, proceeds on the principle that improvement is possible only by stimulating one or more activities, which in turn stimulate others, until all are active in a harmonious way. Sometimes the opposite course is followed, that of decreasing one or more stimuli with the result that all activities are brought into more balanced and harmonious relation with each other.

As civilization increases, the problem of the proper relation of work and play becomes more acute and complex. In proportion as work of a specialized kind increases, there is need for the balancing activities of free play. Some such relief is needed every day. Yearly vacations are not sufficient, although they serve the purpose of giving more or less complete and refreshing change in ways of living.

CULTURE AND HEALTH

Changes in environment made by man and the customs each group form, often have a good deal of influence on health. By wearing clothes the same air is kept in contact with the skin, and less heat is required to keep the body at normal temperature. Shelters have similar effects, especially when there is artificial heating. The latter usually dries the air, and the effect upon sweat glands and lungs is different from that when air moves freely over the skin. Experiments show that most of the bad effects of poor ventilation disappear when the air is put in motion. Normal exercise of the skin as a part of the temperature regulating mechanism is diminished by the culture trait of wearing clothes and living in heated houses in cold weather. This, together with the greater number of germs that thrive in warm houses, largely accounts for the extraordinary prevalence of colds among civilized people. A partial corrective is afforded by another culture trait that has developed, *i.e.* more universal and frequent bathing. Clothing and shelter when used too much, have injurious effects by shutting off the sun's rays, which are now known to be of great stimulating value.

In general, civilized man now has a more permanent home than most primitive people, but means of transportation have facilitated travel so that most men still get a change of air. The air in the neighbourhood of cities when much soft coal is used, is far less clean than that in rural sections.

The culture traits and complexes of modern civilization have greatly modified rhythms of activity and rest. Specialization in industries in this day of machines is often extreme. When one does nearly the same things over and over all day, certain parts of the body are likely to be over-exercised, unless there are periods of rest. Other parts are insufficiently used, and the general balance is consequently disturbed and needs to be restored in play or some avocation. In general, machines have taken the place of muscular force, but have not so much relieved the nerve centres. Fortunately, athletic and sporting traits help to restore the balance disturbed by machines.

It is in the use of foods that culture and culture complexes have made the greatest changes in health habits. Like animals, man's choice of foods depends in part upon its suitability, and in part upon the ease with which it may be obtained. Unlike animals, however, man nearly always makes considerable change in his staple foods, especially by cooking before eating. Most peoples are also influenced by food taboos to refrain from using certain plant and animal foods that are valued by others. Snake meat, pork, snails or dogs, highly relished by some, are under strict taboo among other people because of established customs or religious beliefs.

At the present time, with means of preserving and transporting developed as they are, one may live in any part of the earth and consume food brought from any other portion. Theoretically, an individual might exercise unlimited choice in his eating ; practically, he is largely directed by the customs of his people as to what he shall eat, when, and how much. In homes, each family and individual has some special habits, but in the main these conform in a general way to those of other families in the locality. In all hotels and restaurants there are typical breakfasts, luncheons and dinners offered at certain times, cooked and served in much the same way and in the same quantities. Natural appetite and needs are therefore minor factors as compared with culture complexes in directing times of eating, food chosen and the amount eaten.

SCIENCE AND STANDARDS OF HYGIENIC FUNCTIONING

Previous to the development of the sciences of anatomy, physiology and hygiene, there were many culture traits favourable to health, based partly on more or less correctly interpreted experiences of the group in a given environment, yet often associated with magical or religious customs. Wherever athletic contests have been held, many practices favourable to health are found, but frequently some of them are enforced by magical or religious beliefs. In nearly all tribes there are also customs and beliefs very unfavourable to the preservation of health.

The science of physiology was slow in developing because of the complexity of processes involved and the impossibility of reversing conditions, and also because of changes produced in physiological norms by habit. Early in the use of exact methods, it was established that the usual rate of pulse for adults was about 70 per minute, the normal temperature of the body was a little less than 100° F. ; but what this meant in terms of physiological functioning was not clear, except that much variation from these standards meant disorder, and some sort of treatment was given to restore the temperature to normal.

People who have lived a life of a certain degree of activity at certain temperatures or at certain altitudes for a long time, appear to remain more comfortable and healthy than if they change to lower or higher temperatures or altitudes ; but people with different habits seem to be better off when conforming to different standards.

The best temperature for most office workers and for most mechanical workers has been determined, and may be maintained by using thermometers as guides rather than by relying upon personal opinion. Extensive experimentation has shown that air conditions as regards composition, is far less important than good circulation of air. If a man stands in a room where his skin is bathed in free air, but with his head where much used air is breathed, there is far less physiological disturbance than when he breathes free air, but has his body surrounded by much-breathed moist " dead " air. Proper circulation is, therefore, the most important thing to be secured in a closed building. This may be insured by fans, or by openings to the outside air. The latter is now believed to be the more favourable to health, partly because outside air is usually of more normal moisture and composition than the air heated and confined in a building. There can be no question that man living under artificial conditions may maintain his health better by following rules based on scientific research, than under more natural conditions without the help of science.

People who have become habituated to a certain amount of tobacco, alcohol, opium or strychnine may, with comfort, use quantities which would upset or even kill individuals unused to them. One who has developed resistance to disease germs may be unaffected by their presence, while others sicken and perhaps die, when exposed to them. All of this emphasizes a fundamental truth, that the human organism is extraordinarily self-preservative, and whenever necessary adapts or changes itself in ways that make survival possible regardless, within limits, of temperature, air composition, air pressure, amounts of activity and food. These limits are, however, rather definitely fixed. Unsheltered and unclothed, the endurable extremes of temperature would be less than a hundred degrees apart, and the optimum range one-fourth as great. Pressure variations of a few atmospheres are seriously disturbing, and an active person cannot live on a food intake of less than 2,000 calories, or on more than three or four times that amount. The U.S. Army ration was nearly 4,000 calories, while that of the Japanese was only a little over half as much.

After extensive researches, it has been found that there are standards of health conditions and functioning, approximated by all human beings, but varying with climate, physiological type, amount of activity, physiological habits, and perhaps with race. If a group of men are living in the same physical surroundings and engaged in about the same kind and amount of activity for a number of months, they become more alike, and scientifically established standards of kinds and amounts of food will keep all but a very few in good health. Many soldiers, and students in college dining-rooms, where menus are prescribed by a scientific dietitian, are kept in better health than when they are eating as they wish in their own homes. Animals guided by their natural inclinations keep in pretty good health ; but domestic animals scientifically fed thrive better than their brothers in a wild state. Only after much chemical research and physiological experimentation was this made possible.

WHAT FOODS ARE NECESSARY

First it was found by chemical analyses what substances were needed to supply bodily heat, energy and tissue-building material ; then studies had to be made to find out what ones of these were digestible and readily assimilated. Then it appeared that food must also contain indigestible materials to keep the eliminative organs active. Still later it was discovered that there were food substances not easily detected by chemical analysis, named vitamins, which in very small quantities, were necessary to active, healthy, physiological functioning. A proper diet for individuals of a certain age, living under the same conditions, and equally active, may now be prescribed; but for various reasons individual prescriptions varying slightly from the general standard, sometimes need to be made.

In America, where there are many varieties of food and a large proportion of people with means of purchasing it, most people could get the essential food elements. In some localities, however, customs of eating are found which omit some essential, and consequently health has been improved by education in the freer use of milk, fruits and vegetables.

REGULARITY OF FUNCTIONING

The importance of physiological rhythms and the influence of one activity upon the others, is being recognized. Much research has been devoted to studying the effects of variations in intensity and time relations of activity and rest, and their effects upon health. Researches regarding foods justify the rather general custom of three or more meals a day for adults who are healthy, and vigorously and continuously employed. Babies, young children, invalids and those doing an excessive amount of physical work, are better for frequent eating, although, except in the case of the latter persons, no greater total amount of food is required during the day. Regular intervals of eating give the best results, not only in the way of utilizing the food taken, but as help in regulating other processes, especially those of the bowels, which are thus more likely to form the habit of acting at a certain time each day. Work activities are also more likely to be regulated and efficient, when the eating, as well as the resting process of sleeping, is regular.

Much research has been made to establish standards of work activity in general and in special lines. Activity of a few parts, continued without even the smallest interval between, quickly brings fatigue and inefficiency. No muscle or sense organ can be used more than from a few seconds to a few minutes, without decrease in rate or accuracy of functioning. In most work activities, even in modern industry, there are many sense organs and muscles used in succession, and each set has some chance to rest while others are active. Where several processes are involved, the fatigue of parts is still less.

Besides the parts actually used in any performance, there are always associated contractions which may produce fatigue. For example, many muscles beside those directly concerned in moving a pen, are kept in more or less continuous contraction in keeping the body in proper position for writing. It is for this reason that rather general fatigue may be produced by what appears to be the continued use of only a few parts.

Temporary and local fatigue may be largely avoided by proper intervals of rest, or by shifts to a different set of muscles. Experiments have shown that the amount of work done may be increased and the degree of fatigue produced may be greatly lessened by prescribing intervals when rests are taken, or shifts made.   Men loading pig-iron, when their movements and rest periods were prescribed after scientific study, were able to do three times as much work with less fatigue, than when they worked as they pleased.

Whatever adjustments of activity are made, general and more lasting fatigue cannot be postponed indefinitely.   There must be entire rest in the form of sleep. This is needed every day.   For children and infants more than one period of sleep, and a greater total amount, is required than for healthy adults.   There is sufficient stored energy to enable one to work for long periods without rest, but that, as well as food, must be taken sooner or later.

Experiments show that to work the body as a whole, or any part of it, after fatigue has set in, wastes much energy and ultimately interferes with healthy physiological functioning.

With these truths as a basis, it is possible to determine by experimentation for any group engaged in any type of activity under the same conditions, standard programmes of eating and of work, rest and sleep, that will be most favourable for efficiency and for health. This has already been done in many factories by efficiency and health experts, and to some extent in schools.

HEALTH RULES AND THE INDIVIDUAL

The above scientific truths upon which rules for preserving the health of large groups of people are based, should be known and considered by every individual in maintaining his own health. However individual a person may be, he is in all physiological respects more like the average human being than he is like any other creature. Anatomically he may vary from the usual in many ways, but in the general relations of parts to each other, the balance approximates pretty closely to the average. If he varies in height-weight ratio more than 10 to 20 per cent from the average for his age, his health is not likely to be of the best, and he will usually be benefited by a regimen that makes him more nearly approach the normal. This may mean more or less food, and more or less exercise. In this sense there is some truth in the saying " What is one man's meat is another's poison ". Treatment should *not*, however, *increase individual peculiarities* but should be adapted to maintaining health and bringing about a balanced equilibrium of physiological processes approximating those of the average healthy human being. This truth is of more importance when the individual trait is acquired rather than native. This does not mean that one who has been eating too much or too little, exercising vigorously or not at all, living in the house or out of doors, using stimulants or avoiding them, shall suddenly change and do as others do who are in normal health ; but that he shall change his habits gradually and to the extent necessary to reach a better health equilibrium. A high school or college student who engages in manual labour in the summer, needs to increase the amount of food taken ; but should decrease it again upon resuming his studies or take pains to secure exercise if he wishes to keep in the best of health.

F

BACTERIA AND MAN

Besides keeping all the physiological processes in properly balanced activity as he eats and adjusts directly, and by movements to physical environment, we must live with and adjust to countless living creatures. Many forms of bacteria are essential parts of valuable foods, such as milk, butter and cheese, and swarms of bacteria aid in the digestion of all foods. In addition, there are numerous bacteria and microbes in all decaying substances, many of them dangerous. The air, the soil, and nearly every object touched is permeated with living creatures ; as are also man's own external and internal surfaces with minute organisms that may affect his health. The dangers of associating with the larger animals and with other human beings are acute, not because of what they are likely to do to us, but because of the germs of disease with which they may infect us. Only within the last half-century, and largely through researches begun by Pasteur, has man been aware of the dangers arising from germ infection.

GUARDING AGAINST GERMS

Most germs thrive in warm moist places, usually on decaying substances, or inside of or on living creatures ; although some kinds survive indefinitely, though without multiplying, in dry places or at extreme temperatures. Contrary to early beliefs, infection by means of air is rare. Food and water are the most frequent causes of internal infections, and insects, of those entering through the skin. The human skin itself harbours germs that may produce sores or boils if they get under the skin, unless the germs are destroyed by the corpuscles always found in healthy blood. The chief aim in treating wounds and in surgery is to prevent any germs from getting inside the outer skin. To destroy germs that have penetrated wounds or entered the intestines is difficult without injuring living body tissue, hence antiseptics are now used with more discretion than formerly. Whenever injurious germs begin to multiply within the body, there are usually self-preservative processes set up which check germ activity. Sometimes specific anti-bodies form, and remain in the system after the germ and disease symptoms have disappeared. The individual may thus become immune to a second attack of measles, whooping-cough, smallpox, etc.

One way of guarding against germ diseases in severe form, is to inject blood containing anti-bodies from another person or animal who has had the disease, or to produce a mild infection perhaps associated with injection of anti-bodies. Danger from diphtheria, typhoid fever, smallpox and other diseases, has been decreased in this way. Another method much more desirable whenever practicable, is that used in combating yellow fever and malaria, viz. : destroying all the germ-carrying insects in the region which cause the disease. This method may entirely eliminate the disease, while vaccination and inoculation have the disadvantage of having to be used upon every successive generation, sometimes more than once.

In general, a person who is in good physiological condition can resist the effects of disease infections better than one in poor condition ; but health, however perfect, does not prevent infection and sometimes does not mitigate the severity of the disease. Aside from tuberculosis and some forms of colds, health is therefore not an effective defence against germ diseases, although it may enable one to survive an attack. Sunshine is a partial defence against the last-named disease and some others, not only because it is stimulating to the bodily processes, but because a large proportion of the dangerous germs cannot thrive in direct sunlight. Cold air is endured by lung tissue much better than by disease germs, hence it is helpful in the treatment of tuberculosis and pneumonia.

It is a curious fact that people of equally vigorous health are unequally susceptible to various germ diseases. Measles and whooping-cough are death-dealing plagues among Pacific Islanders, tuberculosis is a scourge to negroes, and intestinal disease works havoc among Caucasians in China. A germ disease new to a people is more fatal than one that has been common to them for generations, probably because immunity is acquired through mild infections by each generation, and perhaps partly because of the survival of those best suited to resist the germs.

Accidents, though very common, do not as a rule directly produce permanent physiological disturbance. The organism recovers quickly from shocks and begins the repair of injured tissues providing no germs enter the wounds. If repairs are impossible, as in the case of specialized tissues, such as that of lungs, kidneys or brain, other parts take on extra functions and a fair degree of health may be maintained with a part of one lung or kidney removed, or even with considerable portions of the brain destroyed. Treatment should always have as its aim, avoiding infection and helping restore normal functioning.

In the case of drowning or asphyxiation the lungs and heart must be stimulated to action. For treatment of burns the skin should be protected from the air instead of exposed to it. Medicines are not usually needed in accidents except in cases of poisoning, when some substance that serves as an antidote to the external or internal poison may be administered with advantage.

PUBLIC HEALTH REGULATIONS

The necessity for health laws and the possibility of formulating them are the result of civilization. The number of diseases and the chances for germ infection are greatly multiplied whenever large numbers of people occupy heated shelters, engage in special industries, and live in close proximity to each other. This makes it necessary to adopt rules and often laws, with penalties, in order that health may be maintained. The number of hours for work may be limited, the physical conditions in factories prescribed, safety appliances required, housing conditions regulated, cases of infectious diseases quarantined, sources of infection mitigated, foods inspected for healthfulness and purity, the sale of injurious drugs prohibited, health inspections of school children required, etc.

Such laws are necessary, not only because of the increased dangers arising from many persons living in close proximity, but because a single individual under such circumstances cannot adequately guard his own health as he can in a sparse population living under primitive conditions. Health of civilized peoples is becoming less a matter of intelligent prudential action on the part of individuals, and more a public affair under the control of experts and officials.

Laws relating to the public health and rules followed in industries, dining-halls, athletic training, etc., may be formulated on a scientific basis with more certainty than those to govern individual health behaviour. The effects of any condition or activity upon a large number of similar persons living under similar conditions may be determined with greater accuracy and assurance than is possible by studying one or a few differing individuals under various conditions. Undoubtedly it is not injurious, and sometimes even advantageous to some individuals to diverge in his own practices from rules laid down for groups similar to himself, because of special physique or special conditions due to habit ; but the presumption should always be in favour of the rules. It is well, therefore, for individuals to conform to the standards established by observation and research as to hours of sleep, kinds and amounts of exercise and food, and in the establishment of harmonious rhythms of physiological functioning, except in minor details, unless on the advice of experts. Each individual should learn by experience to use his own bodily machine so as to keep it as healthy and efficient as possible.

Conditions of life are now such that bodily processes and muscular strength become of less importance as material civilization advances, while the making of intelligent adjustments to situations by the use of machines, organization and other culture facilities is of increasing importance. In other words, the nervous system is used more and the muscular system less as civilization becomes more complicated. These opposite tendencies, if not corrected, produce lack of harmony affecting reciprocally bodily and mental health. There has been a great advance in scientific knowledge of mental disturbances, which shows the part played by unhygienic functioning on physical health, industrial accidents, family troubles and social ills. It is now recognized that the greatest need of modern civilization is improvement in conditions and practices that will be favourable to good *mental* hygiene. This topic will be discussed more fully in the chapter on Individual Psychology.

SELECTED RESEARCHES

"BASE METABOLISM: THE MODERN MEASURE OF VITAL ACTIVITY." By Dr. FRANCIS G. BENEDICT, Director, Nutrition Laboratory, Carnegie Institution of Washington. From *Scientific Monthly*, July 1928. *Quoted by Permission.*

The search of the ancient philosophers for the philosopher's stone or the elixir of life has been fruitless down through the centuries. If, instead of searching for the elixir of life, these men had sought an explanation of life processes, they would have made much greater progress. . . .

. . . Professor Warren P. Lombard, of Ann Arbor . . . devised an extraordinarily accurate balance for this purpose and laid the foundations for the more recent work by the Nutrition Laboratory, in which the loss in body weight from hour to hour and, indeed, almost from minute to minute has been studied.

This invisible loss in body weight, due chiefly to the loss of water vapour from the lungs and skin, has been found to be closely related to the main factors of life processes. . . .

. . . The object of such experiments is best illustrated by considering man as a bank. His food and drink and the oxygen which he absorbs from the air represent his income or his deposits. The urine and feces which are excreted, the water vapour lost from the skin and the lungs and the carbon-dioxide exhaled represent the outgo or the withdrawals from the bank. The balance between these deposits and withdrawals or between the income and outgo can be measured in terms of energy by means of calorimeters. . . . But the most important outcome of these complete balance experiments was the finding that the carbon-dioxide production, the oxygen consumption and the heat output (which Lavoisier had shown to be the result of life processes) are so closely correlated with each other that in order to determine the level of vital activity one need no longer use the complicated, expensive, time-consuming calorimeter for measuring the heat elimination, but can measure the oxygen consumption alone (a measurement calling for a far simpler technique) and therefrom calculate the heat production. . . .

In common parlance no distinction is made between the words " anabolism " and " katabolism ", because almost invariably we are considering katabolism. When we speak of a study in metabolism, therefore, we mean usually a study of katabolism, that is, the breaking down of body material, and it is in this phase that heat is developed.

One of the earliest conceptions of the reason for heat production was that the body must be warm in order to function properly and that heat is produced *to keep the body warm*. The body is ordinarily in an environment much cooler than the body temperature. It is thus constantly losing heat to the environment, and in order to keep the body cells at the proper temperature heat must be produced. This view considers heat production as the *main object* of the chemical processes in the body. Another conception is that heat is a *waste* product, given off *as the result* of muscular motions or chemical transformations arising for an entirely different purpose. . . .

. . . Each animal, even in repose and without food, is continually producing heat—at a low rate to be sure, but at a rate commensurate with the low vital activity under such conditions. This low heat production, measured under certain reproducible conditions, has been called " basal metabolism ". . . .

The oxygen consumption is a somewhat more accurate measure of the heat production than is the carbon-dioxide exhaled. . . .

. . . Is the basal metabolism constant from hour to hour ? From day to day ? How is it affected by sleep, by ingestion of food and by muscular work, all factors entering into everyone's daily life ? These problems can all obviously be studied with one person. But in the broader field of comparative physiology, it becomes necessary to study different individuals, and then the effects of body size, weight and height, age and sex must be determined. More recently race has also been suggested as a potential factor affecting metabolism, and here again the study must be made with numbers and not with a single individual.

. . . It has been found that the basal metabolism of the same individual remains reasonably *uniform* on any one day and likewise from day to day, when the conditions of measurement are the same.

. . . In a typical series of measurements made before and after the *ingestion* of 100 grams of cane-sugar the oxygen consumption prior to the eating of the sugar was 200 c.c. per minute, and twenty-five minutes after the sugar was eaten it had increased to 244 c.c. This finding is of special importance, since it indicates the necessity for avoiding any stimulus to digestion during the period of basal metabolism measurement.

Muscular work has a still more pronounced effect than the ingestion of food. Even small muscular movements affect the basal metabolism, and by severe muscular work the metabolism may be increased tenfold. . . .

. . . " How does the complete withdrawal of food, or *fasting*, affect the metabolism ? " Studies on this point have shown that during fasting the basal metabolism becomes lower and lower each day. . . .

. . . A group of twelve men, who were subjected for four

months to reduced rations amounting to about one-half the normal intake, lost 12 per cent of their body weight and their metabolism fell off 25 per cent. . . .

. . . A great many measurements have been made upon people of widely *different weights*, and values are now available which show that the average new-born baby, weighing 3·5 kg., has a twenty-four-hour basal heat production of 143 calories, the average thirteen-year-old girl, weighing 42 kg., has a heat production of 1,200 calories, and the average man, weighing 70 kg., has a heat production of 1,700 calories. Thus the heat production of the small baby, with less than one-tenth the weight of the thirteen-year-old girl, is considerably more than one-tenth of her heat production and one-twelfth of the heat production of an adult man weighing twenty times as much. The baby, therefore, has a high heat production per unit of weight. . . .

At first it was supposed that two individuals could be compared with each other if they were of the same weight, but it was soon discovered that the *tall*, thin man has a metabolism different from the short, fat man, even if they are both of the same weight. Height is, therefore, another factor which affects metabolism. . . .

. . . How is it possible to interpret the metabolism of a *child* of one year in such terms as to make it comparable with the metabolism of an *adult*? Obviously the total metabolism can not be compared directly. We have just seen that the intensity of the metabolism per unit of weight is much greater in youth than in later years. Comparison on this basis, therefore, is only a crude one. . . .

These same curves enable us to compare boys with girls and *men* with *women*. Up to about one year of age it is seen that there is no difference in metabolism between the sexes. But thereafter the influence of sex becomes pronounced, and the metabolism of men and boys is on the average about 12 per cent higher than that of women and girls. . . .

It is a common experience that severe *mental work* is *fatiguing*. . . . We therefore arranged with the college authorities to have twenty-two students take their examinations, one at a time, inside of a respiration chamber, which was likewise a calorimeter. Subsequently, as a control, each was studied in the calorimeter at a period some time after the examination. To include the mechanical work of writing, the students were told to copy some simple prose which was extremely uninteresting to them. The measurements were not made under basal conditions, but the only factor which differed in the two series of experiments was the mental effort. Under such conditions the specific effect of mental effort, if any, should be noted. The measured metabolism, when the men were under severe mental strain, compared with the measured metabolism during the control period showed no significant effect of mental effort. This is very disillusioning to many of us.

What is the effect of *psychic unrest*, as expressed by mental agitation, distress, anger or unhappiness ?   To plan experiments definitely along this line is obviously difficult.   Incidentally, at the Nutrition Laboratory a few years ago my associate, Dr. T. M. Carpenter, was studying the metabolism of an assistant nearly every consecutive morning, and this assistant had ordinarily shown an unusually uniform heat production.   He was well trained, remained very quiet during the measurements, and there was nothing novel in the situation for him.   One morning when Dr. Carpenter thought he was particularly quiet and relaxed, the metabolism was greatly increased.   Instead of being satisfied with two or three test periods, as usual, Dr. Carpenter made still more and the metabolism still remained high.   There was no fever, and no other cause for the increase was apparent.   Questioning, however, brought out the fact that the evening before the young man had attempted to elope with one of the young ladies in the laboratory and her father had kicked him down three flights of stairs into the street, which resulted in a great deal of physical as well as mental unrest.   The next morning he was experiencing the after-effects in the shape of considerably increased metabolism, which showed even above the seeming muscular exhaustion and somnolence. . . .

We all have days when we feel *below par* and days when we feel better than on other days.   Is this reflected in the basal metabolism ?   The periodic experience of normal women with menstruation is usually accompanied by a feeling of malaise, and measurement of the metabolism during the period of this normal, regular function is perhaps one of the simplest methods of studying the effect of feeling below par.   We have just completed a series of daily measurements of the metabolism with the same woman over a period of two months, in which it is seen that although this normal function causes her practically no inconvenience, there is a distinct tendency for the metabolism to be slightly lower during the menstrual period.

. . . The habits of life during the *summer vacation* are decidedly altered. . . . This effect again has been studied by the Nutrition Laboratory on twenty-two different individuals, both men and women. . . . Greatly to our surprise, however, it was found that in practically all cases the metabolism of these individuals was exactly the same after the vacation as before.   It is astonishing that a procedure which results in such a profound alteration in the subjective feelings, that is, a summer vacation, should not have altered in the slightest the basal metabolism.   This is again a strong indication of the fixity of basal metabolism.

. . . We find that there is a tendency for the metabolism to be lowest in winter, increasing in spring, and remaining unaltered till late fall. . . .

In the Yucatan series, measurements were made upon certain white members of the expedition, both before they left Boston, while they were in Yucatan and after their return to Boston.

Other measurements were likewise obtained on whites who had only recently arrived in Yucatan. These measurements, so far as they go, indicate that the sojourn in Yucatan was without effect upon the metabolism of the whites, thus again emphasizing the absence of effect of a *sub-tropical climate*. Singularly enough, with the Mayas, all of whom were men, the metabolism on the average was over 5 per cent above the northern standards for white men. . . .

. . . It has been found that the oxygen consumption or the heat production increases with exposure to *cold*, as does the heat loss, but not to the degree that one would expect. Thus, experiments were made with the same subject studied in the calorimeter, an artist's model who was well trained to posing without clothing. After lying for fifteen minutes, nude, in a cold room at 11° C. (52° F.) the subject's oxygen consumption was 211 c.c. per minute, as seen from this table. During the next forty minutes of continued exposure there was but a small increase (5 per cent) in the oxygen consumption, although the room temperature was very cold for a nude person. Indeed only when the point of shivering, which is in reality a form of muscular work, was reached, was there any considerable rise in metabolism. This indicates that only under extreme conditions and as a last resort is heat produced to keep the body warm, *i.e.*, when there is an unusually great loss of heat to the environment. Under ordinary circumstances, however, heat production is an end product and not the main object of life. . . .

We know that in *disease* there are great changes in metabolism, even when the individual is lying quietly. In toxic goiter, for example, the basal metabolism is increased 60, 80 or even 100 per cent, and in another thyroid disease, myxedema, it is greatly decreased, 40 or 50 per cent. . . .

Basal metabolism measurements are becoming more and more to be looked upon as the best *index* of the *vital activity* of any individual. To a certain extent the basal metabolism may be considered as the " indicator card " of the human engine, showing its general efficiency, not, to be sure, for muscular work, as in the case of the mechanical engine, but at least for the overhead maintenance of the well-functioning body prior to putting on the superimposed tasks of daily life, whether these be mental or physical. . . . When the basal metabolism profoundly alters, it is usually due either to disease or to some profound change in the general make-up. This change may frequently be a betterment of the organism, or not infrequently it represents a stage of being below par. In this sense, therefore, measurement of the basal metabolism is a splendid index of the level of vital activity, and it is highly probable that in the next decade we will find that basal metabolism measurements will be included in the annual physiological and medical survey which doubtless all of us will consider essential.

Chapter V

IMPROVING THE HUMAN SPECIES, OR EUGENICS AND EUTHENICS

BASIS AND PRINCIPLES

It was inevitable that man, the great changer of his environment and the transformer of plants and animals by domestication, the seeker after a better future for self, and the care-taker of the younger generation, should dream of a superior, improved race of human beings. With the coming of the age of scientific culture, this dream took the form in the mind of Galton of an ideal, and an inquiry into the means that might be used to accomplish it. Since his time, there has been a growing interest in this problem—which is now associated with the name " eugenics ". This science is primarily concerned, not with the improvement that may be made in individuals after birth, but with securing the birth of better types of the human species. Galton considered heredity as the chief direct means to be used in producing a better race.

Subsequent investigations have emphasized the importance of germ inheritance. Since his time it has become clearer that what happens to individuals after birth has little or no effect on the kind of children they produce. The father who has lost a hand or an eye does not produce a child lacking such a member, nor does one who has greatly enlarged the muscles of his arm by exercise produce a child with unusually large arms, nor does one who devotes his life to mathematics give birth to children who can add and multiply without teaching. A man or woman of beauty or exceptional voice may give birth to a child with similar features and voice, but the child will be no more artistic because one or both parents have spent years in the art galleries of Paris, or more musical because they studied music in Berlin.   In other words the traits persons are born with are likely to be transmitted to their children, but those they acquire are not.   If the father learns mathematics easily, his son probably will, but neither more nor less easily according to the years the father devoted to the subject before the child was born.   Nearly all scientific experiments indicate that acquired characteristics are only slightly inherited, if at all.

GERMINAL INHERITANCE

It is now known that the cells which are concerned in the production of young are quite separate from the cells of which the body is composed.   These cells receive their nutriment from the body, but are not otherwise greatly influenced by what happens to the body cells.   The germ cells increase in number by division, and two of opposite sex must unite to produce an individual of the next generation.   Small as these cells are, they cause the nutriment coming to the fertilized cell to organize into a creature of the same species, and having some of the more special characteristics of both parents.

The cells that are to compose the body are separated from the germ or reproductive cells which are to produce the next generation before embryonic development has progressed very far.   These reproductive cells remain in an inactive state until the body in which they reside matures, when they greatly increase in size and numbers.   No matter what happens to the body in which they dwell, they retain their types of potential development, e.g. sex cells of a black rabbit grafted in a white rabbit produce progeny that are black.   Drugs introduced into the body may cause some reproductive cells to weaken or die, but do not usually produce modification of structure.

In the case of all mammals, including man, after two germ cells have united and started a new individual this embryo remains within the body of the mother until it has developed into a new individual of the species, and is able to live without the shelter and nutriment afforded by her body. This period between conception and birth, which in the case of the human species is nine months, is an important one. Although the child is well protected from the outer environment and has no nervous connection with the mother, yet all his nutriment comes from her, and anything which affects that, whether it be poor food or shocks of fear that change the composition of her blood, may check or modify the development of the young life. In the main, the child at birth is the result of the union of the two slightly different cells of his father and mother, although somewhat modified during the pre-birth period. The word " inheritance " is best used to mean the traits produced by the germ cells, while the traits possessed at birth are " congenital ", but not all of them hereditary in the true sense.

Since germ cells are passed on from one generation to another, little affected by the bodies they inhabit, it follows that inheritance is from lines of ancestry rather than merely from parents. In other words, each parent passes on duplicates of the *germ cells* he has received almost regardless of his own bodily characteristics, *e.g.* a blue hen (result of black and white parentage) bred to a blue cock produces black chickens and white chickens only.

HEREDITARY ELEMENTS AND MENDELISM

By means of modern research, it is known that cells are composed of a chromatin and of a plasmic portion, and that the chromatin substance is concerned in the production of hereditary traits, while the plasm furnishes nutriment and perhaps determines species characteristics. This chromatin consists of a certain number of chromosomes in each species. When a female germ cell is fertilized by a male germ cell the chromosomes of the two unite so that the embryo is formed from a union of the parts of both parents.

Chromosomes are analogous to bags of seeds, the individuals of which are called genes. These genes of one parent may combine in any one of several ways with the genes of the other. If they are alike, and concerned with producing black hair pigment, then the child will surely have black hair, but if the genes of one parent are producers or determiners for light hair, and those of the other for black hair, black hair is likely to dominate in all children born to those two parents. The case of grandchildren is more complicated, as they will have germ cells with both light and dark genes or determiners. Germ cells from two such individuals may therefore give different results because of the fact that a dark determiner of one parent may unite with either a dark or a light determiner of the other, and the same is true of the light determiners. If there are four children, the probabilities are that one dark will unite with one dark, one light with one light, while the other two will be a mixture of light and dark. As a consequence, one child will be dark and have only dark determiners in his germ cells. Another child will be light and carry only light determiners in his germ cells ; while the other two will carry both types of cells, but will themselves be dark, because the dark determiner is dominant, and the light recessive. The above relations of dark and light determiners are rather generally found, but there are exceptions due in some cases to diversity in ancestry and the complexity of determiners.

From such truths as these, called Mendelian from their first discoverer, Mendel, we know more definitely why a father and mother who are both dark, may produce one out of four children who has light hair. What is true of hair colour is true of all heritable traits ; hence to know what traits children will have, ancestry must be studied, rather than the appearance of the parents.

INHERITANCE OF BEHAVIOUR AND MENTALITY

There is no question that in physiological characteristics men inherit traits just as animals do. Behaviour traits, as well as form and colour, are distinctly different in varieties of dogs, as shown in the fighting of the bulldog, the pointing of the bird dog, and in the behaviour of varieties of scent and sight hounds. These differences are doubtless due to determiners that control relative size of parts and fineness of structure, and the way in which they are organized for special modes of acting. The special behaviour characteristic of each variety of dog is not itself inherited, but rather a structure and organization favourable to the development of such behaviour. The same is undoubtedly true of various emotional and intellectual traits in human beings.

Evidence of close resemblance in mental qualities to one's ancestors has been rapidly accumulating. Intelligence in the sense of ability to learn without direction, is the mental trait which has been most frequently and most accurately measured. This is found to exist in much the same degree in individuals of the same family. It is not known whether there are special determiners affecting the brain structure and giving a greater or less degree of general intelligence in accordance with Mendel's laws of inheritance, but most of the known facts are not inconsistent with this supposition. Emotional and general mental balance are indicated by studies of many generations of the same family; but what size, quality, and arrangement of bodily structure these traits are dependent upon, is not known. It is clear from the above, that detailed knowledge of the mechanism of human heredity is lacking in many particulars, but that enough is known to justify considering methods of improving the human race by selective matings.

IDEALS AND METHODS OF EUGENICS

At the outset, there are differences of opinion as to what types of human beings are to be produced. On the basis of what we know of all other species, it is safe to say that any variety of men that could be produced, would resemble in essential particulars the type which now exists. Man has not changed the essential nature of any species of plant or animal, and we are not sure that he has produced any variety superior in *all* respects to the original. He has developed cows superior for milk production, and others for beef, and all are of a milder disposition than the original wild cattle.

G

In changing this and other species of animals, he was not trying to improve the species in a general way, but to increase the traits most useful to himself. There is lack of agreement as to what traits in man are of most importance. Eugenists must, therefore, form their ideal in a somewhat different way from the stock-breeder.

It will not be denied that some specimens of humanity are better than others. In general, those who are healthy, long-lived, intelligent, and showing in a moderate degree the usual human emotions, are counted superior to weak, deformed, diseased, short-lived, feeble-minded, poorly - balanced individuals. On this basis of rather general agreement the ideal of the eugenist may be founded. He desires, not necessarily a race of supermen, but one in which there are more individuals of the superior type, and fewer, or none, of the inferior. The general average of such a race would be superior to that existing at present.

Whether it is desirable to have more highly specialized individuals superior in a few traits, or more with general superiority, has not been determined. Theoretically, enough is known of the general principles of heredity to produce either race, though knowledge of many details of *human* heredity is lacking. General improvement would be accomplished by arranging so that the better people in each generation would produce more children than the inferior. To produce specialized individuals of the superior type involves complex problems of selective mating.

It is a general law of biology that matings are usually of those who have more resemblances than differences. Eugenists do not necessarily plan for selective mating other than this natural one.

At present about one-fourth of each generation produce no children, while another fourth produce half of all that are born ; the remaining half producing the rest. If those producing no children were all of inferior germ inheritance and the fourth producing one-half of the children were all superior in germ heredity, the principal ideal of the eugenist of a race averaging much higher than the present one would soon be realized. Statistics show, however, that dividing the population into classes as indicated by intelligence tests, social position, etc., the production of children is in general greater for the inferior classes—college graduates having the fewest children, and the feeble-minded having the most. How to change this situation is only partly a question of making use of principles of heredity. Physiologically, all classes *could* produce more children, but the numbers being produced by all classes are growing less. The problem is to find how the superior persons may be induced to produce more, and the inferior few or none.

It is possible to prevent reproduction among the most inferior classes, the feeble-minded and insane, by custodial care in institutions, or by an operation which without injury to health, makes them infertile. Many states have laws providing for the use of the latter method, but in only one, California, has it been used enough to have any appreciable effect. The first method is used to a limited extent in many states, but no state cares for *all* persons of inferior heredity in such a way as to prevent their having descendants. One reason why this has not been done is because of expense, although in the long run money would be saved by such action. Considerable improvement in average intelligence, and much benefit would follow more effective and more universal use of these two methods by all the states. Many states feebly attempt to accomplish the same results by marriage laws, but in most cases with little effect, because such laws are not intelligently drawn with that end in view.

None of these methods can be readily applied to the moderately inferior classes who are legally competent to manage their own affairs. It is held by some that when such persons are not emotionally unstable, they are easily prevented from giving trouble, and by proper training can be self-supporting and very useful in certain tasks that are disagreeable to intelligent individuals, and hence should be allowed to produce children freely. Their case is somewhat like that of the superior classes. General sentiment would not support any attempt to *force* one class to produce more, and the other fewer children. In both cases, if anything is accomplished it must be by other than forceful means.

EUGENICS AND THE EFFICIENCY EXPERT

Many grades and varieties of ability are useful to the human race. An efficiency expert would say that we should find just what kinds of special talent and what per cent of each grade of ability are needed in all industries and social organizations, and then arrange for the production of that number of each kind of individual. This would perhaps show a need for only one to five per cent of the highest grade to discover, invent and lead; from ten to perhaps twenty per cent of high-grade secondary leaders, and forty to sixty per cent of those of average ability, while the number of the lowest grade would be about the same as of the highest. Such a distribution would not greatly differ from that now existing, except that there might be more persons of specialized talent. From the standpoint of industrial needs such a race of men might be more efficient for a limited time, but conditions change more rapidly than specialized types of workers could be produced by heredity. Any definite efficiency programme of this sort would also be impossible for many psychological and social reasons. Besides, successful human living, individually and in groups, is much more than a matter of efficient performance of industrial tasks. As yet there is no efficiency expert who can figure out the exact grades and varieties of traits needed for individual satisfaction in a well-balanced society, nor one who can tell how long the needs would remain the same.

Men differing in general grade of ability and in special traits have always existed, and until good reason for doing so is shown, the opposite ideal of uniform standardized individuals now used in growing apples and breeding hogs, should not be adopted for human beings. Many grades of human beings means that all but the lowest and highest have the stimulus of adjusting to both superiors and inferiors. It also favours more effective co-operation than is possible when all are alike. The ideal of most eugenists is therefore not usually a superman, not a race of specialists, nor one with no individual differences ; but a race much like that now existing but having more superior, and fewer inferior, individuals.

EDUCATION AND THE EUGENIC PROGRAMME

Since to attain eugenic ends, education of individuals and the employment of various sociological influences are necessary, it follows that the improvement of human beings by applying knowledge of heredity can be carried out only by means that are usually regarded as euthenic.

The higher the ideals of health, beauty, intelligence, etc., people are led to form, the greater the proportion of such persons that will be chosen as mates, and the more difficult will it be for the inferiors to become parents. Enlightenment in many ways needs to be equalized. If all know something of human heredity and the probability of inferior children if they mate with others having the same deficiency, there are likely to be fewer inferior children born. If some know how to control births and others do not, the enlightenment of all will tend to make the birth-rate less unfavourably selective than it is now, when the superior classes are more generally informed. We cannot take the knowledge away from the superior classes, hence in fairness to the individual and for the good of the race, it should be given to all. Everyone should also be instructed in the general laws of heredity and have the help of expert advice when in doubt as to the soundness of health of the potential offspring of a contemplated marriage.

EUGENICS AND SOCIAL CONDITIONS

Various economic and social adjustments have to be made in order that superior persons shall produce as many or more children than the inferior. As it is now, superior persons who are to become leaders spend many years in preparation for their work, and as a consequence marry at a later age than those of less ability. If they produced an equal number of children per generation, the descendants of the inferior who marry young, would after a few centuries be much greater, because they produce four or five generations in a century, while the superior, marrying after thirty, produce only about three to the century.

According to statistics the superior produce fewer children, hence in the course of a few centuries their descendants will be greatly outnumbered if some factors in the situation are not changed. Births among the superior classes are limited for many reasons implied in the terms " forethought " and " ideals ". The superior persons have high ideals as to the advantages which children should be given, and looking ahead, refuse to have children when there seems little prospect of reaching these ideals. An economic adjustment of some kind is needed that would make it easier for superior persons to realize their standards of what they think is necessary. Prohibition of child labour now has some effect upon decreasing the production of children by the poorer classes. Free public schools help to equalize opportunities, but the superior classes would be advantaged by more free higher education. Persons with children have a slight advantage in income-tax exemption, but this has little eugenic influence. Probably there will yet be devised more effective means than now exist of inducing superior persons to produce more children, and care for them in accordance with their higher standards.

If conditions for bringing up children according to varying class standards were made equally favourable and all had knowledge of birth control, then those who most desired children would be the ones who would leave the most descendants. This would tend to decrease rather than increase any tendency to race suicide, so much stressed by opponents of birth control.

EUTHENICS AND ITS RELATION TO EUGENICS

The movement designated by the term euthenics has for its primary objective making conditions more favourable for human living without special regard to the type of people born. Its advocates are less concerned with the direct and indirect effects upon germinal inheritance than with finding what sort of cultural and physical environment is best suited to bring all the powers of individuals to their fullest development. It is quite certain, however, that the conditions of living provided by euthenists, will serve as selective factors helping to determine what type of persons shall leave descendants, and thus be favourable or unfavourable to eugenic ideals. Some have claimed that the result is likely to be unfavourable; a claim not wholly without grounds, especially as social control usually lags behind other advances of scientific knowledge.

If knowledge of health and maintenance of health conditions are used to keep persons of inferior inheritance alive until they are old enough to produce children, and there is no force of social control used to prevent them from perpetuating their defects in their children, then euthenics *may* interfere with the programme of the eugenists. The number of persons susceptible to tuberculosis, for example, may thus be kept greater than would be the case if so many such persons were not brought to maturity by euthenic means. This does not imply, however, that the programme of the euthenists as a whole is opposed to that of the eugenists. It is true that individuals who most readily succumb to germ attacks are weeded out more effectively in places where there are many such germs and little medical care, yet a population freed from the germs of malaria, yellow fever, hook worm, etc., is of greater vigour than one where the disease is more prevalent.

Euthenic conditions discovered in one generation and passed on to subsequent ones are generally favourable for the development of the highest type of human beings, and of disadvantage only in minor ways which may be avoided by enlightened action of society conversant with the eugenic ideals and methods. Better methods of farming give better crops, providing none of the poorest seed is used in planting; and human beings improve under good euthenic conditions providing the inferior individuals are not allowed to propagate. Euthenic programmes that save the lives of persons of tubercular susceptibility and guard against infection of others, will not increase tuberculosis in the next generation if means are used to prevent selective mating of the susceptible individuals.

KINDS OF EUTHENIC ADVANCE MOST VALUABLE

Some kinds of euthenic advance are of much greater advantage to the race than others. To know how to avoid infections and how to eliminate disease germs from the world is of more value than knowledge of how to treat the diseases after they occur. Knowledge of how to deal with criminals of all sorts is of far less value than knowledge of conditions favourable to the development of normal individuals who are co-operative with their fellow-men. A good many humanitarian and benevolent activities are of doubtful value. To feed hungry individuals may preserve the life and health of the individuals, but if it pauperizes them and their children after them, the results are distinctly disadvantageous to the race. If, however, means are found of placing and training such persons and any descendants they may have, so as to be self-supporting, there is considerable advantage to the race from its being relieved of burdensome individuals. The general level of humanity, however, is not raised as it may be if the methods most advocated by eugenists are used, of getting more children born who are normal or above average. Such individuals will not only prove to be no burden to the rest of the race, but will aid in the use of better euthenic methods.

Since man is such a large factor in changing his environment and making it better euthenically, any improvement in the germinal inheritance of the human race insures a permanent advance, even in places where environment is unfavourable. Euthenic advances in the way of inventions, discoveries, customs and organizations, may prove of value to many successive generations, but if in the meantime the germinal stock should become successively poorer, the machines would rust and not be replaced, the customs would become useless forms, the organizations unwieldy, and co-operation ineffective.

Whatever heights a nation may reach by euthenic means, it will decline as soon as there are enough inferior individuals to hamper the activities of those of moderate and superior ability. On the other hand a group of people of superior inheritance will evolve a euthenic environment from almost nothing.

IMMIGRATION AS A PROBLEM OF EUGENICS

The old way of looking upon the free immigration of all peoples of the world to this country as desirable because they enjoyed better living conditions, supplied cheap labour needed for some industries, and promoted prosperity, is no longer satisfactory. It is evident that for the future good of humanity in America, the important thing to consider is the effect the immigrants will have upon the general level of the future population of this country. Intelligent people now recognize that it is a mistake to admit individuals whose ability is below that of the general average of those now here, whatever their race or the immediate advantages gained. Excluding obviously defective persons such as the feeble-minded, the insane, the criminal, and those suffering from certain diseases, is not enough.

Many difficult problems have arisen in this country from the presence of great numbers of the Negro race and some of the Mongolian. It is not yet known whether, if they remain distinct, harmony and co-operation can be secured when such distinctly different races live with each other. To decrease racial differences by intermarriages might bring still greater disadvantages. Immigration of various strains of Caucasians adds to the complexity of the problem. A crossing between two varieties of a species results in descendants many of whom in the first generation and sometimes in subsequent ones, are equal or superior to the inferior parent race, and sometimes to either of the parent races ; but if the differences between the races are great, usually some weak, deformed, or poorly balanced individuals are produced. This means that the crossing of racial stock may increase the vigour of future inhabitants of this country, or may decrease it ; with the chance favouring the latter condition when the races differ considerably, and inferior individuals are not prevented from propagating.

EUTHENIC RESULTS OF IMMIGRATION

On the euthenic side it has been claimed that there are distinct advantages from having the cultures of the various races thrown into the melting-pot of American life, to be fused into something better than that of any one nation. This claim, however, is not well substantiated by the facts. It is true that every group of people *may* profit by coming into contact with another group, whose cultural development has been different. Close contact of people and cultures where there is great difference is, however, often disastrous to one and of no advantage to the other. In this country, in Australia, and in the islands of the Pacific, both the cultures and the original natives have suffered severely from contact with men of the white cultures, and the white men have gained little from the native cultures. The same is partly true regarding the relations of foreign nationalities to the dominant race in this country. Valuable features of the culture of some immigrants have been lost to them, with no corresponding gain to the native population.

A nation often gains most and loses least by less intimate relations. They take what is most consistent with their own culture, assimilate it, and make it fully their own. In close contacts of differing people within a nation, there are sure to be many conflicts and the people whose culture dominates, instead of taking the best of the other, are likely to regard all of it with contempt. It is too early to reach a conclusion as to the final advantages and disadvantages of the mingling of cultures on this continent, but it is safe to say that up to the present time the people of America have gained more from contacts with the *leaders* of other national cultures, both personally and through works of art and literature, than they have from the *immigrants* from the same countries. This is especially true of those differing most widely from us in culture, such as the Asiatic and the Southern European. In the case of Northern Europeans, the results are somewhat different, partly because of similarity of culture, and probably also because a larger proportion of the immigrants from those sections have been of average or superior stock.

INCREASE IN POPULATION AND EUTHENICS

When people have become familiar with their environment, and the means of preserving health are organized for effective co-operation in producing necessary and desired things, more people can live in a given locality and on the whole earth, than when such euthenic conditions are not provided. Not only can more people exist, but also the standards of living may be kept higher. There is a limit, however, beyond which euthenic improvement cannot provide for further increase. When that limit is reached, then further increase of population inevitably means a lower standard of living, and this in turn means in the course of time, poorer euthenic conditions which will tend to increase the death-rate and decrease the population. All species of animals increase when conditions of living are favourable, and decrease when they are unfavourable. Man, however, may succeed in increasing the food supply for a considerable period while continuing to increase in numbers, but not indefinitely. His desires include more than mere food and shelter, and he may halt population increase as soon as it becomes difficult to obtain the means of attaining high standards of living. The number of persons with the highest standards, are, as we have seen, the ones who first decrease their birth-rate. This decreases human population as excessive death-rates decrease population among animals and uncivilized peoples ; but may eliminate superior instead of inferior individuals.

The above truths hold for the whole world, and for any given nation. In the case of a single nation the truth is partly obscured by the fact that a highly civilized nation of manufacturers may increase in population far beyond the possibility of producing all that is needed on its own land. To do this, they must, however, produce articles that can be exchanged, not only for food produced elsewhere, but for other things necessary to maintain living standards at a high level. This may be continued as long as plenty of food is easily produced in other places from which it may be transported. As soon as a nation's capacity to produce exchangeable articles becomes less per person, or when less productive lands of the world must be cultivated, or good lands more intensively cultivated with diminishing returns of the amount produced in proportion to effort expended, then increase of population must cease, or the standards of living of even the most favoured nation must be lowered.

The adjustment is usually made in the most advanced nations by decrease in birth-rate, and in the less advanced by increased death-rate ; but it appears to be as inevitable in one case as in the other. The laws by which increase in numbers of individuals of a species is limited locally and on the earth as a whole, seem to work sooner or later in the human species in spite of the fact that man has great foresight, and much voluntary control over means of living. The greater his intelligent foresight and use of means, the longer may he continue to increase in numbers, but there are limits set by the nature of the world in which he lives and by his own nature, beyond which he cannot go. What these limits of population are cannot now be stated with any certainty. Estimates vary from two hundred to six hundred million people for the United States, and from five to twelve billion in the world.

EUGENICS AND POPULATION

The white race which settled in the United States, because of its superior ability and culture has increased to about 120,000,000, while the Indian, after thousands of years of living here, had, when the white man came, a population of less than a million. The standard of living of this small Indian population was also low compared with that of the white race. Only recently has there been any evidence that Indians may greatly increase their numbers by acquiring the culture of the white man. Probably they could do this more rapidly if they did not have to compete with the white man while absorbing his culture.

This is only one of many historical examples of races occupying successively the same territory, one of which carried the increase in population and in standards of living much farther than the other. We also find certain races showing ability to do this, as they migrate from one portion of the earth to another. It must be, therefore, that certain strains of the human species have greater ability to make their own environment, and to change themselves so as to attain higher standards of living. How much it is due to native differences and how much to cultural advantages already acquired is not known.

If the general level of human ability is raised in any nation, it seems certain that the people will evolve a culture of more euthenic living, will make their environment produce more, and will organize for co-operation in their industries so as to produce more exchangeable goods ; and by these means will maintain high standards of living longer while continuing to increase population, than if the general level of hereditary ability remains the same or is lowered. Evidently the eugenic programme is even more closely related to population growth than the euthenic programme, although each in general promotes the other. The ultimate effects of the two pro- grammes on population growth are slightly diverse. In general, the nation emphasizing the eugenic programme will cease increasing in numbers earlier than the one following the euthenic programme, but will have higher standards of living. The euthenists may get some immediate increase in standards of living, but unless the general level of ability is high, the possibilities of continuing to raise them are not good. On the other hand, more foresight and control is needed to carry out a eugenic programme than a euthenic one, and hence its chances of success are not so great unless a large number of the population are already of a high grade of ability.

SELECTED RESEARCHES

" HEREDITY AND NATURAL RESISTANCE TO DISEASE."
By W. V. Lambert, Iowa State College. From *Scientific Monthly*, February 1929. *Quoted by Permission.*

In many diseases no successful methods of control have been developed. This fact has led a number of workers, in genetics primarily, to undertake another possible solution of the problem, namely, the production of disease-resistant strains. In the plant kingdom this method has been used extensively. . . .

In animals much empirical evidence exists relating to this subject. . . .

. . . In man, also, racial differences have been freely observed. It is a well-known fact that when diseases common to civilized races are introduced into uncivilized or isolated regions, where those diseases have not been present, the mortality resulting among such people is often appalling. The death-rate among the American Indians following the introduction of smallpox and measles is a well-known example of this. Much other evidence of a less clear-cut nature also exists. It is generally considered that the negro is more susceptible to tuberculosis than the white man. Much evidence, largely statistical in nature, has been presented to show that susceptibility to tuberculosis is an inherited trait. Its incidence is significantly greater in certain families so as to leave no doubt that a weakness or inherent susceptibility toward this diathesis is an integral part of the germ-plasm of those families. . . .

If nature has been able to evolve completely resistant lines in naturally inbred species, and has shown a tendency toward producing partially resistant lines in outbred species, it is reasonable to believe that by rigid selection based upon an animal's ability to produce resistant offspring, the use of a moderate amount of inbreeding and with constant exposure to a virulent type of the disease, naturally resistant strains of animals may be produced. With these reasons in mind the problem of producing a strain of chickens having a sufficiently high natural resistance to withstand epidemics of fowl-typhoid was undertaken in the writer's laboratory. . . .

As foundation material healthy mature chickens were selected and each bird was fed the same quantity of a virulent culture of fowl-typhoid bacteria. From the survivors of this group those birds that had shown the least reaction to the disease were selected and used as breeding stock. The next year the chicks from these birds were infected with a standard dose of the fowl-typhoid bacteria, a dose that in preliminary tests had been found to be lethal for approximately 90 per cent of all chicks secured from ordinary outside sources. Concurrently with the infection of the chicks from the surviving parents an approximately equal number of chicks with similar breeding but from an outside source were also infected. The chicks from the surviving parents showed a total mortality of 41 per cent, whereas those chicks that came from non-surviving parents gave a total mortality of nearly 90 per cent. This is a difference in mortality between the two groups of nearly 50 per cent, a difference that certainly cannot have been due to chance alone, since over eight hundred chicks were used.

Thinking that perhaps a large part of this difference in resistance between the above groups of chicks might be transmitted in some manner through the yolk of the eggs of the surviving mothers, typhoid-surviving males were mated to hens of similar breeding that had not been exposed to fowl-typhoid. The total mortality observed in the chicks of these matings was approximately 60 per cent, a figure intermediate between that of the first two groups. In this case the increased resistance of the chicks came from the sires alone, and since numerous experiments have indicated that passive immunity cannot be transferred from the male to his offspring, the resistance must have been due to factors for resistance resident in the germ cells of the sire. The reciprocal cross, namely, typhoid-surviving females and non-tested males, gave approximately the same results.

Not only in total mortality, however, was there a difference in the three groups of chicks. The rate of speed of mortality exhibited the same general relationship. The chicks with double typhoid-surviving ancestry showed a slow rate of mortality; those with single typhoid-surviving ancestry, an intermediate rate; and the group with non-typhoid ancestry, a very rapid rate. This indicates a higher potential of resistance in those chicks whose parents had both withstood an attack of the disease, although, as indicated by total mortality, this potential was not high enough to protect all chicks against death from the infection.

It has been found also that sires differ markedly in their ability to transmit resistance to their progeny, a situation that would be expected if resistance to this disease were an inherited character depending upon a number of factors for its expression. These differences were so marked in some cases that there can be no question of their significance.

The findings reported herein have been accumulated over a period of three years, and the relationships from year to year have been very consistent. This consistency indicates clearly that the hereditary basis for resistance is reasonably constant in any given strain of chickens. It is also shown that the experimental technique is sufficiently accurate to enable us to predict within fairly close limits what may be expected in any given trial.

Another experiment dealing with the same general problem has been carried on in this laboratory, using the rat as the experimental animal. It has been proven beyond question that selection is effective in producing inbred lines of rats having a much greater resistance to the Danysz bacillus than that existing in an unselected population. Furthermore, it has been shown that the second selected generation has a much higher degree of resistance than the first selected generation. ·. . .

This demonstration of the possibility of selection is the main contribution of these experiments to date. Whether selection based upon the above basis will result in the eventual development of naturally disease-resistant animals remains to be seen. The possibility has been clearly indicated, but many unforeseen difficulties may be ahead of its ultimate accomplishment. If accomplished, the value of such experiments will be untold. Chiefly, perhaps, from the practical standpoint, but not alone, for many problems in immunology and bacteriology may be solved only when hosts that can be depended upon to react in a constant and definite manner toward certain micro-organisms become available. And lastly, if they should help in an eventual revival of the idea of constitutional fitness as one of the sound policies of eugenics they may result in vast benefits for mankind in ages to come.

" RACE CROSSING IN JAMAICA." By Dr. C. B. DAVENPORT, Carnegie Institution of Washington. From *Scientific Monthly*, September 1928. *Quoted by Permission.*

. . . In order to make a comparative study of the efficiency of a hybrid race and the two parental stocks from which it was derived, the Carnegie Institution of Washington accepted a gift made to it and undertook a study of Negro-white crosses in the island of Jamaica, British West Indies. . . .

. . . To carry out the programme of the committee in charge of the investigation it was necessary to study carefully one hundred full-blooded Negroes—male and female—called hereafter " Blacks " ; one hundred white people and one hundred mixtures between the two races—whom we may call Browns. To make the two groups comparable it was necessary to take them, as far as possible, from the same social stratum. . . .

Studies were made also on children ; both babies at the crèches, or day nurseries in Kingston, and school children from eight to sixteen years of age. The open-air schools that abound in the island offered good shelter and excellent light for the measurements and tests. . . .

Gene differences between races are recognized as such partly by an important difference in mean size of the trait and partly by the behaviour of the trait in hybridization. If we consider the breadth of the nose we have a trait which is genetically different in the white and Negro races. The hybrids have a nose which is intermediate in breadth, and in later generations, indeed in a mixed Negro population, we find a very great variability in nose breadth, as shown in Table A. An examination of this table shows that the variability of the browns, as the hybrids are called, is distinctly greater than that of the whites and blacks, as the coefficient of variability which is used as a measure of such variability shows. There are no broad-nosed whites and no narrow-nosed blacks, but the browns range all the way from narrow noses to broad noses.

TABLE A

Proportional Distributions of Nasal Breadth in the Three Groups. The different classes of nose width are given in the first column ; in the successive column, left to right, the proportion of each racial group that has a nose of the class of width named in left-hand column.

Class mm.	Whites percentage.	Browns percentage.	Blacks percentage.
30–32	16·0	—	—
33–35	48·0	1·1	—
36–38	26·0	9·7	—
39–41	10·0	26·9	5·9
42–44	—	35·5	23·5
45–47	—	18·3	45·1
48–50	—	1·5	21·6
51–53	—	1·1	3·9

Mean and probable error—34·90 ±0·24   42·61 ±0·24   45·82 ±0·26. Standard deviation and probable error—2·56±0·17   3·44 ±0·17   2·75±0·18.

Another distinguishing genetical trait is that of form of the hair as measured by the diameter of the curl. This is, as everyone knows, very small in the case of the Negroes ; very great in the case of the whites, a large proportion of whom, indeed, have no measurable curl in the hair. The browns are intermediate in respect to hair form. The variability of this hair form, as measured by the coefficient of variation, is seen to be 50 per cent greater in the blacks than in the whites.

Similarly, in skin colour the offspring of two mulatto parents

H

may run the whole gamut from a white skin to an ebony black, like that of the Negro ancestor. The range in variation of skin colours in such hybrids is, indeed, very great. . . .

We have studied about thirty physical traits in the three groups. In some of these the Negroes and whites differ so greatly that it is quite certain that distinct genes are involved. Thus the races differ in length of arm-span and leg, which are both greater in the Negro than in the white. The breadth of the pelvis is much less in the Negro. The lower arm constitutes a relatively greater fraction of the entire arm in the Negro. The Negro's head is longer, but not broader or higher. The distance between the pupils is much greater than in the whites. The feet and hands are longer in the blacks. The outer ear is not so long. There are fewer hairs developed on hand, arm and leg, and such as there are are short. . . .

In the matter of rhythm, also, the blacks are far superior to the whites, scoring an average of 86 to the whites' 78. The browns show a great range of scoring from 50 to 100. . . .

. . . Thus in the cube imitation test in which the subject has to reproduce a certain more or less complicated sequence of movements of the examiner, the blacks get a score of $4\frac{1}{2}$, as contrasted with that of $6\frac{1}{2}$ obtained by the whites. The whites do, therefore, nearly 50 per cent more of the test correctly than do the blacks. The browns are nearly intermediate in their efficiency in this test, although they lie somewhat closer to the blacks than to the whites. . . .

Another test employed was that of putting together six pieces of wood on which are drawn the parts of a man. These were to be placed so as to reconstruct the image of a man. The blacks took longer to make the reconstruction than the whites. Thus, on the average, blacks took forty-three seconds, as contrasted with twenty-six seconds required by the whites. The browns are intermediate, but much closer to the blacks than to the whites in this capacity, and, as measured by the standard deviation, their scores were the most variable. . . .

Another test applied was the so-called Knox moron test, consisting of a board with a hole into which were to be placed blocks of different forms so as completely to fill the hole. The blacks on the average took 119 seconds to perform this test; the whites 87 seconds, and the browns 113 seconds. . . .

The application of the results of the study of Negroes, whites and hybrids between them in Jamaica leads to the conclusion that physically there is little to choose between the three groups, although, on the whole, the Negro makes the better animal, and especially is provided with better sense organs. The browns show much greater variability and, indeed, are put together differently from the average whites and blacks. Thus, whereas the whites are characterized by relatively short legs and long body and the blacks by relatively long legs and short body, some of the mulattoes have an unexpected combination of long legs and long body and others of short legs and short body. Also, while there is a high degree of correlation between leg length and arm length, some of the hybrids are characterized by the long legs of the Negro and the short arms of the white, which would put them at a disadvantage in picking up things from the ground.

But in regard to intellectual traits the conclusions are different. The browns show great variability in performance. They comprise an exceptionally large number of persons who are poorer than the poorest of the Negroes or the poorest of the whites. On the other hand, they show some individuals of a high intellectual quality. . . . A population of hybrids will be a population carrying an excessively large number of intellectually incompetent persons. On the other hand, a population composed of hybrids between whites and Negroes will contain persons better endowed in appreciation of music and in simple arithmetical or mental computations, as well as more resistant to certain groups of diseases, than a pure white population. If only society had the force to eliminate the lower half of a hybrid population, then the remaining upper half of the hybrid population might be a clear advantage to the population as a whole, at least as far as physical and sensory accomplishments go. . . .

SUGGESTED READINGS

The literature of Eugenics, including heredity, has recently greatly increased ; while the problems of Euthenics are extensively treated in all sociological writings, though not usually under that name. Among the best general works are :

CARR-SAUNDERS, A. M., *Eugenics*, 1926.
CONKLIN, EDWIN G., *Heredity and Environment in the Development of Man*, 1923.
EAST, EDWARD W., *Heredity and Human Affairs*, 1927.
GUYER, MICHAEL F., *Being Well Born*, 1927.
HOLMES, SAMUEL J., *Studies in Evolution and Eugenics*, 1923.
JENNINGS, H. S., *The Biological Basis of Human Nature*, 1930.
KELLOGG, V. L., *Mind and Heredity*, 1923.
WALTER, H. E., *Genetics, and Introduction to the Study of Heredity*, 1924.

The best historical study of hereditary ability is that of :

WOODS, F. A., *Heredity in Royalty*, o.p.

Some special studies of congenital deficiencies are :

DUKEDALE, R. L., *The Jukes*, 1910.
ESTABROOK, A. H., *The Jukes in 1915*, 1916.
ESTABROOK, A. H., *Mongrel Virginians*, 1926.
GODDARD, H. H., *The Kallikak Family*, 1909.

Recent studies of inheritance of mental traits are :

BANKER, H. G., " Genealogical Correlation of Student Ability," *Journal of Heredity*, 1928.
ENGLISH, H. B., " Mental Capacity of School Children Correlated with Social Status," *Yale Psychological Studies*, Vol. 23, No. 3, 1917.
PRESSEY, S. Z. and R. R., " The Relation of General Intelligence to the Occupation of Fathers," *Journal of Applied Psychology*, Vol. 3, No. 4.
TERMAN, LEWIS, *et al.*, *Genetic Studies of Genius*, 1926.

See also the *Year-book for the National Society for the Study of Education*, 1928, on " Nature and Nurture ".

The bearing of intelligence testing on immigration problems is presented by :

KIRKPATRICK, CLIFFORD, *Intelligence and Immigration*, 1926.

Chapter VI

AVOIDING WASTE, OR ECONOMICS

WHAT IS ECONOMICS ?

It is a body of knowledge concerned chiefly with acquiring, producing and exchanging material things and immaterial services, with a minimum expenditure of energy, time, and materials. A tribe living where there is an abundance of food and other necessaries all the year round would have little need or incentive to acquire knowledge and habits of economy. Scarcity of food all the time would not necessarily lead to economy, but would merely cause some accumulation of knowledge of the nearest places for obtaining food at a given season, and an amount of searching for it commensurate with the degree of appetite.

The primary stimulus to economy is given by seasonal shortages of food in which it can be had only by previous effort in storing and preserving it. Some animals do this storing, but there is no evidence that they learn to know just how much to store or how to gather it by the least effort. Men, with more foresight and intelligence, do acquire such knowledge, and pass it on to their descendants. The stimulus to gaining such knowledge increases as exchange of articles develops and as they have to be treated in some way before being used or for preservation, or have to be artificially produced or increased. A still stronger stimulus is competition of one group of producers with others.

The more man has increased the earth's products of useful things, learned to utilize its materials in constructing what he needs, and increased his numbers, the more occasion has there been for economy of effort and materials in production. Problems of distribution arise in the necessity for securing effective co-operation and consequent economy in production. Economics as a science did not emerge until the age of machinery. Much was learned of economical practices through experience and passed on to following generations previous to the industrial revolution, but without any attempt to formulate a science.

UTENSILS, TOOLS AND MACHINES AS MEANS OF ECONOMY

Animals use things as they find them, or change and transport them by help of mouth, body and limbs. Man finds things and makes tools for changing them, constructs containers of leaves, baskets, pottery, etc., for transporting and storing them instead of using his hands or mouth and making many trips. Any tool or utensil is a means of economy when the labour of making it is less than the labour that is necessary without it, during the time that it lasts. The same principle applies in making tools for cutting, pounding, etc., to aid in the making of other tools and utensils. Machines are more complicated constructions for doing things than tools, and they free man in part from the exertion of so much strength in a given time (by means of levers, etc.) and from the necessity of directing motions with accuracy. In earlier ages men began saving their own energy by utilizing that of animals and slaves. In modern times both men and animals are relieved of muscular effort by using the energy of falling water, blowing winds, the chemical energy of coal and other substances much of which can be converted into electric energy and transported where it is needed.

By means of these helps the modern American can lift a million pounds as easily as one, and can do in a second what formerly required days. Because of machines, each American has in his service the equivalent of perhaps fifty slaves. This does not mean that he works with fifty times as great economy of energy, because some human energy and much of that supplied by natural forces, must be used in constructing the tools and machines used.* The net saving of energy is, however, enormous. As shown by statistics, the labour of fewer people is required, although more is accomplished every year, in farming, manufacturing and transportation. The men concerned in production are also exerting less muscular force and for a shorter number of hours. In grinding wheat or building automobile frames, one man by the aid of machinery can do the work of hundreds under old conditions.

Many of the forces of nature are inexhaustible and all are subject to more economical use, hence there is no visible limit to the economy of effort man may attain, except that of his own ability to find and use the possibilities of economizing his time and energy.

---

* Chase in *Men and Machines* gives the following figures, showing comparative production of former and recent times :

Ten tractors plough as much ground as 500 men and 1000 oxen.

One girl using machines, spins as much cotton as 300 girls did formerly.

Two men and a crane do as much lifting of stone for the repair of Cologne Cathedral, as was formerly done by 360 men.

To produce one bushel of corn now requires 41 minutes' work, while formerly 271 minutes were necessary.

The same time required to make 500 pounds of nails formerly made only 5 pounds.

One man now thrashes as much wheat as 135 men formerly did in the same amount of time.

In one hour as much sheeting can be made as was made by hand in 106 hours of hand labour.

With modern machines one man can make as many bottles as 18 men without the machinery.

These great increases in production are partly offset by various factors. Ford claims that the tractor is twice as economical as ploughing by horse power, when all allowances are made. The factors to be considered are : (1) labour to build tractor factory ; (2) labour on materials for factory ; (3) labour of constructing tractor ; (4) labour of selling ; (5) repair and maintenance ; (6) labour on materials used in constructing and running it ; (7) depletion and obsolescence ; (8) interest and insurance.

One manufacturer complains that after decreasing cost of production one-half, he was compelled by competition to double his selling costs in order to continue in business.

There has been a general increase in selling cost of goods, and of transportation costs, as production costs have diminished.

HUMAN QUALITIES THAT FAVOUR ECONOMY

Obviously man must have intelligence of a high order to discover how to save energy and to substitute nature's forces for his own muscular exertions, and exactly adjusted machines for his trained skill of hand. Other qualities, analogous to those involved in all kinds of thrift are also needed. Ideas of future situations must influence him, otherwise he would exert himself to satisfy present desires only. The beginnings of economy are exercised when food is gathered while it is plentiful and easily obtained, and stored for future use.

All indirect means of getting results, such as making a tool to exchange for food or other necessity, or the doing of one part of a complex task while others do other parts, the whole to be shared or exchanged, is a necessary trait in all economical production. Persons who lack it will not voluntarily exert themselves in tasks indirectly leading to distant desired ends. Neither will they do more work than is needed to get what they want in the present and immediate future. Many savages cannot be induced to work much because they have few wants, most of which can be satisfied by comparatively little effort. In this country most people have so many desires that they cannot work enough to realize them all.

Men may be driven to work by starvation and cold, or by the whips of a slave-driver, but production by such means has never proved economical. No more is accomplished than must be in order to avoid immediate pain. A free man who is working toward an end anticipated with pleasure, uses his energy with greater efficiency without having to waste the energy of others in keeping him busy.

Another human quality which makes economical production possible is a certain uniformity of behaviour which may be called dependability. In the moving of a heavy object by several persons, the effort of all is likely to be wasted, if any one fails to pull when all are expected to do so. This quality of doing what is expected at the right time and in the right way becomes more and more important in conserving energy as work is specialized, and jobs and industries made dependent on what is being done by others. The failure of one man to do what is expected of him may cause not only loss of time and perhaps loss of limb or life of others in the same shop, but may delay transportation to other shops also, and prevent economical production there and in other related industries. Any worker who is not dependable, whether because of sickness, drunkenness, laziness, instability of character, lack of social adaptability to his fellows, lack of truthfulness in reports or honesty in use of materials, lack of accuracy in skill or accounting, or who acts in ways differing from those expected from members of his group, renders it difficult for others to work economically.

Engineers are studying means of saving materials and power used in production, and ways of substituting nature's forces for human energy, and mechanical devices for intellectual operations. Now one of the chief problems is that of making workers dependable individually, and efficient co-operatively. Efficiency work is now an important branch of engineering and the chief means of further increase in economy of production.

ECONOMIC VALUES

In general, things have economic value only when they have cost some effort to find, produce, transport or make available for use, and when their control can be transferred from one person to another. Ordinarily air and sunshine have no value, being abundant, non-transferable, and needing nothing done to them to make them usable. Water confined and transported for convenient use has value. Land and other things may be of greater or less value according to their location. Beautiful scenery and good climate may thus have an indirect value. Natural products, plant, animal and mineral, in so far as their possession and use is transferable, may have value largely proportioned to the usual amount of work required to make them available for use at the right time and place. Public parks and reservations and their contents are usually supposed not to have economic value, since no one is permitted to acquire individual ownership of them. It has been shown, however, that the total value of a residential tract of land is increased by devoting a part of it to a public park. Service by which physical or mental effort is used for the advantage of another may have economic value, as may also the right or a licence to render it for pay, as in the case of the doctor, the inventor or the author. Friendly aid is usually paid for in kind, and does not have direct economic value. If such help is known to be given for pay, it ceases to be valuable as a friendly accommodation and has only the value of an employment or advertising agency.

Only such things as are frequently transferred can be assigned a definite price. Rare objects, especially those appreciated by one or a few individuals because of some sentiment or association, may have a high value to the few people, yet not be generally saleable. In a place where farms are rarely sold, it is difficult to determine their commercial value.

ADVANTAGES OF TRADE

There are two advantages of trade : (1) greater variety of things obtainable ; (2) greater ease of obtaining goods. If one person or tribe is farming inland, and the other lives chiefly by fishing, each has tools, utensils, knowledge and skill appropriate to his industry and does not have to go far to practise it ; hence much energy is saved for both groups by exchanging their products with each other. Both may also find it more economical to exchange food with the makers of tools, etc., and perhaps also with those who devote themselves to the transportation of goods, than to make tools or transport goods for themselves. Geographical conditions or natural advantages in favour of one industry or another, often make it highly and permanently economical to exchange products of one locality for those of another, *e.g.* it will never pay to raise bananas in the greenhouses of the North, instead of exchanging knives or cloth for them in the South. On the other hand, it will not pay to transport natural ice to the tropics, when it can be obtained more easily by manufacturing it there. In general, there is economy in exchanging one article for another when, allowing for the energy and time used in transportation, the foreign article can be obtained with less effort by producing and exchanging something else for it. Improved means of transportation and of preserving have greatly decreased the advantages of producing meats and vegetables and other necessities near where they are consumed.

Economy in production sometimes depends, not on natural advantages, but upon culture in the form of tools, machines, knowledge, skill and efficient organization, which make it possible to produce goods with less effort than they can be produced where natural advantages are greater, but the artificial means of producing are deficient. In an economical arrangement of the industries of the world the artificial advantages would become located where the natural advantages were the greatest. The chief exception to this general tendency is found when the type of people who are naturally efficient in any industry are also the ones who will never do their best in the climate where natural advantages are greatest. Transporting iron workers to the tropics might cause greater loss of efficiency than would be involved in transporting raw materials and finished products. This means only that in valuing natural advantages, the efficiency of different peoples in different climates must be considered. How far such differences may be overcome by habituation and training is still to be determined. We are not here concerned with the non-economic advantages of trade, such as facilitating the exchange of cultures.

The general effect of tariffs, especially when levied for the purpose of giving some local industry an advantage in the world markets, is to prevent the removal of artificial advantages to the places where natural advantages are greatest, and thus to retard the general world movement toward economy of production. Of this there can be no question. Whether a tariff is a temporary benefit, a permanent benefit, or of no permanent advantage to any particular country, is a matter of opinion rather than of scientific knowledge,

The difficulties in the way of settling the matter are increased by the fact that tariffs are also used as a means of revenue, a substitute for direct taxation. This raises the question as to who really pays the taxes. The claim that it is paid by those who send the goods into a country is no longer allowed. It is certain that part if not all of it is paid by the people levying the tax, not only those using the imported goods, but by all the nation in the form of a general increase in living costs, which may or may not be balanced by greater average incomes. Masses of statistics have been collated without showing conclusively the exact degree of advantage or disadvantage to a nation, of a protective policy in general, or of protecting any particular industry. This, however, is worthy of note : the industries now receiving protection are no longer " infants " but more often " giants ", which have all sorts of artificial advantages. In a democracy such a condition seems inevitable and in opposition to the purpose of protection. If a bonus were given to an industry only while it was acquiring artificial advantages equivalent to those in competing countries there would be less likelihood of such aid being long continued.

MONEY AND ECONOMY

When a man or a tribe must find someone who is willing to barter what he has for what is offered, there may be much loss of time and energy, not only in transporting the goods, but in finding the one who will make the particular exchange desired. Fairs where people gather from various localities at certain times for barter, was the method formerly used, and even yet it is used in some sections. Such a meeting of people did not limit the difficulty of securing, and agreement as to how much of one kind of goods should be exchanged for another. The need for measuring the value of various articles, led to selecting something that was generally desired, and that did not change much with time or vary greatly at different seasons, as a means or standard for agreement on terms of exchange. All sorts of things have thus been used, but a large portion of the world finally adopted silver and gold as the most convenient, enduring, and constant measure of the values of all goods and services offered for exchange. The government stamp on the metal rendered it more reliable as to quality, and did away with the necessity for weighing it, and thus avoided disputes and saved time and energy.

After money thus became a medium of exchange, it was no longer necessary for producers to store up and transport goods to such an extent as formerly. Money was moved easily from place to place, and goods transported only when and where needed. An individual with money could easily supply his needs if he moved to a distant place instead of carrying many things with him.

Money has not as yet become an accurate measure of values. It is not an unvarying measure, because first, the material of which it is made sometimes becomes more plentiful and then it takes more of it to buy what is wanted. It measures values at a given time fairly well, but does not correctly measure the comparative values at different times. Extensive gold discoveries naturally decrease its purchasing power, and prices rise. Goods are affected earlier than wages, consequently the labourer is at a disadvantage at first, but when prices drop he is temporarily benefited. Considerable inconvenience and waste is caused by changes in the purchasing power of money that would be eliminated if an unvarying measure could be found and put into use, as has been advocated by Professor Fisher.

A second reason for variation in the purchasing power of money is the fact that every nation has enlarged its supply of money by substituting paper money in part for metal money. Within each nation, as long as the people are sure that such money may be exchanged for metal money, and consequently for goods, it serves just as well and is usually more convenient to use than coins. How long such money will have the same value depends partly upon how much of it there is in the country in proportion to coined money, and partly upon confidence that the government is stable and, if called upon, will give coin in exchange for the paper.

Within limits it may increase or decrease the total amount of money without changing the comparative value of gold and paper money, but the amount of goods a dollar will purchase decreases as money becomes plentiful.

Money is not a convenient means of *world* exchange because the units are different—francs, pounds, dollars, etc., and people are loath to accept money of another nation because of unfamiliarity and lack of confidence. Gold usually inspires more confidence than other metal coinage and much more than paper, but it is not convenient to use when of unfamiliar units.

BANKS AS ECONOMIC MACHINES

Banks are primarily safe depositories for money. This advantage is least needed when people receive only about what they spend every day. Persons who can save from daily or weekly wages a part of their income for future purchases, are relieved of trouble and anxiety by a bank which cares for the surplus until it is needed. The person who receives large amounts of money at a time, much of which is not spent at once, finds the bank a very great convenience. Banks are also especially useful in helping to transfer money to distant people.

A bank is not only a convenient and efficient depository for money that is not to be used immediately, but it is one of the most effective means of making use of credits. Experience shows that much of the money placed in a bank remains for some time, hence the amount accumulated at any one time is much greater than there is any likelihood of being immediately drawn out. A bank is likely to have to pay out on any one day only a small per cent of what has been deposited with it. By arrangement of credits between banks, whereby if one bank needs to pay out more than usual it can draw upon another that has an extra supply, the actual money on hand may safely be very small.

Money, like machines and people, is most useful when working, and all banks of deposit have opportunities to set idle money to work that individual depositors do not have.

Therefore, the bank, instead of hoarding all money deposited loans it to merchants, manufacturers and others who can use it to advantage, and they pay the bank interest for its use. This enables the bank to pay its running expenses with some profits, and to pay to those who leave their money on deposit for a considerable time, a slightly lower interest than the borrowers are paying. Savings banks and savings departments of commercial banks, and co-operative and building and loan banks, make a business of doing the latter ; while the commercial banks do not pay depositors interest except in certain cases, and may charge people who never have much money on deposit for more than a few days, for the services rendered.

Since money is a great saver of energy whenever it is being used in exchanging goods, and banks keep most of it working when otherwise it would be idle a good deal of the time, and since this in effect greatly increases the total amount of money, it follows that banks have something of the same value as machines in increasing economic production. Nothing so disturbs all the industries of a country as a breakdown or inefficiency in this machine.

ECONOMIC VALUE OF CAPITAL

Capital is usually wealth that is being used to produce more wealth. Much of it is usually in the form of lands or machines that facilitate economical production, but some of it must provide food and other essentials while production is going on. Every labourer needs this form of capital wealth to sustain him until pay-day. A large proportion of manufacturers and stores hire the use of capital to purchase materials and pay helpers until their products can be sold.

Machines are the most important means of increasing production with the same number or fewer workers. Capital is needed not only to purchase these machines, but still larger amounts are required to sell and transport materials and products to distant places, since it is seldom possible to sell all near at hand. Individuals and nations lacking capital must use less economical means of production than those that have plenty. High rates of interest for the use of capital cannot be paid unless it can be used so as to greatly increase production.

STOCKS AND BONDS AS ECONOMIC FACTORS

Stocks and bonds are means of obtaining credit used by nearly all the larger and more efficient producers. Bonds are much used also by cities, towns, states and governments in supplying public needs by credit, when there is no money immediately available. Both are partial substitutes for money.

A *bond* is a promise to pay a certain amount of money at a given time, with interest at a certain rate to be paid at regular intervals. It is as good as money when the promise is practically certain to be fulfilled. Sometimes this certainty depends chiefly on the value of the property upon which it is a mortgage, and it is then known as a mortgage bond. In other cases its value depends upon the prosperity and reliability of the corporation or governmental unit financed. A bond is a convenient form of capital because money may be obtained in large amounts in this way from many who, individually, have only small amounts to loan. Not only may bonds provide the borrowers with capital but those who purchase the bonds may obtain loans on them at the bank. Bonds are also especially useful to banks, nearly all of which keep part of their money so invested, because they can be used as a means of obtaining cash quickly.

Stocks are shares in the business of production that serve much the same economic purposes as bonds. They give the purchaser a share in the capital owned by the company and in all its profits, and in its assets if the company goes out of business. By buying shares one becomes a producer of goods by means of money instead of by personal effort or by giving the use of a horse, a machine or a building. As a partner, a stockholder is entitled to his share of profits if there are any. He does not hire his money out at a fixed rate as the purchaser of a bond does, and hence he is not promised anything in return. If the business prospers, he gets the benefit of it, but if it does poorly he may get nothing. During the last twenty years ending in 1929 holders of common stocks in good companies have realized more than holders of bonds of the same corporations because industries have generally prospered. Preferred stocks have a greater safety feature than common stocks of the same company, since they have first chance after bonds for dividends if the company is successful, and first chance before common stocks for a share in the property if it goes out of business. Common stocks in a very prosperous company are more profitable than bonds or preferred stocks of the same company, because they share in all values after fixed amounts are allotted to bonds and preferred stocks but are less safe and less profitable when the company is only moderately or slightly prosperous.

ECONOMIC VALUE OF PUBLIC MARKETS

As was stated earlier, an article can have a definite, reasonably constant value only when things of its kind are frequently bought and sold. With money and credit as means of facilitating trade it is, in addition, necessary that those who produce one article and buy another, shall have convenient means of selling and buying. The old-time village store exchanged groceries for farm products, using money only as a measure of their comparative values. Prices were uncertain, depending upon local supply and demand. Only when an outside public market was found did prices in any section become stabilized so that the farmer could know in advance the probable price of his products, or the merchant feel safe in buying articles that could not be disposed of in a few days. The broader the market for products the more stable the prices, and the more it became possible to plan for economy in production and exchange. Wholesale stores supplemented the local stores and sometimes producers formed associations for selling. The advantages of the latter have been greatest in the fruit-growing industry where there

I

is great waste if shipment is made to any place in excess of the amount that can be used before it decays.

In the case of cotton and the grains, which do not quickly deteriorate in quality and for which there is a world demand, facilities for storing until needed and for transporting to places of consumption, are important. The farmers and bread consumers on opposite sides of the earth help to determine the price received for wheat and paid for bread in every other portion of the world. Wheat and other grains may have to be stored for a long while, or it may take much time to transport and market them in the form of bread. It is of advantage to the miller to know something of the probable price of flour when he buys wheat, and to the baker to know the price he may get for bread when he buys flour. Such knowledge steadies prices and helps everyone concerned, including railways and banks, to do their work economically. They can plan for busy times, and banks can safely give credit to persons producing and buying goods the prices of which can be counted on to vary little.

This is the basic reason for the establishment of markets for grains and cotton, where a given amount and quality may be offered and bought without the articles themselves being present. In effect markets fix and stabilize prices by means of a world auction, where anyone may buy or sell without handling the goods, but merely on evidence that the seller can deliver and the buyer pay for them. The relation between world production and requirements may be estimated, and a price practically the same in all parts of the world is assured.

These advantages are only partly destroyed by persons who buy and sell for speculation only. Sometimes they over- or under-estimate what a future crop will be, or use artificial means for making the crop seem smaller or larger than it is or will be, or they sell or buy so much that the price is forced down or up suddenly. In general, the large speculator, however, makes more by correctly anticipating future crops and prices and acting accordingly, than by misrepresenting the facts. He may profit by over- or under-stating probabilities, but since many men with money and shrewdness are competing, the true probabilities are approximated in the prices on the exchange. The small speculator occasionally wins, but is at a double disadvantage in that he is less well informed, and has less money, which compels him to sell at a time when it would be most profitable to buy. As a result many people suffer the same economic losses from speculation on the exchanges as from other forms of gambling against experts.

It is of great advantage to have this continuous world market maintained and there is gain from having some who are trying to make money through such a market. They keep it active and, by continually forecasting the future, help to keep prices more constant. It is easy to see, however, that in this field of economic activity, even more than in most industries, there is loss when too many engage in it. It is a waste to raise too much corn or make too many chairs, or to have too many preachers ; but the products, though in excess, usually have some value. Too many buying on the exchange adds nothing of value to the world's products, and decreases general productivity by using men and capital which might be used in producing goods.

The stock exchange provides a world market for representatives of wealth—stocks and bonds—and helps fix prices in accordance with the consensus of opinion, which gives them a known credit value. As this form of intangible wealth is continually increasing in amount, such markets are indispensable. Listed stocks and bonds have a known value, hence they can be used to secure credit much more readily than similar stock not sold on the market. On the other hand, the stock exchange furnishes an opportunity for a large amount of wasteful speculation, much of which is a form of gambling in which the big operator, like the gambling apparatus used at Monte Carlo, has considerably the greater chance of winning than the untrained speculator. To take chances is a natural human trait shown in games and adventures, as well as in gambling. The stock exchange facilitates taking of chances in buying and selling securities.

Employment agencies are markets for labour and have an

economic value similar to, but even greater than the produce and stock markets, since they furnish employment to persons who would otherwise waste their time in idleness or in ineffective search for employment. They are also less usable for gambling purposes.

ECONOMIC VALUE OF ORGANIZATION AND MANAGEMENT

Organization provides for the co-operation of a number of persons in accomplishing the same end. Without organization, there is great expenditure of effort with little or nothing accomplished. With good organization each does what he is best fitted to do, in a way and at a time that will facilitate the activities of others working towards the same ends. No amount of goodwill and industry can take the place of good organization. To be efficient an organization must have individuals for each form of activity suited by nature and training, not only for the industry, but for the particular job. There must be neither too many nor too few for each task, and all must be kept working regularly and efficiently, not only in so far as their own part is concerned, but so that other workers will be helped rather than hindered in their tasks. Since machines can do the work of many men in tasks requiring great strength and accuracy, and in those where the same motions must be made over and over, it is economical to have all such jobs done by machines instead of by men, when the cost of capital to secure the machine is less than the wages saved during its life.

On the basis of facts gained from organizations of many sorts, it is possible to formulate plans of organization and rules of management, that prove much more efficient than it is possible to make on the basis of the experience of a single individual. In organizations in which results are continually measured, such as banks and insurance companies, rules may be developed which are so reliable that failure is practically impossible when such institutions are conducted in accordance with them. The same is true in all industries, but in a less degree; and also in organizations not directly economical, such as schools, societies and governments.

The value of a manager of an organization depends partly upon his knowledge of the truths already known about efficiency of organization in general and in his special field, and partly upon his ability to use these truths in selecting helpers, assigning tasks, training workers, keeping all healthy, satisfied and effectively busy, and in buying machines and adjusting them to the special industry and the special conditions to be met.

One of the manager's most difficult problems is to keep the workers and machines productively active so that there is no waste of power and time. In farming and in many factories, employment is naturally seasonal, and there is much waste of human resources because of idleness and attempted transfers to new jobs. A dairy farm presents less difficulty in this respect than a fruit or wheat farm; and a cotton mill, less than a millinery establishment which must adjust to more changes in style. Some firms having sufficient capital, solve the problem by continuing to produce for future sales, and others diversify sufficiently to have productive work for their helpers all the year, *e.g.* the ice business in summer, and coal in winter.

The larger the organization, the more important relatively becomes the management compared to the workers. A good manager of a business using a half dozen men may add to their production more than an additional helper would, while a good manager of an establishment consisting of a thousand men and a few machines, may have the value of several thousand additional workers in increasing the production. Scientific studies of the tasks performed by men and machines, of the relations of processes to each other, and the employment of personnel directors to select workers and to keep them at their best, have greatly increased production in many industries.

Every such increase demands more specialization on the part of workers, and greater ability on the part of managers. The larger production resulting, and the necessity of selling at a distance, involves great increase in clerical and selling forces. In other words, "white-collar" jobs are increasing in number, while "horny-handed" jobs are becoming fewer. However, the increase in clerical jobs is now being checked by adding machines and other devices which enable one person to do the work of several. The decrease in "horny-handed" jobs is partly, but not wholly offset by increase in machines to be made, since machines are used in making other machines.

EFFECTS OF INCREASED PRODUCTION

The natural result of increase in production by workers is the same for society as in the case of an individual who does as much in three days as he has been doing in a week—there is more leisure time. With the present increased efficiency it would not be necessary for people to work more than a few hours a day for a few days of the week—*provided* nothing was produced except what *must be consumed* in order to keep the workers healthy and efficient. The estimate of two hours' work a day as all that would be necessary is probably too low, because considerable time must be used in constructing machines and in training men, and less than half the population is directly productive. There is no question, however, that every increase in efficiency of production ultimately means the possibility of shorter working hours for all workers.

If there is more leisure time than is needed for rest and recreation, it may be used in sloth or dissipation. These will lower efficiency. If used in agreeable recreative ways, there will be greater efficiency. Such use, however, always makes necessary the production of means of pleasure and recreation, usually called luxuries, since one may live in a fair degree of physical health without them.

The amusement industry now ranks as one of the largest in the country. The proportion of income spent in this country on amusement and luxuries, lies somewhere between one-quarter and one-half, according to whether such conveniences as bath-tubs and telephones are counted as luxuries or necessities. Increased economy of production has therefore decreased hours of labour in general to some extent, but has in a greater degree increased the production of goods to be enjoyed, which add only indirectly to the productive efficiency of the workers.

In some industries such as coal-mining and agriculture every increase in efficiency of production has thrown men out of work. Only about half the number of men formerly necessary is now needed to produce all that could be consumed in this country and marketed abroad, provided only the best coal-mines and the best farm lands were worked in the most efficient ways. Part of the workers in these industries must be idle and forgo all luxuries, or must change to some other industry for whose production the limit of demand has not yet been reached. Every increase in efficiency of production of any kind of goods calls for changes in working time, or for new goods to be produced by those not now needed in their former work.

This situation presents many difficulties of adjustment, but far-sighted men realize that it is, in part at least, self-corrective, providing workers are paid as much or more for shorter working periods than they formerly were paid for the longer ones. With such pay they are not only able to buy what will keep them in physical health, but such additional conveniences and luxuries as will keep them in good mental condition. This furnishes the increased demand for goods, necessary that those thrown out of work by efficiency methods in necessity industries may find work in producing luxuries. A continual adjustment is imperative in order that demand and supply in each and all industries shall be properly balanced, and in order that all workers may be employed a sufficient portion of the time and paid enough to buy what is provided.

The problem of men thrown out of employment by increased efficiency of production is similar to that of industries which are seasonal in character, with slack seasons every year, during which only a fraction of the employees can be kept busy all the time. Failure to provide employment for workers and machines not only wastes energy and capital in the industry concerned, but decreases the buying power of the workers, and not infrequently wrecks families and individuals.

STANDARDIZATION AND ECONOMY

A certain amount of standardizing is an inevitable result of the use of machinery. To make a single article such as a chair of a certain size, shape and marking by means of an automatic machine would be almost as wasteful as going around the earth to get to the post-office. Unless thousands of parts are to be all exactly alike, there may be nothing gained by the use of machinery.

In addition to this compulsory standardizing wherever machines are used, it is a great saving for all persons in industries to conform to certain fixed standards. All railway and automobile manufacturers construct parts to correspond to the standard width of roads ; and use bolts, nuts and screws, etc., that are of standard diameters, length and thread, while screw-drivers and wrenches are made to match. Tyres and many other parts of bicycles and automobiles are of standard sizes and usable on machines wherever made. The same is true of parts of houses, beds, chairs, etc.

The more completely every part is standardized the greater the economy possible in making parts, assembling, and in repairing. The time required to put together the parts of the frame of an automobile has been reduced from days to seconds. Whenever a radical change is made in a " model " much machinery and special skill must be scrapped. Making many new models of automobiles or styles of shoes, and changing them frequently, is a heavy economic waste. Through the action of the government in conference with manufacturers, the number of different models of shoes, beds, saws, etc., has been greatly reduced. Waste is the inevitable price of progress in designing and improving manufactured articles, but the losses are unnecessarily heavy when standardization is made too soon, too late, or in too great detail. There is much loss in changing the standards if the article is one which depends for its usefulness upon the skill of the operator or accurate measurements, *e.g.* keyboards of typewriters, metric units instead of foot-pound units. The waste and inconvenience of changing are so extensive, that it has proved impossible to secure adoption of the more convenient metric system where other systems have long been in use.

Where goods are to be sold at a distance without examination by the purchaser, it is very desirable for selling convenience that they shall be of standard quality as well as size, shape and construction. In the case of farm products there is some waste in selecting oranges, apples, potatoes, etc., of standard quality, shape and size for marketing, but this is more than balanced by the advantages gained in transporting and selling.

ADVERTISING AND ECONOMY

Much material and a large number of trained men are employed in advertising goods. Does it pay, or would it be better if these men were producing instead of helping to sell goods ? The firms that advertise efficiently sell enough more goods than their competitors to give them the advantages of large production and they may thus prosper without raising the price to the public, and sometimes may lower the price. In the last accounting, however, the public must pay the cost of advertising, since without it the price could be made still lower.

Almost without effort on their part the people thus get their compensation in knowledge of time-saving objects and of goods having the qualities they desire, which they may thereafter buy with little waste of time in searching for and testing in order to get what they want. Through advertisements the public learns of improvements that they might not hear of otherwise in many years. This is the greatest value of advertising. After the public has been educated by advertisements and experience with standard products, no time is wasted in examining a given specimen to be purchased. It does not pay to advertise anything which is not pretty well standardized, hence each article of a given make and name is usually very much like every other; and to gain confidence, the manufacturer will usually exchange any that are not according to standard.

Notwithstanding these and other advantages, there is no question that much advertising is a waste of materials and effort, and poor advertising is always a loss. Good advertising of some commodities while of advantage to the firm that succeeds in selling large quantities, is not of corresponding advantage to the public. After the public is once well informed as to the qualities needed in soap, why should it pay for the advertising of particular brands? If the quality was assured by a label, the name of the firm producing it would be of no significance. Yet who can say when an article is so well known and standardized that the firms competing for its sale may not be stimulated either to improve the article or the means of producing it?

ECONOMIC VALUE OF INSURANCE

Insurance of property or of lives does not prevent their being lost to society. Just as a thrifty person saves not to keep for ever, but to use at a time when need is greater, so insurance is a mode of preparing for possible future needs. In the end insurance costs all that is paid for losses, plus the expense of conducting the business.

When fire or other disaster destroys houses, factories or other property, the productive power of the owner is generally seriously decreased, and without insurance to restore it quickly there would be in most cases a long period of decreased production. Even large firms with much capital may suffer from a period of unproductivity and withdrawal of some of their capital in order to restore the loss. A state having much property, located in places where one fire could not destroy all of it, can afford to go without insurance because it can repair such losses by means of credit, or by an increase in taxes not great enough to interfere with the productiveness of anyone. A city is not so safe without insurance, because of the possible disturbance produced by a single fire.

By insuring property, one is exercising thrift economy better than he would be by saving for possible losses. He is protected against loss as soon as he begins paying insurance, while if he saved the same amount each year for future needs, he would not have enough in a score of years to give equal protection.

Insurance in cases of accident or sickness is also a more effective way of being thrifty than by saving capital for such emergencies. Life insurance is primarily a means of protecting the family of a producer from loss of income by his death. As in fire insurance, disability is better guarded against by insurance than by saving, because protection begins at once, while when one saves for the future the protection is slight until after many years of saving. Life insurance costs more proportionally than fire insurance because death is certain to occur some time, and the face of the policy must eventually be paid ; while much property never burns and hence only a small part of the value of the property insured ever needs to be collected from the companies insuring it. This disadvantage in life insurance is, however, partly compensated for in two ways: (1) the family will ultimately get back all that has been paid ; (2) since the money paid every year is put on interest, this provides for the expenses of the insurance company and leaves something to be added to the face of the policy.

Endowment insurance is a combination of life insurance for the family, and of building up savings by the insured. A thirty-year endowment policy taken out at forty years, would be insurance for the family, and an old-age savings for the insured. A ten-year endowment policy taken out at twenty years of age would be largely a means of saving, since chances of death during that time are slight compared with the longer and later period of from forty to seventy. Endowment insurance is also a means of saving for a special purpose at a certain age, *e.g.* travel at fifty years, or sending children to college.

In no field has the scientific use of statistics been of greater economic value than in the organization and conduct of insurance companies. On the basis of past experience it is known what charges must be made, and how funds must be handled in order that protection shall not fail when most needed. In the case of mutual companies, any excess collected to insure safety is returned to the individual from time to time, thus equalizing advantages instead of giving profits above expenses to stockholders. Individuals, families and society are saved from disastrous shocks by these scientifically devised and conducted safety and thrift organizations.

In many fields there is not a sufficient number of classifiable facts upon which to base rules for regulating insurance. We do not yet know the best forms of sickness and old-age insurance, or the most nearly just ways of providing against unemployment, dishonesty and inefficiency, by insurance. The probabilities of events dependent upon natural forces may be figured with greater accuracy because more measurable, and less affected by human variability. There has been enough data collected regarding automobiles, other than thefts, but not yet enough relating to airplanes, to give a safe basis for calculating risks.

THE SPENDER AND THE SAVER

The one who spends as fast as he produces is not providing against economic losses to self and society which may result from disaster, sickness, unemployment, early death or a non-productive old age ; and a community of such persons cannot be permanently prosperous. On the other hand, a miser who saves all the money not necessary to keep him alive and puts it in a stocking, is not an efficient producer because he is continually making useless to society all that he produces ; and a community of such persons could never use the more economical means of production through which the hours of labour are shortened and the luxuries of life obtained.

Suppose, then, two other types of individuals, both of whom keep themselves efficient and provide for future needs by insurance and saving, but one, when he has a surplus, spends it in so-called luxuries, while the other saves the additional amount and perhaps never uses it. If he puts it in a bank, it is likely to be used as capital to produce more goods. The difference would be that the first would furnish an immediate demand for the additional goods produced, while the other would supply banks with money to be used for producing them. A community of spenders would produce and use more things that men desire than one made up of savers. Too large a proportion of persons carrying saving to an extreme would slow down economic activity, even if they placed their money in banks. Those who save in order to purchase later things of permanent value may, however, contribute to economic prosperity as much or more than those spending quickly but less wisely.

HIGH WAGES AND ECONOMICS

Some manufacturers in choosing their help select those who are intelligent and well trained, though the wages paid must be higher. Statistics show that in many industries the cost of production with such workers is less than with poorer-paid labourers.

Another phase of the question has recently been stressed by economists. The intelligent workers are likely to be buyers of luxuries and to work regularly in order to be able to buy them. This buying of luxuries creates a demand for goods that is not found among unintelligent labourers, or among superior workers who are paid low wages. The men not needed in the industries which are becoming more efficient, can be used in producing these additional goods, and by their buying power help keep economic conditions prosperous. Economic expansion and high wages are related, therefore, and are usually shown by increased use of luxuries, although there are a few individuals even in this country who work less time when paid high wages.

SELECTED RESEARCHES

(Quoted from manuscript by courtesy of the author.)

Economists have usually claimed that free competition will generally insure that the prices of the same quality of goods will not greatly differ in the same market. The need for a factual as well as a theoretical study of this and other supposed economic truths is indicated by the following researches of Rosamund Cook, Professor of Home Economics Education of the University of Cincinnati.

" Samples of sheeting 45 inches wide bought in the open market were judged by 150 consumers and 9 experienced sales persons and tested in the laboratory as to tensile strength, thread count and weight."

The character of the laboratory tests are indicated by the following description.

" The material was conditioned in a desiccator for five hours before testing for tensile strength in order to secure uniform dryness of the material. The tests were all made at one time under constant room conditions. Atmospheric temperature and relative humidity were not recorded, since the test was for comparative purposes only. Neither would they be necessary to anyone repeating the test, since with conditions kept constant the final comparative result would be the same.

" The 1″ strip method was used in testing for tensile strength and a hand-operated dynamometer was used : jaws 1″ wide, distance 1″ between jaws. The strips were ravelled to 1″ width and were 6″ long. Six tests each for warp and filling were made and the results averaged to give the tensile strength.

" The thread count was made with a microtome. Each set, warp and filling, was counted three times and on three different parts of the sample, each count checking with the other.

" A 2″ square was the unit of size used for weight, the balance being checked by a second person for each weight.

" The results of these tests were mathematically combined to give a quality-rating for each piece.

" The last step in the procedure was to combine the three rank order numbers for each piece of sheeting, average, and make a final rank order numbering.

" The ranking of the samples A to I by consumers, sales people and by the laboratory tests was as follows :

Sample.	Consumers' Rating.	Salesman's Rating.	Test Rating.	Price.
				Cents
C	4	5·5	1·8	36
B	7	7	3·5	35
E	5·5	1	3·6	86
G	2	5·5	3·8	36
I	1	4	4·1	42
F	5·5	3	5·3	26
D	3	2	7	44
H	8	9	7·8	36
A	9	8	7·8	31 "

It will be seen that there is little relation between quality and prices.

An extensive study of hosiery quality and hosiery advertisements by Prof. Cook and students of Home Economics Education Dept. of University of Cincinnati also proves that quality and prices are not closely correlated. Consumers are not concerned with quality only or chiefly, as economists suppose. The words of an advertising chief: " Make your ads beautiful, make the words sing. Heavens, there isn't a woman in the world who cares about facts," are possibly nearer the truth regarding the psychology of buying and prices than the assertions of the economists who have the narrow point of view of the " economical man " who is supposed to act always so as to get the greatest financial advantages for himself.

" THE WESTERN ELECTRIC COMPANY EXPERIMENT."
By ELTON MAYO, in *The Human Factor*, January 1930. *Quoted by Permission.*

During the past two years, Elton Mayo and officials of the Hawthorne Works of the Western Electric Company in Chicago, have been conducting experimental investigations of rest periods, working conditions and other influences affecting workers. . . .

The investigators showed, at least tentatively, and in highly mechanized and repetitive operations, that

1. Total daily output is increased by rest periods and not decreased.

2. The conditions of work during the working day have more effect on production than the number of working days in the week.

3. " Outside " influences, *i.e.* conditions not directly relevant to the task, tend to create either a buoyant or depressed spirit which is reflected in production. A distinct relationship is

apparent between the emotional status of the workers and the consistency of their output.

4. The method of the supervisor is the most important single " outside " influence. Home conditions may affect the worker and his work ; and a supervisor who can " listen " and not " talk" can in many instances almost completely compensate for such depressing influences.

5. Pay incentives do not stimulate production if other working conditions are wrong.

The most important and significant result is that dealing with the method of supervision. It was found that " bully-ragging " methods of supervision not only depressed workers but their production. It was found that workers came to increase their liking for their jobs with the new kind of supervision which substituted sympathetic " listening " for officious " talking ", with a consequent increase of production. The new type of supervisors listened not only to talk about shop but about home and personal affairs. . . .

" AN EXPERIMENTAL STUDY OF EFFICIENCY OF WORK UNDER VARIOUS SPECIFIED CONDITIONS." By PITIRIM A. SOROKIN and others, Univ. of Minnesota. From *American Journal of Sociology*, March 1930. *Quoted by Permission.*

. . . I tried to apply the experimental method for the clarification of the problem whether the communistic or individualistic organization of labour is the more efficient. . . . Providing that all other conditions remain constant, and only the investigated condition varies, does the efficiency of work depend on, and vary with, different systems of remuneration, such as " individual " and " collective ", " equal " and " unequal " ; remuneration of the worker himself and that of his good friend ; finally is the overt-pure-competition not remunerated by any material value, a factor of efficiency ? If each of these factors influence the efficiency of the work, in what way and how ? Such were the problems of the experimental study. You can easily see their theoretical and practical—even purely economic—significance, especially for our age of a reconstruction of the capitalistic system, rationalization of labour organization, and Communist, Socialist, and Equalitarian tendencies.

(*a*) THE TECHNIQUE OF THE EXPERIMENTATION
AND THE HUMAN MATERIAL

Experimentation was first made with a group of pre-school children, from three to four years of age, in the Child Welfare Clinic of the University of Minnesota ; later on with three high-school boys from thirteen to fourteen years of age; and still later on with the group of kindergarten children. . . .

The first series of experiments was made during April, May and June 1927. The work which was done by the pre-school children was running and carrying marbles from one corner of the yard of the Child Welfare Institute and the hall of the kindergarten to another; picking up small wooden balls or pegs of a definite colour from a box filled with balls, squares and triangular objects or with pegs of various colours; filling cups with sand, carrying them a certain distance, and emptying them there. The work of the high-school boys consisted in carrying pails of water from one place to another; in filling a pail with sand and carrying it to a certain place; and finally, in computing a list of points on paper and in performing the operations of addition, subtraction, multiplication, and division of a series of arithmetical problems given in a specially prepared list. . . .

The next point to establish was " the equality of all other conditions " except those which were studied. This was easily done through the identity of the kind of work done, of the children working, of the time of the work, of cups, of distance, of boxes, etc.

More difficult was an elimination of the effects of fatigue and practice. Their elimination was reached through a series of repetitions of the same work and alternation or reversal of the order of the work under each pair of conditions studied. One day the children started the work with an " equal " or " collective " remuneration and passed to the work with an " unequal " or " individual " remuneration, while the next day the sequence of the work under these conditions was the reverse. Under such circumstances the effects of fatigue, practice, and similar factors are likely to be eliminated, and the total amount of work done in a series of the experiments under each of the conditions studied may be reasonably ascribed to the difference in the method of remuneration. . . .

As the " remuneration " to the children for the work I used various kinds of children's toys, and, later on, pennies. . . .

(b) EFFICIENCY OF WORK OF THE PRE-SCHOOL CHILDREN UNDER " THE COLLECTIVE OR GROUP " AND UNDER " THE INDIVIDUAL " REMUNERATION

This is shown by Table I. By the " collective or group " remuneration is meant that the toys were not allowed to be " taken home " as an individual possession of the children but were given to their collective " play-house " where every one of them could enjoy them, as a " collective possession ". By " individual " remuneration is meant that the child who earned his toy could " take it home " and do with it whatever he would like to do: he had a full right of property over it. The results

K

of the table are clear. They sum up as follows : in all the experiments, with the exception of that of Number 7, " individual " remuneration stimulated a greater efficiency in the work of the same children than " collective " remuneration. . . . The difference for the first four experiments in the efficiency under both systems of remuneration was that between fifty-six and sixty-one units of work for a total period of work time 15 minutes 30 seconds ; for the next four experiments the difference was fifty-nine and seventy units of work for a period of time equal to 33 minutes 30 seconds. Taking into consideration the shortness of time, the difference in efficiency was rather remarkable. If we imagine instead of 33 minutes 333 days and instead of four or two workers, forty thousand of them, then the above difference would grow to an enormous amount quite important from the economic standpoint. . . .

The next problem, related to the above, was to find out whether there was a difference in the efficiency of work when remuneration for it was given to the working child himself and when he worked for another child in the working group while the other child worked for him. . . .

The table shows that the efficiency of work for " himself " was greater than for a fellow co-worker. The difference between 232 and 212 units of work indicates the stimulating rôle of " egotism " in work. . . .

(d) Efficiency of Work under " Equal " and " Unequal " Remuneration

The next problem was to find out whether the efficiency of work was the same when the members of the working group were remunerated " equally " and " unequally " in proportion to the work done by each member, the total amount of the remuneration for the whole working group being the same in both cases. . . .

The data below clearly show that an " unequal " remuneration stimulated more efficient work than an " equal " one. Practically all the experiments, not to mention their total series, show this. Thus, though total remuneration for the whole group in each of the cases of the " equal " and the " unequal " remuneration was the same and all the other conditions remained equal, a remuneration according to effort and work done or an unequal distribution of the remuneration within the group stimulated greater exertion in work-efficiency than an equal distribution of it. This is true in regard to the children as well as the boys.

In contrast with the results where the work was physical, in a purely intellectual work (computation of the points and solving of arithmetical problems) the difference in efficiency of the work under " equal " and " unequal " remuneration was practically insignificant. . . .

STRIKES

This preference of the system of " unequal " remuneration has, however, its own drawback. While in all the cases of the " equal remuneration " we did not have any single case of " a strike " among the working children, we had them several times in the cases of the " unequal remuneration ". . . .

. . . I wished to determine more exactly the stimulating rôle of a pure competition not followed by any pecuniary remuneration. For this purpose a series of experiments was made with the children of the Child Welfare Institute and with those of the kindergarten. . . .

The table shows that as far as manual work is concerned the work under the " pure competition " was more efficient in all five working teams of children than the work under the equal remuneration. . . . Only in the half-mental work of picking pegs was the work under the pure competition less efficient than that under equal or unequal remuneration. I am not prepared to explain this last result at present. But the results in their total are rather remarkable in their witnessing to the great incentive power of the non-pecuniary-competitive-situation. They testify that human efficiency may indeed be stimulated through pure competition—in this case through a mere speech-reactional incentive : " we want to see who can beat ". . . .

SUGGESTED READINGS

Economics has been organized on an analytical and theoretical basis, rather than developed from inductive studies of wealth activities. This makes very clear exposition possible, such as is found in most of the following typical books :

BYE, RAYMOND T., *Principles of Economics*, 1924.
CARVER, THOMAS N., *Elementary Economics*, 1920.
CLAY, HENRY, *Economics for the General Reader*, 1918.
FISHER, IRVING, *Elementary Principles of Economics*, 1926.
MARSHALL, ALFRED, *Principles of Economics*, 1920.
SEAGER, H. R., *Principles of Economics*, 3rd ed., 1923.

Works containing more statistical facts are :

BYE, RAYMOND T., *Applied Economics*, 1928.
CARVER, THOMAS N., *The Economic World and How it May be Improved*, 1928.
CHASE, STUART, *The Tragedy of Waste*, 1925.
SEAGER, H. R., *Practical Problems in Economics*, 1923.
SMITH, EDWIN S., *Reducing Seasonal Unemployment*, 1931.
TAUSSIG, FRANK W., *Tariff History of the United States*, 7th ed., 1923.
WELD, W. E., and TASTLEBE, A. S., *A Case Book for Economics*, 1927.

Typical studies of special industries are :

HAMILTON, WALTON H., and WRIGHT, HELEN R., *The Case of Bituminous Coal*, 1925.
SELIGMAN, E. R. A., *The Economics of Installment Selling, with Special Reference to the Automobile*, 1927.

Insurance is clearly discussed in :

RUBINOW, I. M., *Social Insurance*, 1913.
WOODS, EDWARD A., *The Sociology of Life Insurance*, 1928.

The human factor in Economics is presented in :

TEAD, ORDWAY, and METCALF, HENRY C., *Personal Administration, its Principles and Management*, 1926.
WILLIAMS, WHITING, *Mainsprings of Men*, 1925.

And in articles in the *Survey Graphic* by AMIDON, April 1, 1929 : BRUERE, February 1, 1927 : KELLOGG, March 1, 1928 : and in the *American Economic Review Supplement*, by DOUGLAS, March 1926.

GUILFORD, in *American Economic Review*, September 1929, and COBB, in *American Journal of Sociology*, May 1927, show how the methods of inductive science may be used in studying all phases of economics.

CHAPTER VII

MEANS OF CONTROL, OR POLITICAL SCIENCE

ORIGIN AND FUNCTIONS OF GOVERNMENT

WHENEVER individuals come in contact some of their acts may be of little significance to each other·; but many acts necessarily assist or interfere with others. Every individual learns to modify his behaviour so that others will not block his efforts to get what he wants. There may be much conflict but the tendency is for individuals to adjust behaviour to that of others. Some seek to obtain their ends by force, others by stealth. As the association continues habits develop and each expects a certain type of reaction from the other. One is likely to be surprised or offended when companions act in unexpected ways, and there is usually an attempt by the persons most concerned to make the offender conform. This often results in fights and the consequent disturbance of persons not concerned in the affair. When it becomes customary for many of the disputes that arise between individuals to be settled by one or more representatives of the group in accordance with accepted ways of behaviour, then the group has in fact developed a government.

According to Rousseau's social contract theory, governments were formed by individual men coming together and agreeing each to give up some personal liberty in exchange for certain advantages which society, in the form of government, could offer. Of course no such meeting or contract was ever formally made in organizing a government, but human beings have always acted in the way that such a contract implies.

One of the prominent needs leading to the formation of a government is that for security. Danger may be the result of physical surroundings, but is more often felt because of the actions of individuals within the group or by threatened conflict with the people of another group.

Political economy as a science is not primarily concerned with what governments *should* be, but with a study of what they *are*, what they *do*, and the *results*. In its applied form it is the business of the science to discover what functions governments can and do perform with less waste of human energy than individuals or other types of organizations may accomplish by their independent, competitive, or limited co-operative action. Whatever functions are usually better carried on by governments than by other means are properly assumed by the State. " Better " here means two things : (1) more satisfactions of common desires, and (2) greater efficiency in obtaining the objectives.

Government in the sense here used is distinguished from other forms of control such as imitation, custom, and the work of special organizations, by the fact that it is the strongest and most universal director of *objective behaviour* of the group by more or less forceful means. Religious or other organizations may arouse the emotions and direct the *thoughts* of men, but governments are supreme in controlling *objective* behaviour by organized effort.

The fact that government is in its very nature the dominant power in controlling the behaviour of a group, does not mean that it continually uses force to prevent or change the actions of individuals or organizations. Any government that needs to continue to overcome strong opposition in order to survive is inefficient ; it is either working toward ends not generally desired, or is using unwise means of securing them. A permanently and effectively strong government is one that is in harmony with general desire and with the approved customs of its people. Such a government may temporarily oppose the efforts of certain individuals or classes, to maintain or change old customs ; but unless its policies are of such a nature and executed in such a way as to ultimately give more general satisfaction than had been previously experienced, both common sense and science will condemn it as inefficient.

The subjective satisfactions attained by means of government are to be determined scientifically not so much by direct study of mental states as by objective results, such as reduction of the need for force partly indicated by decrease in crime ; and by positive facts, such as improved economic and health conditions. Efficiency in these respects is measured by comparison with previous conditions in the same country, with conditions in other countries, and with instances where similar functions are being carried on· by private individuals, societies or corporations.

LIMITATIONS OF GOVERNMENT

It is human nature to resent interference with one's acts when they are of little or no significance to other persons. Where acts are clearly of this type it is always a waste of effort for a government to try to compel the individual to change his conduct, even though it is pretty certain that the required behaviour is for his own good. Such laws are usually resisted or evaded and poorly enforced. The results of laws to control the individual in matters of food, clothing, health, recreations, etc., if based on the welfare of the individual whose acts are restricted, are rarely successful. Each individual adult usually assumes with reason that he can look after his own interests better than anyone else can do it for him. A vaccination or other health law, is not justified by advantages to the one vaccinated, but, if justified at all, it is on the ground that the public generally is thus protected against more frequent exposure to infection. Laws regarding pure food and sanitation are justified because under modern conditions an individual has not sufficient knowledge and power to protect himself.

In the last few centuries there has been much more recognition of personal liberty which must not be violated by government control than in former times, but on the other hand conditions have been changing to such an extent, especially in cities, that great numbers of acts formerly of a purely personal nature are now of vital significance to others. We have, therefore, a growing acceptance of the *idea* that governments must not interfere with purely personal affairs, and, on the contrary, changing *conditions* which render formerly personal acts of great significance to others, *e.g.* keeping poultry in a crowded section, driving an auto on the highway, building according to one's own notions, etc.

There are many religious and social beliefs and customs, formerly generally accepted and assumed to be of public concern, which are now regarded as personal affairs. All laws regarding church attendance, Sunday observance, and many sex relations, are now regarded by many as personal matters with which the government should not interfere. It is not difficult to convince most persons that there are advantages to all in the continuance of the family as an institution, which justify some legislation giving it a reasonable chance for survival; yet it is equally evident that this does not necessarily involve the regulation of all sex relations by law. What laws interfering with personal liberty are justified on the ground of protection for others and for the preservation of material and social conditions favourable to satisfactory living by all, can be reliably determined only by scientific investigations of facts and conditions.

Differences of opinion arise not only as to what objectives are of advantage to all, but as to whether these objectives can be more efficiently realized by means of laws enacted and enforced by government, or more effectively brought about by educational effort on the part of the government or of individuals and voluntary organizations. In many instances, such as in the development of recreational facilities, it has worked well to have the facilities and modes of conducting playgrounds provided and tested by voluntary organizations, before asking governments to undertake to provide and supervise such activities.

When material conditions of living are changing rapidly and social customs are also being modified by intercommunication and social contacts, it is inevitable that personal liberties will be too much emphasized in some directions and that, on the other hand, many unwise restrictive laws will be continued or enacted. All the help that scientific research can give is needed in framing laws, and studying how they work under various conditions and policies of enforcement.

In general, government control follows other forms of control, defining approved behaviour more specifically and providing penalties for variations from it, *e.g.* highway regulations for right-hand passing, etc. In the present state of rapid changes, new laws, if not too much opposed to what have been, often help to produce customs and attitudes quite different from those that formerly existed, *e.g.* requirement that no special rates for freight and passenger transportation shall be made to individuals or corporations. Every law should be regarded by the political economist as an experiment, the direct and indirect results of which are to be carefully studied as they appear, and the truth thus learned used in modifying old laws and drafting new ones.

FORMS OF GOVERNMENT

Autocratic government in an industry or in a state may for a while be very efficient and a democratic government quite inefficient. The latter is likely to be true when a democracy is established among a people who by nature, tradition, and training are not prepared for it—as witness the former failure of South American republics having governments similar to our own. A one-man government is not likely to care for the interests of all concerned ; and however able the ruler may be he cannot surpass the sum total of wisdom and ability of all the people. Neither is he likely to continue to improve nor to be followed by a succession of able men working for the good of all. The people he trains to obey will also become less and less fitted to take control. However benevolent and able an autocrat may be, he cannot be of advantage to future generations unless he abates his autocracy sufficiently to give training in government to leaders, and to the people generally.

A democracy, if it is efficient enough to avoid wasteful rebellions, is almost sure to develop better means of adjusting conflicting desires and utilizing and correlating diverse abilities than autocracy. An autocratic government may be much more efficient in an emergency than even the best organized democracy, but if it becomes oppressive there is no way of improving it except by revolution.

The type of national government is not always indicated by the name given to it. The English government is a monarchy but has always been partly democratic, and is now distinctly so. The Magna Charta signed by King John was chiefly an agreement on his part to govern in accordance with former customs, which in principle were rather democratic.

ANARCHISM, SOCIALISM, COMMUNISM

If it should ever be demonstrated that a large group of people without a government would by individual and voluntarily organized non-forceful action so adjust their behaviour as to decrease crimes, increase wealth, health, and means of enjoyment to an extent greater than is usually attained where there is some form of government to direct and compel in accordance with general desire, then there would be scientific justification for doing away with government as is advocated by the philosophical anarchist.

The more enlightened people become and the better the customs they form, the less need is there for control by government ; yet there always have been individuals or classes of people who were not inclined to act as the majority think proper. A few such persons may make it difficult or impossible for others to behave satisfactorily and efficiently without some form of government to compel conformity. It is conceivable that offenders might be induced to conform by example, teaching, and persuasion without the use of force, but it is doubtful whether mankind will ever have sufficient patience to generally adopt such methods and forgo all use of force. The ideal, however, is worth considering and may ultimately approach realization.

Although increased goodwill decreases the need for a government by force, yet in modern society it is not enough that individuals shall mean well. Life is constantly becoming more complex so that it is more and more necessary that persons and organizations shall direct their actions not only with reference to their immediate neighbours, but in such a way that the actions of all other persons and societies in the nation will be facilitated rather than interfered with. Every specialization in occupation and every invention such as the automobile, telephone, or radio is made more useful by regulations as to the ways in which it is to be used. Some centralizing authority is needed to make the regulations, but if no force is used it may be impossible to get the rules into effective operation.

One of the chief reasons for forming and strengthening governments has been the danger to the group from outside enemies. As long as there are wars or fear of wars, governments will continue. If all fear of war were eliminated it is conceivable that a highly civilized group of people with few individuals differing greatly from the mass might prosper without a government using forceful means of control.

The ideals of *socialists* are in some ways the opposite of those of anarchists. Their belief in the need for general co-operation and in the efficiency of governments in securing such co-operation, is so great that they hold that the sphere of government should be extended to many, if not to all forms of group activity. Such control of mails and schools is now generally accepted and in operation, and its extension into economic, recreational, and other fields has been proceeding rather rapidly ; but individual and co-operate control of most activities still continues.

The ultimate test of every increase in government control is the extent to which satisfactions are thus secured more completely and with less waste of wealth and human energies than by non-governmental means. The greatest difficulty in the way of the success of socialistic attempts is in securing the same energy in public service as in private enterprises, and in the proper placing and utilizing of diverse talents. The success of socialistic enterprises, if permanent, must be secured largely by other than forceful means. Hence although socialism and anarchism are in many ways opposed to each other yet the practical success of each depends upon the development of means of control other than those of force. To attain success for anarchistic ideals there must be great improvement in individual ability and character ; while socialistic ideals require improved organization and better managed governments.

Communists emphasize equality of human beings and seek equal and common advantages for all. Some seek to secure this result by force directed toward the strong, and others by the development of attitudes of brotherhood. Small groups of select communists animated by the same ideals have sometimes maintained their existence for decades with economic success, and considerable social satisfactions: *e.g.* the American colony in Jerusalem ; but they are usually disrupted by more individualistic persons joining the organization. Strict communism has never been continued for any length of time on a national scale. Russia's partially forced communism is being modified in order that it may survive.

Much may be learned of political economy by studying experiments in anarchism, communism, and socialism, but nothing permanent is gained for the science by discussing their ideals and theories only. The problem is one of determining the facts as to possible adjustments of human beings to each other and the effectiveness of the various means used. It would be rash to say how far human groups may ultimately adjust ; and the failure of a given type of individuals under certain conditions does not prove that another type of persons, or the same type after several generations of development of social attitudes as a part of the mores of the group, may not succeed. Some phases of the Utopian states that have been created by imagination are already being realized.

ESSENTIALS OF AN EFFICIENT GOVERNMENT

There must be a set of fundamental laws as a basis for the establishment of any kind of government that is to endure after the death of the individuals principally concerned in forming it. These fundamental laws may consist almost wholly of traditionary customs and institutions as is the case in England; or of a definitely formulated and adopted constitution, as in the case of the United States. In the latter instance the written constitution must be in general harmony with the traditions of the people, or it is not likely to work well. The United States Constitution is successful in this country where we have inherited many English customs and attitudes and have almost completely adopted English common law. Constitutions similar to our own have been far less successful among people with a different social inheritance.

In a democratic government there must be (1) machinery by means of which the people may indicate their wishes and effectively direct policies; (2) there must be provisions for administrators or executives to carry out policies; and (3) there must be a judicial system to interpret and apply constitutional and legislative enactments. In America these departments are separate and only one of the functions is usually performed by the same individual or department. This arrangement avoids many dangers, but not infrequently makes rapid, vigorous, unified action impossible.

1. In a democratic government, policies are more or less definitely endorsed by the majority of the people before being put into operation. Prominent men lead in supporting or opposing proposed measures and usually there is a division into two and sometimes more groups or parties that in the main continue to stand for the same policies. In this way government by parties usually develops without special provision for it having been made in the constitution.

After parties have existed for some time, often as much or more interest in the success of one's party develops as in securing the adoption of certain national policies and having them carried out with efficiency. When there are possibilities of obtaining honours or wealth by working for the party rather than for the good of the country as a whole, much corruption and inefficiency results. To some extent this is naturally prevented from going to extremes if the two parties are nearly equal in strength, and each is liable to lose an election through exposures which could be made by the other party.

Constitutional and legal enactments also serve as more or less effective checks to extreme and long-continued party dominance and corruption. In our own country two of the most notable legal enactments to serve as checks were the provision (1) for secret balloting and the correct counting of votes, and (2) the establishment of a civil service system making persons in government service independent of party selection or control.

It is often difficult to arrange for the people to indicate definitely by their votes what policies are desired. Not infrequently a vote is cast for a candidate because he is personally acceptable or stands for policies most approved. Similar difficulties are encountered by a legislator who may believe in one policy, his party endorse another, and the people who elected him ask for still different action.

Laws providing for initiative and referendum are helpful in determining acceptable policies since they allow certain questions to be submitted to direct vote without relation to party or persons upon whom the responsibility of administration may rest. Unfortunately, however, the questions submitted are often not so much what shall be done, as some technical detail of a law to be enacted, the suitability of which can be determined better by experts than by the average citizen.

It is highly desirable for legislative efficiency that governments shall be conducted so as to secure results in accordance with the desires expressed by the people ; but it is just as necessary to employ experts to prescribe the means, as it is to employ doctors, architects, engineers, etc., to show how health may be preserved, satisfactory houses built, safe bridges constructed, etc. From ten to twenty thousand laws are enacted in the United States each year. Many of these are not more intelligently read by the average person than are doctors' prescriptions, or engineers' formulas. Some of these laws are like bread pills in their harmlessness, while others may be as disturbing to the social fabric, as strong drugs are to the body.

Only a few stimulate and direct actions favourable to the carrying on of vigorous, harmonious living together.

This situation is being partly corrected by appointing commissions to investigate conditions and to find the best ways of bringing about improvements. These commissions often call in specialists to advise in the planning of means and the formulating of laws that will be effective in giving what is desired. Aid is also rendered by scientists who investigate the working of laws previously passed.

2. After policies have been decided and given definite form and force by legislation, it is the function of the executive officials to carry them out. This can usually be done most efficiently when the details are not all prescribed, but are left to the judgment of the administrators. The people may be supposed to know in a general way what they want, and legislators, assisted by experts, to know how to formulate a law and provide a suitable means of carrying it out ; while the executive is continually faced with special problems and the need of adapting to many situations that could not be foreseen by either people or legislators. There is, therefore, a growing tendency in this country and England to give each administrator or commissioner the authority not only to decide in individual cases, but to formulate rules for his department which shall have the effect of law in so far as they are not contrary to legislative enactment. This in general promotes efficiency, providing the detailed regulations are not applied to subordinate divisions and administration, or to heads of smaller units of governments such as cities and towns. Departments may become unbearably dominated by bureaucratic conservatism and hampered by red-tape regulations applying to every sort of detail if all rules are made by a central authority leaving minor and local administrators no initiative or discretion, *e.g.* Berthelemy reports that one local official in France had to wait two years to buy a box of pins, the request having passed successively through the hands of twenty-five or thirty officials.

Such centralization of control is much worse in some lines than in others. In the field of education it is especially objectionable, while it is less so in the management of prisons. Parents and other inhabitants of cities and towns are directly concerned in the support and success of schools, and hold the local administrators responsible ; while there is no one directly interested to see that county jails and poorhouses are well managed.   Surveys have shown that the latter institutions are generally wretchedly managed, while in towns and cities with a large amount of local control the public schools are generally superior to those managed and supported chiefly by the state.   In general a central authority has more facilities for gaining and using scientific and expert knowledge of various kinds, but local people know special conditions better, and when directly interested in what is being done, may be expected to look after details of administration better than central officials.

The central authorities may best formulate a few general principles, while local officials are left to apply the general principles to the special situations that arise.   The United States Bureau of Education is a useful organization without power to control education in any state, city, or town.   It performs the functions of carrying on research and distributing information regarding education in all parts of this and other countries.   State educational departments that devote most of their efforts to studying the results of different educational practices in various cities, and little to actually directing education in local communities, are in general the most efficient.

In this, as well as in other fields of control, it is possible to get quicker results by issuing orders and seeing that they are carried out, but continued successful and improved functioning is then wholly dependent upon the ability and effort of the few in the central office.   Also there is little utilization of local abilities and interests, and limited opportunity for comparison of methods used in one locality with those used in others.

3. Judicial specialists are needed chiefly for two reasons. (1) Human interactions furnish so many varieties of conditions and motives, involving near and remote consequences that

it is found absolutely impossible for general laws as to what may or may not be done, to be so formulated that they can easily be applied to all cases that arise. (2) Persons concerned in disputes are not generally in an emotional condition favourable to accepting the application of any law which is unfavourable to their interests or to that of their friends.

Hence, judges are needed to supplement their own knowledge and wisdom in applying the law to a particular case, by principles of common law and by the decisions of other judges in similar cases. They are not necessarily keen observers of facts or good judges of the character of the individuals brought before them. A jury of plain unspecialized persons is often utilized for the performance of this function in which every one who has had much experience in dealing with other human beings is something of an expert.

A judge learned in the law and a jury alive to the human interests involved, neither of them personally interested in the results or prejudiced against any of the parties concerned in the dispute, is supposed to be the best combination for giving just decisions. In order that the law precedents and all the facts pertaining to the case shall be brought to the attention of judge and jury, lawyers are usually employed by each contestant.

There is, however, much complaint against the workings of courts. On the one hand judges are charged with being prejudiced, and, on the other, with violating common sense by too close observance of technicalities and precedents. By training, judges are governed more by the past in making decisions than by consideration of the present and future conditions and changes, which may make old principles no longer applicable, e.g. Legislation limiting working hours and conditions called for by modern conditions were long hampered by court decisions based on old principles of assumed freedom of contract.

Juries have also been subjected to a variety of criticisms on many grounds, but the tradition is strong that a man may be surer of justice from a group of his peers than from a specialist in legal procedure, and so the right of trial by jury

L

is likely to be continued, although judges are often better fitted to decide many types of cases.

The belief that courts are not generally efficient in doing their work has been growing, and investigations made by experts confirm this belief. The establishment of the juvenile court and more use of its procedure, which is largely freed from technicalities, is an advance. The most important needs are to secure more prompt and consistent judicial action, less controlled by technical procedure, and more responsiveness to social changes without sacrifice of old and valuable principles of common law.

GOVERNMENT AND FORCEFUL CONTROL

A government develops and becomes strong in proportion as it successfully settles disputes and enforces accepted modes of behaviour. The stronger a government becomes the more force it may use in compelling action in conformity with laws. The more efficient the government, the less is it necessary to actually employ more than a small fraction of its potential power. It acquires prestige so that resistance by individuals is rarely made. Thousands may be directed and controlled by a few individuals who represent the overwhelming power of the government. Lynchings and other non-legal means of using force indicate either that the potential power of the government is not great, or that it is inefficient in its use of the power it has. The city or nation that preserves the peace with fewest police and least actual exercise of force, is, other conditions being equal, the one where the government has gained prestige because of its demonstrated efficiency. A government is a failure in the use of force unless it either employs so much force that nothing more than momentary resistance is possible, or has acquired such prestige that all offenders yield without resistance to its representatives.

Governments are not necessarily efficient merely because little or no open resistance is offered to its representatives. It is a general principle that weak individuals, animal and human, when confronted with strong ones, resort to deception and stealthy means of securing their ends. Thieves and other non-conformers work in secret, using all kinds of devious methods of getting what they want without suffering penalties. Wealthy men and corporations also utilize all sorts of technicalities to avoid punishment without offering actual resistance to the government. An efficient government needs, therefore, to be wise as well as powerful.

To severely punish a few of many criminals is shown by psychological studies of both men and animals, to be a very inefficient means of controlling behaviour. Certain and quick punishment of slight intensity for undesired acts, and rewards for approved ones are scientifically proved to be much more effective. Intelligent governments, therefore, are now seeking to increase the promptness and certainty of punishment, and to provide positive advantages for conformity instead of adding to severity of penalties, as was formerly done. There are growing doubts as to the wisdom of punishing criminals any more than is incidental to their being prevented from injuring others. There is so much waste of human energy and human sympathy, and so little gain from pain and the fear of pain, that it is a question not yet settled by scientific investigation whether punishment as such has much, if any, value in decreasing crime. When theft was punished by death and the people gathered to see a thief hanged, pocketbooks were never safe.

The idea of government chiefly as a substitute inflictor of vengeance is waning, and the more scientifically based idea that it should get results in the way of diminishing criminality by the best means offered by common sense and science, is gaining. As in medicine, more effort is now being devoted to the prevention of undesirable conditions than to their cure. The promotion of economic welfare and the offering of educational and recreational facilities have been shown to be effective in reducing crime.

In summary, then, governments are more efficient than individuals or societies in the use of force because they potentially possess the greatest power, and may acquire the prestige which renders little force necessary. To use this force in controlling the conduct of individuals demands acuteness in discovering changing behaviour. Since the use of force is always wasteful of human energy, governments will become more efficient in preventing and correcting unapproved behaviour in proportion as they use non-forceful means.

GOVERNMENT BY DIRECTION AND ENLIGHTENMENT

One of the necessary functions of government is to prevent unfair practices by individuals and corporations. This is analogous to the function of an umpire of a game. Every game is played in accordance with rules which are revised as the occasion requires. Umpires see that players observe these rules, inflicting appropriate penalties when necessary. The more perfectly developed the game as to rules and standardized equipment, the less necessary is it for the umpire to interfere with the personal movements of the players or to make difficult decisions. The equipment used in playing baseball, for example, is such that it is not necessary for the umpire to prevent the batter from striking as hard as he wishes or running as fast as he can. His difficulties are in deciding facts as to arrival of ball and players at bases. In basketball and football there are rules about personal contacts which are difficult of control by players, and of decision by the umpire ; and the difference between an act bringing a penalty and one leading to a victory is often slight and not easily distinguished. The more a game admits of fouls difficult to avoid and judge, the less perfect is it as a game. In a perfect game, players are not continually under the direction of a coach or trying to deceive the umpire, but while observing the well-known rules of the game are using all their skill and initiative in trying to surpass their opponents. A government, in exercising its great function of making and administering laws so as to secure fair competition among individuals and institutions, is efficient in proportion as it avoids unnecessary interference with personal and corporation liberties, and needs to make few difficult and doubtful decisions as to what are fouls in the business world. As a rule for the game of business, the Sherman Anti-Trust Law is not wholly satisfactory.

The building of roads, and regulations regarding their use have generally been better done by governments than by individuals. With the development of railways, telegraph and telephone lines, power companies, etc., it has been found that government regulation is necessary if they are to function economically and for the general good. The same is true of banks, insurance companies, and many other corporations affecting many people. All are now regulated and supervised to a greater or less extent by state or national governments. Not all such control has been wisely exercised, but it has been demonstrated that governments are better suited to do some of this work than are single individuals or corporations. Further researches are needed to show just what functions may better be performed by the government, and what left to individuals and corporations who compete or co-operate for special advantages.

The government may do two things: first, make and enforce needed regulations that cannot be made effective in any other way ; and second, preserve fair competition while conserving the interests of the general public. The most important success of governments up to the present time is in controlling the issue of money and the regulation and supervision of banks and insurance companies.

Modern governments have undertaken to conduct scientific researches upon the most effective means of doing all sorts of things, and giving individuals, corporations, and industries the results of the investigations. This has been especially well done in the Department of Agriculture, and the Bureau of Standards, of our own country. At present both national and state governments are carrying on investigations not only in sciences related directly to industries and to welfare— e.g. weather—but also in pure science. In addition, commissions are frequently appointed to investigate special problems such as those of the coal industry, the valuation of railways, means of caring for deaf persons, etc. Such investigations, more or less scientific, give knowledge of great value not only to individuals and industries, but to the government in carrying on its own functions, and as a help to the smaller units of government. The chances of wise legislation and efficient management are thus increased by the aid of experts in various fields. Not only legislators and administrators, but judges also, are beginning to avail themselves of such aids by calling in experts to testify or to report on researches. A very promising development of governmental research is now being made in the interest of more efficient departmental organization and the selection of employees for various departments by the civil service experts.

Government officials may often profitably spend their time in educating the people regarding what is best to do, instead of using force to compel necessary action. Education may take longer, but the results once gained will be more lasting, and more effectively carried out. In emergencies, however, autocratic control may be the only way of preventing disaster.

Education, especially of all children, as a preventive of poverty, disease, and crime, is more economical than to deal with these conditions after they occur. It is an important problem of government to decide on the means to be used. Parents, school officials, churches, and other organizations, are working for the same ends and are often in a better situation to do many of the things necessary than are government officials. It is probably best for the state to compel schooling for all, and to prescribe in a general way the education needed by all citizens, leaving details to school officials and administrators. Negative prescriptions as to what shall not be taught are of doubtful wisdom.

In the matter of adult education it should be recognized that in a democracy it is necessary that the majority shall rule if the government is to continue, and it is equally necessary that the minority shall have freedom of speech and press in their attempts to secure a majority in favour of their interests and beliefs. Not only should the majority not use force in suppressing such means of adult education, but it is a question how far they may wisely go in promoting, at government expense, propaganda in favour of government policies or even in emphasizing the assumed superiority of one's country over all others in the attempt to give patriotic education. In publicly supported universities whose students are mentally adults, it would seem wise to give them ample opportunity to hear both sides of every disputed question as a necessary training in helping to decide public policies.

In secondary and elementary schools it would also seem to be in the interest of efficient government by the people for training to be given in getting facts and weighing evidence on all sorts of questions. The whole trend of democracy and of scientific method calls for this rather than for the acceptance of whatever is presented by authority. Neither teachers nor representatives of the government may, in a democracy say, " Believe this because I say so ".

FREEDOM OF SPEECH AND PRESS

Language is an invention which greatly facilitates the mental picturing of objects and events. Discussions are a form of competitive struggle, but the possible happenings occur only in the minds of the individuals and in their language expressions. By means of words, a vivid picture of the results of a proposed policy may be produced, then displaced by pictures of opposite results. By talking and reading, the nature and probable results of any policy may be carefully examined during a period of months or years, before being accepted and put into execution. If freedom in language expression is restricted, no such preliminary study can be made, and the consequence will be that the policies selected and acted upon will often be found to have unanticipated results, some of which may be serious and irremediable. Men are much more likely to judge wisely after full discussion, than when they act quickly, or after hearing only one side of a question.

It is true that words are a preliminary to acts, and when addressed to an already excited group of people may be like a match to powder. When words are likely to have such an effect before there will be time for opposing words to be uttered, it may be in the interest of free speech to prevent the first utterances. In a London park where curious crowds gather to listen to the soap-box orators on all sorts of questions, it is found to be quite safe to permit an anarchist to demand that the king be killed and the government be destroyed. The act cannot be performed at once, and there is abundant chance to hear other demands. If rival orators in the park abandon words and resort to blows or a crowd attacks the speaker, then the police may properly suppress the disorder, and speech may be resumed later. On the other hand, if an excited crowd gather around a child killed by an automobile and someone begins advocating the lynching of the driver, it is in the interest of fair discussion as to what shall be done to him that such talk shall be stopped at once. In the absence of both the driver and the excited crowd, however, any sort of a policy may be advocated without danger.

Sometimes when a hostile crowd gathers to attack a speaker advocating an unpopular cause, he is not allowed to talk. This is not in the interest of freedom of speech. This would demand that the crowd be required either to go away or to remain quiet while the speaker is allowed to continue. On the other hand, if there is a crowd gathered for a legitimate understood purpose and some one interrupts with something irrelevant or objectionable to which no one wishes to listen, the intruder should be silenced and the audience protected in listening to such discussions as it desires. It should never be regarded as disturbance of the peace to speak to citizens who are willing to listen, and who are not likely to act without time for consideration. Under such circumstances society is not in danger, no matter what ideas may be set forth. The above statements must, of course, be understood as referring to instances where the persons concerned are supposed to be capable of exercising the functions of citizenship. Some limitations of freedom may be necessary when the audience is composed of defectives or of immature children, although the latter should have some experience in choosing between opposing policies.

What has been said of speech applies even more to the

Press, because rarely can printed words excite to immediate action without the chance of considering results and alternatives. To prevent freedom of speaking and publishing usually results in secret propaganda by means of which individuals are often induced to act in ways that would not have seemed justifiable to themselves if the same words were freely circulated and there were opportunities to see how they were received and replied to by others. Secret propaganda is thus more likely to produce unwise action than any possible free publications can. With freedom of oral and printed discussion the best ideas thrive in the free air of public decision, while those of little universal appeal grow like disease germs in the comparative darkness of censorship.

SELECTED RESEARCHES

"SHOULD THE TAX LAWS BE ENFORCED AND EN-
FORCEABLE?" By Professor FRED R. FAIRCHILD, Yale
University. From *Scientific Monthly*, February 1927. *Quoted
by Permission.*

. . . Today a law which does not have the approval and
support of the great majority of people is difficult or impossible
of enforcement, simply because the old idea of enforcement by
main strength against a hostile people has been abandoned and
the government has come to rely upon the goodwill and co-
operation of those to whom the law applies.

. . . To a very considerable extent the taxpayer is asked to
assess the tax against himself. . . . He is willing to pay his
share and even ready to aid the assessor in determining exactly
what is his share under the law. All this, however, on the
assumption that the taxing authorities are playing fair with
him, and that what they ask of him they also ask—and require—
of others; in short that the tax law is enforced.

. . . And just as soon as failure is generally known comes the
end of the assumption upon which the taxpayer co-operates in
enforcing the law against himself. . . .

. . . Assessors are provided by law, charged with the duty
of preparing these tax lists. The category of taxable property
includes in most states, not only real estate, but such forms of
tangible personal property as household furniture, books and
libraries, musical instruments, jewellery, and intangible property
such as notes, bonds, credits and book accounts, money on
hand, deposits in banks and sometimes shares of corporation
stock. To aid the assessor in the obviously difficult task of
discovering and valuing all these classes of property in the
possession of each owner, the law calls upon the taxpayer for
co-operation, to the extent generally of rendering at least a list
and description of all his taxable property. . . .

. . . In general the assessor accepts the taxpayer's statement
with little or no question, scrutiny or check. . . .

Not so long ago I had occasion to test the assessment of
jewellery and watches in the city of New Haven by an inspection
of the records of the probate court. In the inventories of seventy-
one estates examined the total value of jewellery and watches
was $123,042. The late owners of this property in their last
tax lists had reported as the value of this property (in excess of
the legal exemption of $25) just $3,900. Of the seventy-one

owners, thirty-two had filed no tax list whatever ; of the rest, twenty-eight had listed nothing under this head ; eleven had listed something less than the true value ; while three had made a correct return. Of these three paragons of civic virtue, two were women and one was an insane man. . . .

. . . Yet few taxpayers having incomes even moderately complex are able to make out their own returns without the aid of lawyers, tax experts and accountants. Students of the problem are becoming increasingly alarmed at the situation which has been created by the almost unbelievable complexities of the income tax law. . . .

Thus I arrive at the answers to the questions which stand as the head of my essay. The tax laws should be enforced. Any other situation is intolerable. But the reason the tax laws are not enforced is that they are not enforceable. Let no one think that enforcement is to be obtained by giving greater powers or higher pay to the taxing officers, or by increasing the severity of the penalties for tax evasion or by starting a popular hue and cry against " dishonest taxpayers." In only one direction is the remedy to be sought. The tax laws must be made enforceable. How this is to be accomplished is another question, one which may well enlist the utmost skill of the tax students and experts and the patient constructive thought of the taxpaying public. . . .

"OUTDOOR RECREATION LEGISLATION AND ITS EFFECTIVENESS." By ANDREW G. TRUXAL, Ph.D., Columbia University. 1929. *Quoted by Permission.*

. . . The study here undertaken divides itself sharply into two parts. The first part constitutes a summary of the American legislation of the past twelve years (1915–1927) making provision for public outdoor recreation. . . .

The second half of this study is in the nature of a scientific exploration. Much has been written but little has been done to discover whether or not the provision of recreational facilities is worth the effort, in terms of the general welfare. A small segment of one problem was chosen for analysis. The question raised was whether or not the occurrence of recreation areas is associated with the incidence of juvenile delinquency. The field of investigation was Manhattan Island. The territory was divided into a number of play districts, in each of which the amount of play space in use in 1920 was related to the number of arrests for delinquency in the same year. A mathematical statement of the amount of this association for the island as a whole was arrived at, and further evidence was gathered concerning certain environmental factors which are supposed to contribute to child delinquency : racial composition of the population, child density per acre and police regulation. The material collected on these latter factors served to check up the conclusions reached by the former comparisons, which revealed a certain amount of association between the presence of supervised play areas and the absence of juvenile delinquency.

. . . Minnesota had a law passed in 1885 and applicable to St. Paul, requiring that real-estate men making a plat of twenty acres or more had to set aside one-twentieth of it for a public park. The experience of the city under this law was that real estate operators " having more than twenty acres to plat made two plats or three if necessary and filed them at different periods in order to get away from the park dedication clause." The law, having become of no effect, was repealed. With regard to subsequent legislation, Mr. Herrold continues :

Our platting laws adopted in 1887 are rather crude and meagre, but we have been able to do a great many things by persuasion, and since the adoption of our zoning ordinance we can, of course, refuse any plat where the lots do not give the area required under the zoning ordinance for the various zones. . . .

Paragraph 33 of the law reads :

Before the approval by the planning board of a plat showing a new street or highway, such plat shall also in proper cases show a park or parks suitably located for playground or other recreational purposes. . . . ; and that the parks shall be of reasonable size for neighbourhood playgrounds or other recreational uses. In making such determination regarding streets, highways and parks, the planning board shall take into consideration the prospective character of the development, whether dense residence, business or industrial. . . .

What some of the realtors are doing voluntarily to meet this problem will be apparent from a few selected illustrations. . . .

. . . in Greensboro, North Carolina, there is an average of 14·6 per cent set aside for this purpose ; the Bayonne Housing Corporation of Bayonne, New Jersey, has devoted 22·4 per cent to the public for playground purposes ; of the Red Acres Subdivision in Memphis, Tennessee, 44·5 per cent is reserved for recreation and other public uses. . . .

SUGGESTED READINGS

Political Science, like economics, has been based chiefly on observation and theory, but recently scientific methods have been used more in the study of governmental functioning. General works are :

BEARD, C. A., and BEARD, WILLIAM, *American Leviathan : the Republic in the Machine Age*, 1930.
CLARK, JOHN M., *Social Control of Business*, 1929.
DUNNING, W. A., *A History of Political Theories*, 1924.
FOLLETT, M. P., *The New State : Group Organization and the Solution of Popular Government*, 1918.
HOCKING, WM. E., *Man and the State*, 1926.
KALLEN, HORACE, ed. *Freedom in the Modern World*, 1928.
KELSO, ROBERT T., *The Science of Public Welfare*, 1928.
KENT, F. R., *Great Game of Politics*, 1930.
LUMLEY, F. E., *Means of Social Control*, 1925.
PITKIN, WALTER, *The Idea of Social Justice*.
SEYMOUR, CHARLES, *The Story of the Development of Elections*, 1930.

The nature and development of law are presented in the following :

ALLEN, CARLETON K., *Law in the Making*, 1927.
LOWIE, ROBERT, *The Origins of the State*, 1927.
POUND, ROSCOE, *The Spirit of the Common Law*, 1921.
WIGMORE, JOHN H., *A Panorama of the World's Legal Systems*, 3 vols., illus., 1928.

The possibilities of non-violent means of control are shown by C. M. CASE, " Non-Violent Coercion : a Study of Methods of Social Pressure," 1923.

Significant factual studies of governmental institutions and laws illustrating the use of scientific methods follow :

Administration.

BRECKENRIDGE, SOPHONISBA, *Public Welfare Administration in the United States. Selected Documents*, 1927.
GLEUCK, SHELDON, and GLEUCK, ELEANOR T., " Predictability in the Administration of Criminal Justice. Mental Hygiene," Oct. 1929, reprinted from *Yale Law Review*, Jan. 1929.
PATTERSON, ERNEST M., " Federal *versus* State Jurisdiction in American Life ", *Annals of American Academy of Political and Social Science*, Jan. 1927.

SMITH, D. K., *United States Civil Service Commission ; its History, Activities and Organization*, 1928.

TELFORD, F., "Report of the Director of the Bureau of Public Personnel Administration for the Fiscal Year Ending June 30, 1929," *Public Personnel Studies*, 1929.

WHITE, L. D., *Public Administration*, 1926.

WILLOUGHBY, WM. F., *National Budget System (Institute for Governmental Research)*, 1927.

Cities.

GARFIELD, JAMES O., "Laboratory Work in Municipal Citizenship," *National and Municipal Review*, Oct. 1928.

GRIFFITH, ERNEST S., *The Modern Development of City Government in the United Kingdom and in the United States*, 2 vols., 1927.

WALLACE, SCHUYLER C., *State Administrative Supervision over Cities in the United States*, 1928.

WOODRUFF, CLINTON R., "The City Manager Plan," *American Journal of Sociology*, Jan. 1928.

Courts.

Cleveland Foundation Survey of Criminal Justice, Cleveland, 1921.

POUND, ROSCOE, "Causes of Popular Dissatisfaction with the Administration of Justice," *Report of American Bar Association*, vol. 29, page 395.

POUND, ROSCOE, "Reform in the Administration of Justice," *Annals of American Academy*, vol. 52, No. 141, Mar. 1914.

Public Ownership.

CRECRAFT, EARL W., *Government and Business : A Study in the Economic Aspects of Government and Public Aspects of Business*, 1928.

PECK, H. W., "An Inductive Study of Publicly Owned and Operated, Versus Privately Owned and Regulated Electric Utilities," *American Economic Review Supplement*, March 1929.

STATTEN, F. A., "Fort Atkinson, Wisconsin : a Case Study of Public Ownership," *Journal of Land and Public Utility Economics*, June 1929.

Public Opinion.

CAMERON, MERTON K., "Experience of Oregon with Popular Election and Recall of Public Service Commissioners," *Journal of Land and Public Utility Economics*, June 1929.

HAYES, E. C., "Formation of Public Opinion and Popular Government," *Journal of Applied Sociology*, Sept.-Oct. 1925.

RICE, STUART A., "Differential Changes of Political Preference Under Campaign Stimulation," *Journal of Abnormal and Social Psychology*, page 297, 1926.

RICE, STUART A., *Quantitative Methods in Politics*, 1928.

Success of Laws.

CLAPP, MARY A., and STRONG, MABEL A., *The School and the Working Child*, Massachusetts Labour Committee, 1928.

FIELDMAN, H., *Prohibition : its Industrial and Economic Aspects*, 1927.

GOSNEY, E. S., and POPENOE, PAUL, *Sterilization for Human Betterment*, 1929.

HALL, FRED S., *Medical Certification for Marriage ; an Account of the Administration of the Wisconsin Law as it Relates to Venereal Disease*, Russell Sage Foundation, 1925.

HERVEY, JOHN J., " The Anti-Trust Laws of The United States," *Annals of the American Academy of Political and Social Sciences*, Jan. 1930.

KIRKPATRICK, CLIFFORD, " Capital Punishment," Committee on Philanthropic Labour, Yearly Meeting of Friends, Philadelphia, 1925.

CHAPTER VIII

HOW MAN BEHAVES, OR GENERAL PSYCHOLOGY

WHAT IS PSYCHOLOGY ?

PSYCHOLOGY is a body of knowledge concerned with the ways of acting common to most of the human species. The bodily anatomy and physiology by which life is carried on is the starting-point of psychological study. Psychology is, however, chiefly concerned with the kinds of acts performed in response to environing stimuli. The processes within the body are primarily dealt with by physiology.

The above describes the field of objective psychology now becoming prominent as scientific methods are used in studying mental states. Human beings, however, do not act merely in response to environing stimuli, but are conscious of the objective acts and of how they feel before, after or during the performance of many of them. This consciousness is most prominent in voluntary acts in which there is usually anticipation of what is to happen, and comparison with what does happen. For example, one anticipates dusting the books on a shelf, and after it is done is conscious of realization, but he is not necessarily conscious of each motion made in the process. The conscious or subjective phase of human behaviour (that phase of which only the performer knows) may be quite prominent when some acts are performed and be almost or entirely absent during others. There are undoubtedly these two phases or sides of the acts of human beings—the objective, which others as well as the performer may observe, and the conscious or subjective, which only the performer may perceive.

In watching the acts of other persons, although it is impossible for us to know except by inference what the facts of the *conscious* experiences of the performers are, one naturally thinks of them as existing, and being much like what he himself would experience if he were performing the acts. Rarely do we observe others in a purely objective way, but our usual attitude is to question " What is he trying to do ? " Then " Why does he do it ? ", and only later do we observe closely the exact objective motions made, and decide whether they are suitably adapted to the end to be gained. It is easier to understand and react to people by thinking of the subjective phases of their acts than to confine attention wholly or even chiefly to its objective details. If a person suddenly moves toward us, the important thing to know is his purpose—to assault or to greet us, and the idea of purpose prepares us better for an appropriate response, than if we noted objective movements only. It is not strange, therefore, that the early psychologists studied the conscious side of behaviour chiefly and gave to the continued complex of conscious or mental facts the name of mind, and then defined psychology as the science concerned with the study of the mind or of conscious states and their relations to each other.

The more experiments were used and exact measurements made in studying animals, children and men, the more evident it became that reliable and exact facts could be much more surely obtained by studying the objective phases of behaviour than by trying to find out what the subjective facts were. The result is that now psychology is being more frequently defined as the science of human behaviour. As such it can become an exact science in many particulars. A science of conscious states can never become so exact, yet by common-sense experience and by studying conscious states under carefully determined objective conditions, a considerable body of knowledge that is understandable and of a fair degree of reliability, has been accumulated. In this chapter truths from one or the other sides will be given according as one or the other is more understandable and verifiable.

M

The parts of the body most directly concerned in behaviour acts are muscles and nerves, although all the internal organs have some influence upon the vigour with which these mechanisms function.

The muscle fibres are like rubber bands that may expand or contract.   Many small bands or fibres are arranged in groups called muscles, and frequently muscles are arranged in pairs so that one contracts and produces motion in one direction while the other relaxes.   The process is reversed when the opposite motion is made.   In sleep most of the muscles are relaxed, but when awake nearly all of them are slightly contracted, thus keeping the parts of the body steady in whatever position it may be.   The sensations of these muscular tensions probably serve as a constant background of consciousness, but the chief function of muscles is to move the various parts of the body.

The nerves have for their function the receiving and carrying of messages from the outer world and from all parts of the body to a centre, and from that centre to various muscles and glands.   Each nerve consists of a bundle of fibres.   The motor nerve fibres end in a little pad or coil in a muscle fibre, while sensory nerve fibres, after branching, sometimes end free, but more often in some specialized type of end-organ. These specialized endings probably render the nerve more sensitive to certain kinds of stimuli such as heat, pain or light.

Nerve ends are so close together in the skin that in many parts a needle cannot be inserted without touching one or more of them.   Those most sensitive to contact are near the surface, and those for pain deeper, while there are still others for heat and cold.

There are in the mouth, besides the same kind of nerve endings found in the outside skin, others especially sensitive to taste stimuli, and in the nose, endings sensitive to smell. At the back part of the eye in the retinal layer are nerve endings especially sensitive to light, and in the basilar membrane of the ear those sensitive to sound vibrations.   In the stomach and other internal organs are endings similar to those of the skin.

In the case of the eye and the ear, we have very complex organs by the action of which the effects of light and sound are greatly increased. If one of these is defective or injured without affecting the nerve endings in the retina or in the basilar membrane, mechanical correctives or substitutes may be used to help these senses. The normal eye and ear may also have their range greatly increased by mechanisms that focus or intensify the stimuli. If, however, the nerve endings themselves are destroyed they cannot be repaired and no mechanical device will restore sight or hearing. The other senses have no such specialized organs for adding to the effects of stimulus to end organs, and cannot readily be helped by mechanical means.

Every nerve fibre leads to, and is really a part of, a nerve cell, hence every sensory nerve ending and every muscle fibre is connected each with a special cell body. This cell body in turn is connected by fibres or by minute projections with other cell bodies. A group of cell bodies is called a ganglion. The brain and spinal cord are composed of many ganglia, all connected with each other.

In the outer surface or cortex of the brain are many cell bodies that are not connected directly with either muscles or sensory nerve ends, but are probably connected indirectly with every portion of the body, and are themselves the means of making such connections. When an object, e.g. a dog, is seen, then heard, cells in the back part of the brain are made active by the impulses coming over fibres connecting with the retina, while brain cells in the temporal region are made active by impulses brought from the ear by auditory nerve fibres. Nerve centres lying between the visual and auditory centres are also made active and some of them may send impulses along motor fibres to muscles, causing them to move. Others register the effects of the excitement and when the same object is seen again, may pass on the impulse and excite motor cell bodies and also the cell bodies in the temporal region, making them all act as they did when they were

directly stimulated by impulses from the auditory centres, so
that the sight of a dog causes one to image the sound of barking
and perhaps imitate it. Thus the brain has special parts for
doing special things, so that whether we see red, feel pain, or
hear note middle C, depends upon the special cells that are
connected with the nerve endings in the eye, the finger, and
the ear. If the connections could be changed we might hear
with the finger and see with the ear.

If there is loss of sensation or motion in any part of the
body and the sense end organs (or receptors) and the muscles
(or effectors) and the nerve fibres (or conductors) are in good
working condition, the trouble can usually be located in the
spinal cord, in the inside of the brain, or in its cortex. The
brain, however, is supplied with duplicate parts in its two
halves and often nearly the same act may be performed by
apparatus in the spinal cord and within the brain. The
cortex has so many connections with the upper and lower
centres that considerable portions of the brain may be wholly
destroyed and after a little time it may work nearly as well
as ever. Some experimenters on animals and on human
brains have been led to say that each part has its special
function to perform, while others have been sure that the
brain functions as a whole. The brain is composed of about
eight billion cells and is probably a million times more complex
than any machine ever constructed by man, hence it is not
strange that complete knowledge of just how it works is
lacking. We really know more of the subjective states
associated with brain functioning than of the physical processes
involved.

Muscles, nerve fibres and cell bodies are excited by electricity,
by touch or pressure, by heat and cold and by acid, and
some by other stimuli, the mouth and nose by chemical stimuli
of many kinds, the eye by rays of light from objects, and the
ear by vibrations of air or other medium. The results of
stimulating by any of these means is shown objectively by
contraction of muscles, and subjectively by sensations. These
sense stimuli are means of knowing and reacting to the world
in which we live. The nerve endings within the organs of

the body are means of knowing the condition of our bodily mechanism as regards health, hunger, etc. The nervous system unifies all the sensory and motor activities involved in reacting to the surrounding world, and in satisfying needs.

Some disorders of vital physiological organs, such as the lungs and heart, have little effect upon the working of the muscles and nerves which are chiefly involved in behaviour, except to limit somewhat the vigour of muscular activity. The stomach, intestines and liver, and several ductless glands such as the thyroid, that affect the quality of blood going to muscles and nerve centres, have, however, important influences upon emotional attitudes and the degree and kind of behaviour activities. What is known as temperament and disposition is believed to depend more upon peculiarities of glandular action than upon special differences in nervous and muscular structure. The effects of excessive glandular secretions upon mental states is sometimes as great as the influence of drugs, which, as is well known, may, like ether, depress nervous activity or, like strychnine, excite it. On the other hand, changes in nerve excitation may greatly influence the action of heart, lungs and all the vital organs, as in fear or anger, when, as Cannon has shown, breathing and heart-beat are quickened, and digestive processes stopped, and the composition of the blood modified.

Although some serious physiological diseases do not greatly hamper the action of the neuro-muscular system, and may even stimulate mental action, yet in general well-balanced functioning of the whole body is favourable to normal behaviour. The muscles are especially affected by changes in physiological condition, and the brain cells in a less degree.

Some of the phenomena of great significance to psychologists as well as physiologists are those resulting from long-repeated activity of any kind, known as fatigue. This is indicated by decreased vigour, accuracy, and regularity of performance. The whole neuro-muscular system appears to be subject to fatigue, although the parts in which it can be clearly demonstrated are the nerve endings and the muscles. It is possible to fatigue these in seconds or minutes ; while hours of work do not seem to decrease the efficiency of nerve fibres in carrying impulses, and the evidence that cell bodies become fatigued is not decisive.

Intense activity of one part if continued results in activity of associated parts. If one taps with the forefinger rapidly for two or three minutes, the muscles of the jaw and other portions of the body are brought into action by the effort to continue tapping. If the hand is allowed to come up from the table the muscles of the wrist or forearm will execute the tapping, thus allowing those of the finger to recover. This is the reason the same action may sometimes be performed for a long time without fatigue, since the same muscles are not continuously active. On the other hand, when the eye and other muscles are used continuously the effects extend to other parts of the body, sometimes to the point of producing a nervous breakdown.

The intervals between contraction of muscles have much to do with the onset of fatigue. If the pauses are long enough, there will be no fatigue, but if the stimuli to contract are given so rapidly that there is no chance for the muscles to relax in an appreciable degree, fatigue comes on quickly, as one will find by trying to hold the arm extended at exactly the same height. The passenger in a taxi worried lest he be late, who keeps his muscles tense, may be more fatigued than one who walks to the station with confident alternating movements of the legs.

In general, efficiency of body and mind is favoured by the complete relaxation of all the muscles during a period of sleep each day. This period is helpful not only because of relaxation, but because of changes which take place in the way of removing waste materials from the blood, and of carrying to the various tissues materials which during sleep are built into the structures that have been exercised. Activities of all sorts are most efficient when the reserve energy stored up in muscular tissue is kept at a high level by sufficiently long periods of rest and sleep.

In practising to acquire skill it is economical to have periods short enough so that the parts most concerned are only slightly fatigued, with intervals for recovery between. One or sometimes more such periods a day give the best results in the early stage of learning anything. The periods must be short if the same parts are used all the time, and if the one practising is young or new at the task; but may be longer if the activity is complex, the person mature, or already used to that sort of work or play.

Each end organ and nerve cell and muscle has a certain amount of inertia that may be overcome by a stimulus of a certain measured degree, and one that will just overcome this inertia is known as the minimum for light, heat, etc. Several stimuli, however, of a less intensity, if applied successively at proper intervals, will cause subjective sensations or objective muscular contraction—a phenomena known as summation.

A stimulus that is too strong paralyses, *e.g.* a blinding light, deafening sound, a hard blow. A moderate stimulus is one in between the minimum and maximum, at the degree that gives the most muscular contraction and relaxation, or most clear sensation. Time as well as degree is of importance since a weak stimulus continued for a tenth of a second may produce as much effect as a stronger one for a hundredth of a second. In experimental work, when performed with great accuracy, not only the strength of a stimulus is measured, but also its duration and the time elapsing between it and others, since the effects of a stimulus are modified by other stimuli. For example, the knee jerk may be increased or decreased by stimulating some other part of the body at appropriate intervals, before the tap on the knee.

EFFECTS OF STRENGTH OF STIMULI ON BEHAVIOUR

The comparative intensity and time relations of stimuli are very important factors, not only as regards vigour of action, but also as to what is done in a given situation, *e.g.* an object which is both bitter and sweet may be swallowed or ejected according to which of the two stimuli is perceived first or most intensely. The comparative strength of initial stimuli is especially important in determining behaviour. The comparative brightness of a snake's head and of a strawberry, may fatefully decide one's action as toward or away from the reptile. A loud voice may repel a child attracted by a smiling face. A slight difference of emphasis in the words directed toward a companion may determine whether the response will be friendly or hostile.

This influence of more or less intense stimuli on behaviour and consciousness is correlated with passive or involuntary attention. The following laws have been established by experiment. If objects are alike in every respect except size, the larger one is likely to get the attention first. If they are alike in size and in all other ways except brightness, the brightest one will be seen first. If they are all alike except in colour tone, red or orange is likely to be seen first of all the colours. In general, the strongest of the various stimuli being given any sense organ gets the attention, as advertisers now know well.

Since strength is relative, any feature of a page may be made an effective stimulus to attention by leaving a blank space around it, nearly as well as by making it large or bright. Because attention is limited to one or a few related features, the maker of a poster who tries to have *all* objects give a strong stimulus fails because each is likely to conflict with and decrease the effects of the others.

A changing stimulus is more effective than a constant one of equal intensity and, within limits, the attention is the more surely attracted the more rapid the change. The gradual coming of daylight attracts little notice, while the sudden blazing of a match startles. If the water is heated slowly enough a frog may be boiled without causing him to move.

The influences of intensity are not limited to present action, but have far-reaching effects upon future behaviour. The stimulus that produces movement toward or away from a new object will have thereafter power to produce the same reaction to similar objects, unless a stimulus to an opposite movement of considerable intensity quickly follows. What gets our favourable attention once, continues to get such attention if there are no unfavourable results. After much experience of the same thing in the same surroundings, the attention to it may not be conscious, but it is still effective, because we miss it if it is absent or replaced by another. A new stimulus is, however, subjectively stronger by its contrast with the usual. The most effective poster or other complex stimulus to attention in any form, is one that presents an old stimulus often attended to with satisfaction in a new setting. On the other hand, if the old has often been disagreeable in itself or in its accompaniments, we are likely to turn away from what otherwise seems attractive. The announcement of the name of the author of a poem may determine how the poem is received. Our likes and dislikes of persons, places, names and things are the result of the stimulus which made us actually or mentally turn away from or turn toward them in the first few experiences we had with them. After such an habitual attitude has been developed, only a very strong stimulus of an opposite type will change it. For these reasons most adults are likely to cherish old possessions, old places, old friendships, old societies and customs, old ideas, and old prejudices, although they are occasionally attracted for a time by the new.

HOW WE ATTEND AND ACT VOLUNTARILY

Voluntary attention and the acts that sooner or later follow, are partly controlled by images or ideas. You find a lost article not because it gives your senses a stronger stimulus than other things, but because as you voluntarily look for it you hold an image of it in your mind, and this added to the stimulus of the object, makes you see it. Generally, therefore, voluntary attention is successful because an image makes a weak sensation strong. We may thus hear a whisper in spite of louder sounds. By voluntary effort we direct the muscles so as to favour the stimulus to be strengthened.

Ideas get attention because of their greater strength, and sooner or later induce action toward their realization. In much of our conduct an idea of an objective is aroused by something in the environment, and we at once close the door, attend to the furnace, or write a letter, the act being carried out partly by automatic movements and partly directed by voluntary attention to means of attaining the ends. In some cases, however, ideas of means and ends are not in harmony, one stimulating to the action and the other against it, behaviour being determined by the strongest one. In some instances there is a prolonged competition between ideas associated with several means and ends. The idea that proves strong enough to remain in consciousness when action begins, controls not only for the time, but is frequently dominant in directing one's conduct.

In voluntary acts it seems as if the self takes part in the contest, weakening some ideas and strengthening and holding others. This feeling has an undoubted basis in the fact that one's past experiences, as well as the particular actual and imaged situation of the moment, *are* factors in the choice of means. The individual attends, decides and acts as he does today not merely or chiefly because of what is stimulating action at the moment, but because of past acts of attention and will. Unnoted muscular contractions add to this feeling of the self as doing the willing.

So strong are the tendencies to act in certain ways developed by years of consistent action, that a person may decide without effort to tell the truth, although he knows it will bring disagreeable results, while a frequent liar would have to make intense effort in order to avoid lying. One's ability to attend to a lecture or article on a certain subject while affected by the present sensations of tone of voice, gesture, etc., will vary greatly with the readiness with which ideas gained by previous study do or do not support those suggested by the speaker's words. If the speaker arouses related ideas in the mind of his hearers along with the ones he presents, he may thus control the attention of hearers who could not otherwise pursue such a line of thought.

NATIVE AND ACQUIRED BEHAVIOUR

Parts of the reacting mechanism are connected at birth and ready to function. If the child's stomach is empty and the insides rubbing together (this is probably what causes hunger sensations) and his lips are touched, they curl around the nipple, the tongue does the same, while the muscles of breathing produce suction, and when the milk touches the throat, swallowing occurs. These acts improve somewhat with practice, but not a great deal. Reflexes such as closing the hand around a finger touching the hand, or closing the eye when the lids or eye are touched, or the instinctive act of jumping at a loud sound, continue to be performed in much the same way as at first.

The chief changes in behaviour as age and experience increase are in the ways in which activities are started and various ones combined to accomplish ends. After a baby has seen a bottle many times and then felt it in his lips, the sight alone excites him. After he has seen an object approach his eye several times, he responds to the sight of it by closing the eye *before* receiving the touch stimulus. Such acts are called " conditioned reflexes ". Before a child is a year old he has formed many conditioned reflexes and acquired connections between sensations direct and indirect with various groups of muscles used in securing desirable results. He can hold himself erect, direct his two eyes toward a block on the table near him, move the hand toward it, clutch the block with his fingers, and bring it to his mouth or pound the table with it.

In general, every series or combination of movements in response to initiating and associated stimuli are such as to accomplish certain objective changes and produce subjectively agreeable results. In reacting positively or negatively to objects, movement is likely to continue and vary until results that give satisfaction are gained, or, in objective terms, until equilibrium or balance of the various stimuli and muscular contractions are restored. In an infant, this may occur when, after several attempts, he gets a smooth object pressed against his lips, or a bitter or a rough object out of his mouth.

After several experiences of this kind, images of the results to be gained are formed, and they seem to aid in producing those results more quickly and surely. Purpose thus becomes an important factor in behaviour. A sight, sound, touch, or other sensation arouses an image of end results to be gained, and this helps to co-ordinate the movements that are then made toward that end. All voluntary behaviour is of this general type, although with increasing age and experience the matter becomes very complex. At first actions toward or away from objects are largely influenced by native sensitiveness, paths of connection, and by excess responses of a random character ; while after experience, images of results are prominent and are more complex and better co-ordinated.

In all voluntary movements the idea of the end to be gained seems to have the co-ordinating influence which hastens the process of learning how to get one result and avoid others. After an end has been secured a number of times by the same means, the idea of what is to be gained is enough to insure the appropriate movements with little or no attention to the special kind and order of movements required. In writing one's name, attention may at first be given to fingers and pen, and to the exact motions to be made ; but after much practice, no attention is given to the feel of the pen, and little to the exact movements involved in writing. In general, therefore, the development of human behaviour is from simple native reactions, accompanied and followed by conscious sensations, to complex reactions with conscious imaging of results to be gained and little consciousness of the special movements involved.

In most cases there are intermediate stages in which special sensations caused by combination of simple reactions are prominent in consciousness and continually compared with nearer and more remote results imaged. In the regular daily activities of adult life, ideas of results are chiefly in consciousness, while the sensory motor adjustments involved in doing, are made almost automatically. This leaves the consciousness freer to image past and future experiences.

It appears to an individual that his conscious states are the *causes* of what he does, but the fact that at first acts are involuntary and unanticipated and that later habitual acts of great complexity are performed under the usual stimulating conditions without being consciously initiated (or even contrary to intention, as when the author knowing that the electricity was turned off and that it was of no use to try to turn on the light, found himself trying to do so) leads some people to doubt whether conscious states do really cause reactions or direct them in any way.

No absolute proof that conscious states are causes of changes in objective acts can be given, neither can it be demonstrated that they are merely resultants of sense and muscular activities determined independently of consciousness. It is probably as near the truth, and certainly a matter of convenience, to think of there being an objective and a subjective side to most functioning of the neuro-muscular system. In our experience, sometimes one side and sometimes the other is most clearly perceived. In learning new things the subjective is prominent and seems to be selective and directive as the activities are being co-ordinated for securing the end. It is convenient to describe acts of persons as if this was the case. Native reflexes and instructive acts appear to occur without conscious control, while automatic and habitual acts such as breathing and walking are often performed without perceptible consciousness.

LANGUAGE AND MENTAL FUNCTIONING

In many ways the behaviour of higher animals such as dogs, cats, monkeys, is very much like that of human beings. In reacting to objects and situations actually present, animals are often as successful (or " intelligent ") as men. This way of adjusting to things may be called sensory-motor intelligence.

Animals may be conditioned so that any given adjustment of this kind that they have learned to make will be made in response to a signal or word. Thus language may seem to play a considerable part in the behaviour of animals. A horse naturally takes up his foot, then puts it down again when his shin is kicked or rapped with a stick. By conditioning, he will do this when he sees the stick move quickly toward his shin, or sees a change in his master's face or posture that has previously preceded such a motion, or when he hears a sound or word that has been frequently uttered just before striking his shin. He may then be started to pawing at a gesture, look or word, and be made to stop at another. He may now be exhibited as a horse of intelligence who can count the number of people present by pawing the proper number of times, or even add two and three, or find the square or cube of two. In reality, however, he is not responding to the sentences uttered by his master, but to special signals he receives for beginning and stopping. He may become so acute as to see these signals when human observers looking for them are unable to do so. If a screen is placed between him and his master, however, he can no longer answer the questions.

Animals have been trained to respond to sentences, but careful study reveals the fact that special tone, emphasis or accent are the conditioning guides in most cases, rather than the words themselves. The same is true of young children, but older ones respond appropriately to sentence meanings, however the words are uttered, or whatever the type of print or script words used. Such responses to word symbols are never made by animals.

Words are conditioning stimuli which may become effective in other places and at other times than when first experienced. A child who has been frightened by a dog and heard the word dog uttered, may later act the same when he hears the word when no dog is present. Animals sometimes thus respond to a single significant word, but cannot understand sentences as a child may, as " It is a little white dog we saw at Johnny's last week, and not the big black dog that frightened you on the street ".

Word symbols may also be used as the sole means of learning

to perform new acts. This is not possible to any animal other than man, and demands a special type of intelligence—one making much use of concepts. Without language such intelligence is of little use, as is shown by the condition of deaf persons who have acquired no language.

Delayed responses are much more prominent in men than in animals. For example, a dog that has learned to go to the place where a red light appears for food, does not readily or surely go to the right place if the light is turned off and he is not allowed to move toward it till a period of several minutes has elapsed. A person may do this after hours or days of delay. It is easy to describe this difference as being due to the fact that the human being can form a memory image that serves as a guide in the absence of the actual presence of the red light. This ability to image a situation or sensation, and to act as if it were present, is a form of intelligence in which man greatly exceeds animals, and one that is cultivated by the help of language. It corresponds to what in behaviour terms is called delayed reactions.

When we think how words serve to arouse such images in man, and see what tremendous advantage man has in being able to adjust mentally, to objects and situations not present, we realize something of the importance of language in human life. Animals do not lack the ability to retain impressions so that they behave as they did at some former time when in the same situation, e.g. a horse gets frightened when he comes to a turn in the road where he was frightened long before, and the person does not to the same extent because he can image the dangerous object separate from its surroundings. Animals seem unable to picture the essential element in a situation as existing in another time and place or with different associates. Animals live and act chiefly in the present, while persons with the aid of images and word symbols are able to use widely separated experiences of the past to realize purposes of the future.

Not only do words arouse images, and images take the place of sensations in attaining ends, but words may come to stand for classes of things and for elements in many situations and activities without the necessity of imaging particular sensations, objects or complexes. The word " dog " does not necessarily call up an image of a large or of a small dog, nor of one with long or short hair, nor of a specific colour, especially if one is asked to define the word. We realize that the word may serve not merely in the place of an image of a particular dog, but of any animal having certain fundamental characteristics in common, some of which differ from those of any other species of animal. When words or any sort of symbol may be used to indicate general qualities instead of particular objects or acts, it is possible to act mentally with great rapidity, and to direct actual behaviour very successfully. The architect, by a series of conventional drawings and symbols, mentally constructs a house and conveys to the builder what is to be done. This may take hours or days, while to actually erect the structure in accordance with the indicated plans, may require the work of many men for months or years.

The acquiring of general word symbols and the ability to combine them in ways corresponding to the possible combinations of things, adds immensely to the possible accomplishment of human beings. When we reflect that not only the essentials of one's own experiences may be grouped around words and arranged to help direct action now and in the future, but through the understanding of words and symbols one may make use of the experiences of others, we are led to conclude that no tool or machine invented by man has added so much to his power to deal successfully with situations as the invention of language.

It is largely because of ability to make use of words that the child learns what his animal companions in the same home never acquire ; and why animals live as their ancestors did millions of years ago, while each new generation of men is guided by the experiences of all his ancestors.

The value of words in themselves is, however, sometimes over-estimated. Children in school without adequate experience of things indicated, or who are slow in getting their significance, gain nothing of value from memorizing words and their combinations. The ability of some persons to use words as tools in dealing with the essential elements of things and situations not present, is limited, and cannot easily be developed beyond a certain point. The continued attempt to teach such people by means of words is often wasteful of time and energy of both teacher and pupils. It has been found much more profitable to give them more opportunity to deal with real things, since progress in proportion to effort expended is so much greater. Many who cannot advance in book-work beyond the fourth, fifth, or sixth grades, frequently become quite successful in dealing with actual objects and situations, and not infrequently, in getting along with people.

ECONOMY IN LEARNING

When two neuro-muscular elements have been active in succession, stimulating one of them, especially the first, serves as a partial stimulus of the other. The forming of conditioned reflexes and all associative learning is dependent upon this fact. The more intense the activities thus linked with each other, the greater the number of times they have acted together or in succession, and the more satisfactory the results, the more surely will the first activity produce the second. The earlier repetitions have the greater effects, perhaps because intensity and consciousness are then usually of a higher degree. If the word " tool " is heard, most people will respond with the words " hammer " or " saw ", because of early experience and greater frequency of association of the word " tool " with those implements.

There is a law of association that often brings results contrary to the law of frequency. It is called the law of recency, although in reality it is simply a phase of the law of effect first described. The passing on of the effects of a stimulus given to the first of a series of responses to the second, is greatest immediately after it has occurred. If one has just been using a screw-driver he may say that word when " tool " is named, even though " hammer " has been associated with the word many more times.

Economy in learning and also in unlearning, is to a considerable extent a matter of taking advantage of the laws

N

of repetition, intensity and recency. To learn economically, repetitions of what is to be learned must not occur at such long intervals that the effects of the former repetitions will have disappeared. Neither must there be enough repetitions in rapid succession to produce fatigue.

In memorizing a series, such as learning to repeat a verse of poetry, the first word not only helps in recalling the second, but also the third. The last word in the line is remembered not merely because the one preceding it helps to recall it, but because all the words preceding it help to do so. Even a small child learns to go back and repeat the beginning words of the line or verse as an aid in remembering the line or verse. Experiments have shown that in learning a poem of several verses, not only are words associated with those that follow, but lines are associated with lines, and verses with verses, and the parts are more surely given if the whole poem is learned by repeating it in order each time. If each part is repeated separately until learned, the last line and word of the first verse is repeated several times just before the words of the first line, and only a few times just before the beginning of the second verse, and as a consequence there is likely to be difficulty in remembering the order of verses. The accumulative effects of repetition are best realized, therefore, when the order is the same throughout.

To repeat at different rates or rhythms does not have as much effect in memorizing as uniform repetition. Many people can sing hymns which they cannot recite in an ordinary voice.

Learning a poem by sound makes it easier to say it, but learning by sight makes it easier to write it. Combined hearing, seeing and saying gives quicker and more permanent learning than doing one of these at a time. If, instead of having repetitions of one or more kinds follow each other, they are alternated with recall or mental repetitions of it, a poem can be recalled at will with less time spent on learning it.

It is easier to memorize words with known meanings than nonsense syllables, and to learn words in sentences than when they are in an unconnected series. It is also easier to memorize an unconnected series of words if one images or thinks what they stand for, than if they are repeated as if they had no meaning.

Familiarity with words and sentence forms adds to the ease of learning similar ones. This is one of the chief reasons why high-school students can greatly surpass second-grade children in reproducing sentences, but are only slightly superior in reproducing a series of strange forms such as Greek or Chinese letters. A person who has played baseball can learn to play tennis much sooner than one who has had no experiences with balls, because he has had experience in noting the successive positions of a moving ball and can anticipate where it will be at the next instant.

Learning is, therefore, most economical when previous associations are most used in learning every new thing. News regarding home people is remembered with a single repetition because of what is already known of persons, places and events ; while to learn the same facts about strange people in another community would require long study. A student of American history learns new facts of our past with greater ease than similar facts of German history. A biologist easily adds to his knowledge of biology, and a physicist to what he knows of physics ; but neither would be able to learn as fast in the other's speciality. An order of learning either subject-matter, or of skill in doing, which makes each part already known help in learning the rest, is the most economical.

Although the above holds for all types of learning, yet the application of the principle is not the same for rote learning and habit uses, as for purposes of thought and invention. In learning to spell words the letters must be seen, heard and made in the same order every time ; and to be most effective should be written as a part of a sentence, rather than as a mere exercise. In gaining meaning for a word, one should not repeat its definition over and over in the same words, but should see and hear the same word used correctly in many *different* circumstances and word combinations. A fact of history or science is best known, not when it has been expressed in the same words over and over, but when it has been related to other facts, events, persons and places. To gain skill in making all sorts of letters, varied practice is best, but in learning for the sake of ordinary use, the sooner a single style is acquired and practised until it is produced automatically, the better.

In all learning, improvement is greatest in doing exactly the same thing in the same way and under the same circumstances ; and less in doing the same thing under different circumstances or in a different way, or in doing a similar thing. If a new set of number symbols such as ├ =0, ⌐ =1, ⌐ =2,

⌐ =3, ⌐ =4, etc., taken from the diagram

$$\begin{array}{c|c|c} 1 & 4 & 7 \\ \hline 2 & 5 & 8 \\ \hline 3 & 6 & 9 \end{array}$$

is practised in order as far as 20 = ⌐├ , there is great improvement in speed in that order. There is less improvement in writing them in reverse order, still less in writing odd numbers only in order, and very little in writing such a series as 6, 1, 5, 2, 7, 4. If an attempt is made to use the new number symbols in working problems, the person who has practised writing them in order for three or four minutes does as well as the person who has practised thirty minutes. To practise parts of an act separately, especially in the same order, beyond the point necessary to avoid errors is always uneconomical. Such practice is justifiable only when necessary to acquire the correct way of doing, since repetition of errors increases the tendency to make mistakes.

As many things should be practised at once as can be done successfully together. Often it is well for a portion of a series to become automatic in order that more attention may be given to the new part being attempted. In learning to drive a motor-car, shifts may be practised with the engine not running until they are made easily ; then the use of the accelerator, clutch and brake as if starting and stopping the car. After that, all the acts necessary for backing, stopping, starting forward, and shifting, may be performed partly or wholly in imagination, a number of times before the engine is started and the thing really done. Such a procedure avoids too much practice of parts on the one hand, and of too great demand of attention to many things at once, on the other ; and above all it helps to prevent the discouragements of numerous failures.

Attention plays a large part in the economy of learning. It has the same effect as increase in intensity of an influential stimulus, hence it is requisite that too many things requiring attention shall not be attempted at once, and that there shall be attention to the right thing at the right time. In preparatory learning to play tennis, attention may profitably be given to holding and swinging the racquet, but as practice continues, handling the racquet should become automatic, while attention is given to the ball and where it is to go. In explaining when not practising, it is sometimes helpful to call attention to right and wrong ways of doing in order to make the right way clearer by contrast ; but just before and while practising, attention should be focused on what to do and how to do it, and *never upon errors to be avoided.*

If both speed and accuracy are to be gained (which is desirable in all cases in which the act is to be performed frequently in much the same way), it is always best to work for accuracy first, and later to speed up while preserving accuracy. If the reverse process is attempted there is almost always much waste of time and energy caused by making and repeating mistakes. Practice does not necessarily make perfect, as the old adage says, but merely insures the kind of doing which is practised, not infrequently leading to increased imperfection. This is often true when there is much rapid writing required outside the penmanship period.

In changing a habit, *e.g.* putting a pen in an inkwell on the right, instead of putting it in on the left, intensity must be stronger than frequency the first time the left-hand well is used. Each recent repetition of using the left-hand inkwell decreases the need for intensity. A dozen such repetitions may for the moment balance hundreds of motions to the right made weeks ago, and the left-hand dipping of the pen may require no voluntary attention. Upon resuming writing after an interval of a few days, however, unless there is conscious voluntary attention to dipping the pen, the hand will go to the right in accordance with the law of frequency. If it does, this gives the right-hand motion the advantage of recency. This is the reason that in changing a habit, it is best to give voluntary attention whenever it is needed, otherwise the occasional repetition of the old act will greatly delay the change to the new.

UNIVERSAL TYPES OF REACTIONS

In all ages men everywhere have not been steadily running mechanisms, but have occasionally been in a stirred-up condition in which for a time the intensity of action is increased while co-ordination is decreased. They have been disturbed to hunger by lack of food ; to fear by unusual situations ; to anger by hindering situations ; to love by the opposite sex ; to care-taking by helpless children ; to imitation and competition by companions ; to curiosity by new things ; and each individual has sought companions, laughed, played and prayed. These are the most striking examples of universal instinctive and emotional characteristics of man as a species.

Purposes are formed as the result of these instinctive and emotional experiences, while learning and intellectual development take place in the process of correlating these strivings.

Extreme variations in food supply and in temperature and other conditions produce considerable variation in muscular and glandular activities, with intense states of consciousness that are lessened as activities are co-ordinated in attaining satisfactions. The conscious self is most prominent whenever these sensory motor activities are out of equilibrium or are in process of being brought into equilibrium. The shorter this process the briefer the emotional state.

Necessity for eating, its pleasures and the uncertainties of food supply, and the efforts made to obtain it, have given to emotions associated with food a dominating drive in individual and social activities. Economic activity is primarily conditioned by food needs and desires, and these have to a large extent influenced inventions, migrations and wars. In some parts of the earth, the need for clothing and shelter has played almost as important a part in economic development.

The emotions and drives associated with mating and care of children have been leading factors in the life of individuals and in the development of institutions. Governments and other organizations grow out of life in the primary group, the family.

EMOTIONAL STIMULI AND REACTIONS

The attempt to direct activity in a co-ordinated way causes an emotion to decrease. The securing of food or more comfortable conditions brings in new sensations giving satisfaction, which gradually decrease in intensity as the stimulating effects of contrast and unsatisfied desires are lessened.

Unusual or strong stimuli cannot be immediately adjusted to, and as a consequence there is a convulsive movement of withdrawal and the stirred-up condition of fear results. If the stimulus does not come again, or if well co-ordinated movements are made, the fear gradually dies down, especially when curiosity is aroused and movements of approach are made instead of retreat. When activity toward some end is blocked or interfered with in any way, there is a sudden heightening of imperfectly directed activities and the emotion of anger. Removal of the obstruction or the successful co-ordinating of activities toward some end, quiets the emotion. If the harmless character of the interference becomes evident, laughter may ensue and relax all the tense muscles upon which the feeling of anger partially depends. Both fear and anger if long continued, affect glandular action and the composition of the blood.

In all these cases not only varied intense sensory and motor activities are involved, but often unsettling images play a large part in the emotional state. Probably no animal ever worries about hunger and dangers that are past, or that may come in the future, but is affected chiefly by the present situation ; while man is worried, frightened or angered, by representations of what has or may take place years away from the present day. Even his emotions at the moment when frightened by a sound or angered by a blow, are due partly to images of previous experiences with the object or person arousing the emotion.

The time that emotions last may be increased or decreased by images according as the attention is occupied with those arousing it, or with those of an opposite character. If both images and movements are directed in a co-ordinated way, fear, anger and other emotions disappear. Continued suppression of the outward signs of these and other emotions, while reacting inwardly as before, is likely to prove a severe strain on the nervous system and may lead to a variety of emotional disturbances.

Intense unbalancing emotions are less likely to continue if one seeks to realize varied rather than single interests. Curiosity and humour are especially valuable as weakeners of other emotional states.

The mating instinct in man is more continuous than in animals and involves æsthetic and other emotions. It stirs imagination and therefore often arouses not merely appetite, but æsthetic feelings and love for the exciting mate. This, and the care-taking instinct result in more permanent attitudes toward mates and helpless young in man than in other animals. Human family life as lived and remembered has an importance not found in any other species.

In no other species does group life play such a large part in the behaviour of individuals. Each is stimulated actually and in thought by others, to imitation, rivalry, and to adjustment of his acts to match those of others in gaining individual and group ends. Very persistent emotional attitudes arise from relations of men to each other, and thus are customs and ideals relating to home, country, friends and religion formed.

Men not only act as animals do so as to preserve their bodily life, but also so as to preserve their ego or conscious self. This conscious self is greatly affected by acts and words of approval or disapproval by companions. In all ages, therefore, the emotions and behaviour of men have been determined to a considerable extent by the natural and acquired behaviour of other persons. The customs of a group into which a person is born are perhaps more important than hereditary traits in determining the character and behaviour of individuals. This truth is of especial importance in Social Psychology and in Sociology.

SELECTED RESEARCHES

"LEARNING AND GROWTH IN IDENTICAL TWINS."

By ARNOLD GESELL and HELEN THOMPSON. From *Genetic Psychology Monographs*, July 1929. *Quoted by Permission.*

THE TRAINING OF TWIN C (53–55 WEEKS)

Comparisons of the behaviour of the twins were made at various stages of the primary experimental period, as will be indicated in the discussion of the findings. At the end of this period (age 52 weeks) the results proved so interesting that it was decided to widen the range of comparison by subjecting the control twin, C, to a brief course of training in stair-climbing. This course began when Twin C was 53 weeks old, continued six days a week for two weeks, each session being 10 minutes long.

The purpose of this special training period was to check the results of the previous experiment by determining the trainability of *Twin C at a more advanced age than Twin T.*

The conditions of the training period for Twin C were similar to those already described for Twin T. . . . Since, however, the training did not include creeping, standing, and walking, the actual amount of time devoted to stair-climbing was equal to that used for the same purpose in the locomotor training sessions of Twin T. Within a durational period of two weeks, therefore, the amount of direct stair-climbing opportunity was for the two twins fully comparable. . . .

Twelve consecutive records . . . together with the various clinical and observational reports and motion-picture records of C's behaviour, furnish the basis control data which will make possible some interpretation of the influence of the more prolonged training and conditioning regime upon the developmental progress of Twin T. . . .

. . . The three tables which follow (Tables 6, 7, 8) afford a summary view of the progress :

TABLE 6

POSTURAL AND LOCOMOTOR BEHAVIOUR OF T AND C (BIRTH TO 46 WEEKS)

Birth : T more active than C.

6 weeks : Both make alternate stepping movements when held in standing position with feet in contact with floor. . . .

28 weeks : Both show peculiar but identical behaviour when placed in seated position, snapping body back in rigid extension. Similar reactions in prone and standing postures. . . .

36 *weeks* : Both maintain balance in free sitting position, T showing somewhat less wavering. No rhythmic extension or stepping movements in standing position. Prone reactions very similar with slightly more tendency to progression in T. . . .

40 *weeks* : T's reaction in standing position more advanced. Supports weight holding side rail. Both strain forward in prone position to secure bell ; T is more vigorous and strains first with the right then the left arm, and to this extent more nearly approximates creeping. Prone posture similar. . . .

46 *weeks* : Each twin lifts one foot when placed at bottom of staircase, but neither goes further in an effort to climb. Each walks if held by both hands. Each pulls self to standing position. No apparent difference between T and C in locomotor performance.

TABLE 7

CLIMBING BEHAVIOUR OF TWIN T DURING TRAINING PERIOD
(46 TO 52 WEEKS)

Age (Weeks).	Date	Day of Week.	
46	May 21	Mon.	No record.
	May 24	Thurs.	*Three* times up ; 2nd, spontaneously lifted foot ; 3rd, needed less assistance than before.
47	May 28	Mon.	*Three* times. Stairs climbed with difficulty and needed considerable assistance.
	May 31	Thurs.	*Six* times. Drags up one foot after E placed first. More tendency to left foot.
48	June 4	Mon.	*Five* times. Slow and difficult at first. Looked out of window. Cried when placed on steps fifth time.
	June 7	Thurs.	*Three* times. Slipped back.
49	June 11	Mon.	*Four* times. Feet move faster than hands.
	June 14	Thurs.	*Four* times. Moderately well.
50	June 18	Mon.	*Five* times. Needed a little stimulation at first. (r.k., l.f.)
	June 21	Thurs.	*Ten* times. Very intent in creeping and walking. (r.k., l.f., r.f.)
51	June 25	Mon.	*Six* times. Given a seventh trial, but more interested in creeping.
	June 28	Thurs.	*Four* times. (r.k., l.f. predom.)

(r.k. = right knee. l.f. = left foot, etc.)

TABLE 8

CLIMBING BEHAVIOUR OF TWIN C (53 WEEKS TO 55 WEEKS)

Age (Weeks).	Date	Day of Week.	
53	July 9	Mon.	*Seven* times.
	July 12	Thurs.	*Seven* times. Tends to fall back. Gets caught on last step. *Time :* 40 sec.
54	July 16	Mon.	*Six* times. Less tendency to fall back. 18 sec.
	July 19	Thurs.	*Eight* times. Well motivated on whole, occasionally became weak (walk down) (l.f., r.f.)

. . . It will be noted that in the early stages of the training period, T mounted the stairs only three or four times during the 10-minute session, with fluctuations which could be clinically explained.   Well-defined enjoyment in climbing came into prominence in the fourth week.   The number of successful scalings per session increased until it reached the maximum of ten on the 25th session during the fifth week.   This record may be taken to represent the peak of her performance, regarded from the point of view of spontaneity and of speed.   All told, she had, at this particular session, scaled the stairs 115 times.   At the end of the six-week period, the total number of successful scalings increased to 156.

Turning now to the record of Twin C, it will be noted that she scaled the stairs seven times at the very first session, *even though she had not been trained at all.*   Her maximum record of ten successful scalings was reached in a week and a half, at the ninth session.   It took her from 10 to 18 seconds to make each successful climb.   This time record is approximately equal to the time record of Twin T, who did not, however, attain that score until five weeks of training had elapsed.   It will be noted that all told, C scaled the stairs 81 times in a period of two weeks as contrasted with T's record of 55 times in the first two weeks (May 24 to June 6) and of 156 times in six weeks.   This quantitative difference carries with it many implications regarding the growth factors in the process of learning locomotion, which will be touched upon in a later analysis of the data.   The ratio of total performance (scalings) to total duration (weeks), in the case of T, is as 26 to 1 ; the ratio of performance to duration in Twin C is as 40 to 1—a palpable difference in the efficacy of deferred training.

Perhaps the most striking event which happened during the course of this investigation was the successful climbing of the stairs by Twin C at the age of 53 weeks, without previous specific training and without any environmental opportunity to exercise the function of climbing. . . .

SUGGESTED READINGS

For a brief, clear exposition of what is most generally accepted by psychologists of today :

DASHIELL, JOHN T., *Fundamentals of Objective Psychology*, 1928.
WOODWORTH, R. S., *Psychology*, new ed., 1928.

Behaviouristic Psychology is best presented by :

WATSON, JOHN, rev. ed., 1930.

The Gestalt psychology is advocated by :

KOFFKA, K., *The Growth of the Mind*, 1927.

The various applications of psychology are set forth by :

POFFINBERGER, A. T., *Applied Psychology*, 1929.

In physiological psychology LADD and WOODWORTH is still a standard work. The newer developments in that field are set forth in :

HERRICK, C. J., *Neurological Foundations of Animal Behaviour*, 1924.
LASHLEY, K. S., *Brain Mechanism and Intelligence*, 1929.

The Freudian psychology which has had such a popular vogue, although presenting many theories and shrewd guesses, and helping to develop the art of psychoanalysis, has made little use of the more accurate objective methods of science. ADLER, A., and JUNG, have made some improvements in this direction.

HEALY, WILLIAM, and BRONNER, AUGUSTA, and BOWERS, ANNA MAE, *The Structure of Psychoanalysis as related to Personality and Behaviour*, 1930, presents the most valuable of these theories.

In child psychology a much used text recently revised is :

KIRKPATRICK, EDWIN A., *Fundamentals of Child Study*, 4th ed., 1929.

The pre-school child has been most scientifically studied by :

GESELL, ARNOLD, *Mental Growth of the Pre-School Child*, 1925.

In abnormal psychology ROSANOFF, ARON J., and MEYER, ADOLPH, are authorities. In the study of feeble-mindedness GODDARD, H. H., and KUHLMANN, FRED, have been leaders.

CHAPTER IX

PERSONALITY DIFFERENCES, OR INDIVIDUAL PSYCHOLOGY

I

PERSONALITY

Individuality

Of the billions of the human species who are living and have lived on this planet, no two were ever exactly alike. All have the distinctive qualities of human beings yet these are so combined that there is never precise duplication of personalities as wholes. In a less degree this wonderful sameness in the species and infinite variety in individuals is found in plants and animals. A study of the variations in number of vertebra in the human species and in other mammals indicates that man varies less in fundamental structure from the type than most of the higher animals. In mental characteristics, however, he varies a great deal more.

The more prominent sources of variation in individuals are, first, in the combinations of the genes or unit characters that take place when the germ cells of two ancestral lines unite. This determines the anatomical structure, and as a consequence the general type of physiological functioning. In identical twins (those formed from the same egg) the structures are likely to be as nearly the same as are the two sides of an individual, but in non-identical twins (those formed from separate eggs), the differences are greater.

The second most important cause of variation is the special type of environment, which can never be exactly the same for two persons. In a favourable environment all grow to a greater size than in an unfavourable one. Variations in food, especially in vitamins, and variations in stimuli to muscular and mental activity, may cause more growth of some structures than others, and greatly modify the general type of feature and behaviour. Two groups of individuals much alike in original structure and behaviour, may, after long exposure to environments differing in character, seem to be distinct varieties of the human stock, yet in fundamental traits, including the mental, they are much alike. " Mrs. O'Grady and the Colonel's lady are the same under the skin."

The third factor in producing individuality is in the special relations of original structure of the person to the various phases of the environment in which the person dwells. If two members of the same family differ, the same environment will have a different effect upon them, and even if they should be nearly alike, it is not probable that they will get exactly the same stimuli, or at the same time. In either case they may develop in quite different ways, each increasing most in the way in which he is already the strongest either by original nature or because of some early or special experience. With children differing at first and never having exactly the same stimuli at the same time, it is inevitable that even identical twins differ. Original structure seems to be the most essential factor in individuality. Identical twins placed in different environments develop much the same, while twins originally unlike, become quite different in an environment as nearly the same for both as is possible. Tests of orphans indicate that their intelligence quotients are more closely correlated with parental intelligence, than with that of foster parents.

PHYSIOLOGICAL CHARACTERISTICS AND BEHAVIOUR

To the superficial observer all babies are alike when born, except that some are larger and plumper than others ; but nurses and mothers notice differences in their behaviour almost at once. Some hold the head up much earlier than others or show more vigour in all movements, and are more or less responsive to sounds or to sights. One gazes at the lamp or window, and the other avoids the light by closing his eyes or turning away from it. At six months individual differences in general ability are so great that a specialist like Dr. Gesell, after observing and testing, can form some idea as to whether a child will be intelligent enough to succeed in college, or be more likely to fail before he gets through the grades. Before the close of the first year various special peculiarities are evident, such as more use of one hand than of the other in the more difficult reachings. Nearly all children make much progress in walking and in talking during the second year, but differ greatly in rate of progress in one or other of these two important forms of behaviour. Great differences in irritability of temper, or persistence in action, and of independence, are also to be noted.

It is common to speak of individual differences in temperament or disposition, but no attempt at classification of individuals according to temperament has been very successful. Several varieties of temperament are easily describable and occasionally found in individuals, but rarely are *all* the supposedly typical qualities combined in the same way in many individuals. Educators and psychiatrists are now making less effort to classify according to type, and giving more attention to the way in which a certain combination of qualities of an individual is likely to harmonize in a given environment.

Disposition and temperament vary so much with general physiological functioning, especially of glands, that the relationship of these to temperament and behaviour cannot be questioned. Glandular treatments are more likely, however, to be successful in restoring to normal, than in changing the general disposition of normal individuals. With the latter, training will probably continue to be the best means of improvement.

PHYSIOLOGICAL FUNCTIONING AND CONSCIOUS PERSONALITY

The sense organs within the body, stimulated by variations in muscular and glandular activity, are continued sources of impulses carried to the brain. The sensations they give vary

o

with habit rhythms and for special reasons, but are generally more constant than those arising from stimulating the special sensations of sight, hearing, touch, taste and smell. They, therefore, form a sort of background for the special sensations, which though little noticed except when there is intense discomfort in stomach, head or muscles, are important factors in conscious personality. As a mass they give one the feeling of well-being or lack of it, and give a feeling tone to the special sensations for which they are the background. Changes of mood are often due to variations in this background of conscious experience. Temperament is probably largely due to constancy of this background associated with comparatively uniform, yet distinctive, physiological functioning of each individual.

Each person learns to know himself in much the same way as he distinguishes others. When *he* does things, however, there are sensations of muscular tension not experienced when the same actions are performed by someone else, and this distinctiveness is also fostered by oft-recurring images. When images and ideas are used in voluntary direction of motion, they are associated with the physiological background. Thoughts are always accompanied by contractions of numerous small muscles and are thus identified as one's own. These experiences give one the feeling of being an active force when imaging or thinking as well as when dealing with real things. Present and past experiences are also continually being linked in memory with each other, on the common background of bodily sensations. Ordinarily there is enough constancy in the bodily sensations and the memories to give the impression of continued existence of the same personality.

Severe accidents or marked periods of divided attention, unusual surroundings or behaviour, may cause division in the mental life, so that one seems to have a different, and perhaps a multiple personality. If common memories are lacking the separation is likely to be complete. A victim of an accident may recover consciousness but recall nothing of his former life, although many of his acquired and automatic abilities remain. After a period of days, months or years in which he gains a new set of conscious memories, he may awaken with none of this intervening life remembered, but with all of his life previous to the accident, intact.

The probability of a shock or other cause producing such double or alternating personality may be the greater because of early childhood experiences. Most children act quite differently when with their companions from the way they act when with their elders. They often play at being someone else for days. Again, children also allow their attention to be divided for considerable periods of time. It is common for persons to behave unusually when sick or angry, or to do one thing automatically while attending to another consciously. In such cases there is temporary and partial development of separately functioning units of behaviour and consciousness. In dreams, day-dreams, and hypnotic states, still more complete separation of memories and behaviour may occur or be induced. Consciousness of former almost unnoticed experiences may be amplified, while present sensations and memories of earlier events are decreased and blocked. In such a state the individual, especially if hypnotized, may ignore real sense stimuli, and act in response to imaginary ones. Nearly everyone has the possibility of manifesting one personality at one time and another, partly or wholly different at another time. It is also possible to have a split-off complex acting separately from one's conscious personality, as is shown in automatic writing and drawing, so extensively studied by Dr. Morton Prince.

In general, however, persons of normal health who do not suddenly change their environment and mode of life, and whose purposes and actions are congruent with each other, develop a unified set of correlated experiences, held together by common memories and general background of physiologically produced sensations, and seem to themselves and to others to remain the same person, notwithstanding the great changes that the years bring.

Some people have a many-sided personality that often seems to others like more than one person in the same body, yet real separation is the exception, and considerable unity of thought and conduct is the rule. In securing such unity the general bodily sensations and the muscular sensations are large factors supplemented by common memories and much experience of connecting past, present, and future in the realizing of purposes. Material objects may be studied separately, but there is no such thing as a sensation except as the experience of some person, neither can any phase of human life be adequately studied apart from the unified personality experiencing or producing it. This makes individual psychology different from any other science. The objective and subjective original and acquired traits are so variously combined and modified in a person, that exactly the same traits do not have the same meaning in various individuals.

Science's usual procedure of analysing for elements, classifying into groups according to certain prominent elements, and then finding general truths for each group, does not work successfully either from the scientific or the practical standpoint. To say that a young man is of Jewish parentage, a college graduate, a blond, of average height, and of artistic temperament, does not tell an employment manager what occupation or job shall be offered him, nor a doctor how to prescribe for him, nor a psychiatrist how to treat him, even though it is added that his is a case of dementia præcox. Such facts are of some value, but no one, and occasionally not even all of them together are adequate guides. In every case the individual must be given special study, his past history as well as his present attitudes and condition taken into account, in order to make any use of the class terms applied to him. The more advanced thinkers in every field of personality study now hold that science and practical needs demand a better technique of individual study and of individual treatment, if science is to be as useful in dealing with individual human beings as it has proved to be in dealing with groups.

CONSISTENCY OF CHARACTER

Personality is the original individual as developed and modified by his environment. Character is largely what the individual has made of himself by his voluntary actions. A well-balanced neuro-muscular structure and constant healthful physiological functioning are good bases for a consistent character. An environment which remains much the same for years, is also favourable. A regular place of abode, and above all, one or more persons with whom one lives as a part of a family group, help give continuity to life's experiences. In addition it is necessary that certain types of activity shall continue during a considerable period, although they may alternate with others not incongruous with them, without disturbing unity. A child whose surroundings and associates are frequently changed, and whose family relationships are disturbed and uncertain, or one who is induced to act in accordance with one set of standards at one time, and to a different set at another time, does not easily develop a unified character. A person, however, who is vigorous and persistent, and who continues to be active in realizing distant and consistent purposes of his own, may develop unity of character in spite of lack of unity and consistency in his environment and treatment. Where there is extreme variation in bodily functioning, especially variations due to certain diseases such as encephalitis, marked changes in personality often result. When there is lack of consistency in both bodily functioning and environment, the chances for a single, strong, consistent personality are very poor.

A strong character is not difficult to develop if the favourable conditions named above are existent, and the individual's interests and dominating purposes are few, and consistent. A person with many interests and opposing purposes that alternate in controlling conduct, finds the development of unity of character more difficult. Of no one perhaps, was this more true than of Goethe, who, with few if any exceptions, was the most gifted of men. Rousseau possessed less varied gifts, but on account of unfavourable conditions in childhood —more unfavourable than in the case of Goethe—failed even more completely to attain unity of character. In both cases, physiological irregularity and unadjusted family life and varied companionships, were important factors in preventing consistency of behaviour and consequent unity and strength of character.

Every individual has more desires and capacities than can ever be realized and utilized. If he tries to attain the same ends by means that are not antagonistic to each other, success and unity of character are promoted. If the means are entirely antagonistic, such as seeking power over the same persons alternately by force and fear, and by sympathy and love, unity is not easily developed. When there are many ends to be gained, harmonizing by some all-inclusive purpose may give unity to behaviour and character.

Strength or weakness of character is the direct outcome of the laws of habit. An individual who has for years made the attainment of wealth the dominant motive of action, becomes more and more certain to act so as to get money, rather than to get ease or comfort. If he consistently tries to get it by honest methods, he will become almost incapable of getting it in any other way. All his past life impels him to attain his ends by such means. If he has alternated between honesty and dishonesty, then part of his past helps in the present, and part hinders. An individual who has to put forth great effort to refrain from taking a five-dollar bill that does not belong to him, lacks the help of past habits of action in the present emergency, while the one who refrains without effort, has that assistance.

Temporary states of mind direct the formation of habits, but habits once formed are likely to be less changeable than emotional states ; hence a stable character can be developed only by frequent action in accordance with certain purposes and as attained by certain means. By long-continued consistency in action one develops a character which continues to behave in much the same way in spite of changes of environment and unsettling experiences of success and failure, joy and sorrow. Such experiences test the inner strength and unity of an individual, and often reveal the importance of some experience, associate, or group custom, in maintaining what seems to be strength of character. One who has persistently sought to meet every situation as successfully as possible instead of being merely dismayed, irritated or stirred up about it, is likely to maintain unity of character whatever vicissitudes he may meet. Much experience of having carried on a line of action to its conclusion, in most cases with success, is the best means of developing a strong character.

INDIVIDUAL DIFFERENCES

The earliest accurate measurement of differences in human beings were anatomical. Excluding a few giants and near giants, and midgets and near midgets, the individual variations in height of the tall and the short are not great, one being less than ten per cent above the average, and the other the same per cent below the average, or a total difference between extremes of less than twenty per cent. Differences in weight are about twice as great. Differences in size of special organs vary, but in general are rather less than in total body weight. Not more than one brain in a hundred weighs less than 40 or more than 50 ounces. Normal temperature is almost the same for everyone, while differences in pulse-rate under normal conditions are comparable to those of height. The individual differences in muscular strength and in amount of food, sleep, and sex requirements are much greater than the more elementary anatomical and physiological ones named above.

The greatest extremes in men are found in the sphere in which they differ most from animals—the mental. In simple sensory motor reactions the extremes above and below the average after equal practice are comparable with differences in size, but in general verbal intelligence tests, which involve images and ideas as symbolized by words, the extreme range is from zero or 100 below, to about 100 above average. In almost any schoolroom of forty children the I.Q. range will be from 75–125, and occasionally from 60–140. In special forms of practised mental activity, mathematical, musical, etc., the genius is widely separated from ordinary persons, and especially from persons deficient in those lines.

One of the most striking things brought out by modern

scientific investigations, is that, generally speaking, individual differences within groups are greater than between the averages or mediums of groups, *e.g.* grade 4 averages differ from grade 6 averages less than individuals in grade 4 differ from each other.   For the surgeon and the physician the races of men differ less radically than do individuals within the same race. The psychologist and the educator find only slight differences in intelligence and scholastic attainments in the averages of racial groups, and wider extremes within the group.   Even in a school where all are of the same race and have had the same school instruction, standardized achievement tests show that the best of the fourth-year students (as high as 25 per cent) are equal to the poorest 25 per cent of the eighth-year classes. In tests in single subjects like reading, the differences between grades are barely evident, while the best individual reader in a grade often makes a score four times that of the poorest. Even when pupils have been carefully classified according to mental age, and members of each group have received the same teaching, still the best score in a group is often twice that of the poorest.

In emotional and volitional activities and in a variety of personality traits of which as yet there are no accurate measures, the differences seem to be as great as in more purely intellectual abilities.

Not only are there extreme differences in special characteristics, but there are infinite ways in which they are combined. An individual testing high in a few mental tests is more likely than otherwise to test high in all ; but there are occasionally combinations of extreme strength and weakness.   There is never certainty, but only probability, that one trait in a high or low degree, will mean the presence or absence of any other special trait in the same degree.

Stability of personality is more likely in persons whose variations from the normal are all in the same direction, than in those who are much above the average in some characteristics and below in others.   Even when intelligence tests only are used, those who consistently test high or low on all tests at all times, are more likely to be normal in behaviour than those who make good records in some and poor in other tests, and especially than those who make variable records on different days.

SCIENTIFIC STUDY OF INDIVIDUALS AND VOCATIONS

Because of the fact that the finding of one trait of an individual does not insure that he will possess other traits, it is difficult to generalize from the study of many individuals and classify them into groups according to certain prominent characteristics. There is a slight probability that the larger children of the same age will do better in mental tests, yet the dullest in a given class may be the largest of the group, while the smallest may be the brightest. There is a probability that those high in mental tests will be more successful in manual constructions, yet the one at the top in language intelligence tests, may do far worse constructive work than the one at the bottom. The intelligent individual is more likely to be energetic, but may be the laziest.

So common are exceptions to earlier generalizations as to traits likely to be found together, that it is now recognized as unsafe to assume that because an individual has one trait, he will have certain others. Inconsistencies of all sorts are found not only among the insane, but among the sane. Scientific research in spite of these facts has, however, made the study of individuals much more intelligent, exact and practically useful. It has shown that certain traits are *usually* correlated with others, and norms of such relations have been established with which individual records may be compared, *e.g.* intelligence scores and school successes. Strength and weakness, and their probable influence upon success or failure in general or in special lines, are thus ascertained. Harmony and balance in traits found are more significant than the single variations from the standard norms.

When certain traits are known to be of importance in a vocation, it is possible to discover by experiment what measured results of several tests will show a high degree of probability of success in that field. By such means it is possible to state after giving a few well-selected groups of tests, the probabilities of an individual's success in high school in general, or in particular subjects such as algebra or stenography, or whether he will be successful in certain vocations such as driving a taxi, or in manual occupations such as sorting balls. In industries, special tests are successfully used to discover probabilities of efficiency in various types of work. Success in taking high school and college courses and in training for professions involving much book preparation, may be shown to be very improbable when general intelligence test scores are below a certain minimum.

It is not at all certain, however, that those making the highest grades will succeed best. Success will be great or small according to other traits than the intellectual. If there is intelligence and energetic persistence, what might seem to be insurmountable physical obstacles may sometimes be overcome, as witness the achievements of the blind and the deaf, and of a few like Helen Keller, with both senses lacking ; or the instance of a one-armed man winning a tennis match, an armless man driving an automobile, and a one-legged man successful in playing basketball.

Exact predictions of success of one or failure of another in a limited field of action may, after sufficient experimentation, be made as ten to one, or one in ten. When it is a matter of predicting that an individual's life as a whole will be a success or a failure, science cannot answer with such certainty. Men of great abilities and opportunities may fail, while others of moderate abilities and apparently few advantages may succeed as judged by colleagues, or by posterity. The brilliant individual may engage in the work for which he is unfitted, or fail to use the means which employ his best powers ; or he may undertake too many things, or use means not in harmony with each other.

Often success or failure depends, not upon the situation and the suitability of his aims and plans to his own powers in the chosen field, but in his success in getting co-operative help from others, or upon the opposition he arouses. Chance and luck also play their part in every life, but in general the outcome depends more upon how the individual habitually reacts to situations and individuals, than upon the situations themselves, or his native abilities alone.

The help of scientific methods in placing men in the right jobs in large establishments, and in advising children and youths as to their probable success in various grades and various occupations, is already of great value and is rapidly increasing. When as reliable tests of interests, will, and other personality traits have been developed, as we now have of physical ability and general intelligence, the aids available will be still more effective.

Accidents in industry occur to some individuals more frequently than to others. Monotony in industry is often more trying to intelligent persons than to less intelligent ones. However, an intelligent person can sometimes make the operation entirely automatic and can then occupy his mind in interesting ways while doing his work. Others may engage in a low form of thought or reverie concerning little annoyances, and as a result become non-adaptive. Transference to another department or working part of the day on one specialized process and part on another, sometimes increases output and helps promote normality in workers.

PERSONALITY STUDIES

The most difficult application of scientific methods to individuals is in personality development. Such studies are now being extensively made in hospitals, institutions for the insane, prisons, juvenile courts, industrial establishments, and in a number of schools and colleges. With added experience, more reliable methods of getting significant facts are being used, but it is being realized more and more, that although generalizations can be made as to single traits or conditions, and their effects upon most persons, yet it is unsafe to prescribe for an individual without studying how he has been reacting to the situations he has met. There is always something special in the individual and his surroundings that may make him behave differently from well-founded expectations. Every one of a dozen boys arraigned for theft may need a different prescription according to the causes found to have been most influential in producing that type of conduct. Every individual must be studied in various aspects, not only as to his present behaviour but also his past history. General principles of psychology and of normal functioning will be helpful in evaluating the facts discovered, and in determining the causes of present conditions. Advice as to what will be most likely to restore normal functioning will be based upon these general principles and the special facts of the case.

The most important truth found by researches in this field is that more individuals are restored to normal by positive than by negative means. Also what is good for normal persons is in general good for the exceptional individual if proper adjustments to his abilities and his former attitudes and interests are made. In a subsequent section of this chapter the general principles of what makes for normal functioning are given.

Security is necessary at all ages in order that there may not be uncertainty, fear and worrying. It exists partly because of confident dependency on others who are always on the job and never fail to care for one, as in early infancy, or because of individual ability to meet situations presented successfully, as is the case in successful maturity. In personality development a proper balance should be maintained so that as dependency decreases, competent independence may develop without much regression to dependency, in order to maintain security. This means that as far as possible the child should attempt independent action in cases where he has been dependent whenever conditions are favourable for success.

The problem of directing normal individuals so that they will make the most of their lives is so complex that no one is justified in attempting it guided only by science and his own ideas. It is safer to arrange conditions as far as possible so that the individual shall have opportunities for and stimuli to normal development along many lines, leaving the direction of development largely to his own natural responses and choices. Changes in environment and activities, and an attitude of sympathetic understanding, are generally advisable whenever an individual is believed not to be developing as well as his capacities make possible.

II

MENTAL HYGIENE

Physical Peculiarities

Lack of normal physiological apparatus and functioning does not necessarily and directly interfere with good mental hygiene, but it does often produce difficulties in the way of making successful mental adjustments. An individual who is physiologically deformed, a weakling or different in any marked way from his fellows, cannot easily adjust his behaviour to that of other people, and this is likely to disturb his mental adjustments. A blind person tends to become dependent, a deaf person, unsocial. The greater the effect upon his behaviour and that of others toward him produced by his condition, the less well balanced and normal is he likely to become. In the best institutions for the blind and deaf, the inmates are now treated as nearly as possible like normal persons, and expected to behave in the same way. This has resulted in great improvement in the mental normality of the graduates.

It is possible to maintain mental balance when there is a marked physiological disorder, as witness the lives of some invalids ; but on the other hand, slight physiological or other peculiarities may result in a seriously diseased mentality. For example, a hare-lip may prevent an individual from ever becoming well adjusted to people. Persons of mixed race who are not handicapped in the slightest degree physically or intellectually are usually at a serious disadvantage in their association with people of other parentage, because of the attitude and behaviour of these people toward one who differs from their race. Giants and dwarfs are treated differently from average people, and are therefore handicapped in making proper mental adjustments, but sometimes not more so than persons not quite so extreme in size, who are expected to conform more closely to group standards.

It is a very fundamental truth of nature that the normal individual of the species is hardier than the one who diverges in a marked degree from his fellows. This truth of biology and physiology is reflected in the *mental* attitude of human beings toward each other. A large proportion of human beings are alike in all essential particulars, and learn how to behave in much the same ways toward each other. The few persons of unusual traits may be more or less interesting or disgusting, but are generally regarded with doubt and disfavour. One is slightly disturbed by a one-eyed person, an individual with an extra finger or with a mutilated member, or one with a prominent birth-mark. This fact makes it difficult for the peculiar individual to adjust as ordinary individuals do to others. The mere fact of being unusually large for his age may prove an insurmountable difficulty to a boy in the maintenance of good mental hygiene. Unusual mental quickness or slowness often hinders the process of attaining mental balance in reacting to others. It is true that the " freak " in biology or among human beings sometimes proves vigorous and is the means of developing a new variety of the species or, in the case of human beings, of changing the social customs of his people in a marked degree. The chances, however, are always against the very unusual individual, plant, animal, or person, and only one of many usually succeeds in making normal adjustment.

In view of these truths it is clear that the problem of securing good mental hygiene is greater for any individual who differs in any way, by nature or training, from the people with whom he associates. It should be equally clear that it may be more difficult for normal individuals to adjust to the customs of some peoples than to those of others. Conventions that require everyone to spend many hours in prayer, days without food, to become completely continent, or that make women dependent servants, may be difficult for normal human beings to conform to, and yet failure to do so may present still greater difficulties of social adjustments. There are, therefore, social problems analogous to those of public health regulations that present special difficulties to individuals.

KEEPING MENTALLY NORMAL

Some of the more important characteristics of normal behaviour and attitudes favourable to maintaining mental health, may be enumerated.

(1) The general attitude toward life of normal human beings is that of striving to preserve one's individual life and to increase its experiences, especially those that give satisfaction. This means that it is normal to be optimistic rather than pessimistic in behaviour, even though pessimistic theories may be held. The behaviour of most people shows this characteristic, and the ones who act as if life was not worth living, are those who are not in a good condition of physiological and mental health. A healthy attitude of this kind does not require a fatuous expectation that everything will be all right, but a profound instinctive drive that makes it seem worth while to strive for whatever seems desirable even though not easily attainable. Whenever one begins to say, " What is the use ? " he is showing signs of falling below the normal standard of living, which finds some of the various activities of working and playing, social and religious conformities, etc., worth while doing. Some of these may be undervalued because other ends seem so much more important, but for purposes of mental hygiene an individual needs to preserve an attitude toward life similar to that shown by most people in all ages, which is that of " carrying on " in a more or less optimistic way. To be interested in nothing indicates low vitality, and to be interested exclusively and continuously in one thing is likely to lead to lack of mental balance.

The beginnings of unhygienic states are, therefore, indicated by marked variation in behaviour from the usual type of human action. Refusal to act in special ways as others do in his group, may be a healthy reaction against unnecessary artificial restrictions, yet persistence in such conduct with resulting opposition and disapproval of companions, makes it difficult for the person to remain normal. The pacifist in war-time becomes a social outcast. The boy who shows contempt for athletics with their accompanying cheers, emblems, etc., will find it hard to adjust himself socially to his fellows. If he smokes where the sentiment against it is almost universal, he has difficulties in adjusting to the people of his group ; but if he refuses to smoke when all his fellows do, it is scarcely less difficult to maintain a satisfactory relation with them. In such instances the strong individual may retain his mental balance among people who differ from him in many forms of behaviour, and yet adjust in general to his companions.

Anyone, however, who varies markedly in interests and behaviour from those common to people in all ages, is not likely to be well adjusted in his own personality, even though he is talented and even admired by certain peoples, *e.g.* the religious ascetic, or the hermit or the philosopher who have no interest in bodily comforts of eating, resting, no interest in exercise or playful pursuit, no love for mates or children nor desire for friends, nor sympathy for unfortunates, no interest in life, death and the phenomena of nature. Whatever the achievements of the great philosophers and religious leaders who have lost these human interests, the fact remains that in general their attitude is not favourable to healthy mental balance.

(2) Not only is a normal attitude toward life as indicated by interests needed, but also a mind which works as the minds of others do. This is closely associated with acquiring a common language by means of which minds are adjusted to each other, and rendered orderly in their reactions. The mental peculiarities and twists of a deaf person disappear in proportion as he gains control of a language by means of which he may adjust his thoughts and actions to those of his companions. Children having all their senses, sometimes show considerable mental disturbances because of speech defects, or on account of difficulties in learning to read or write.

Vigorous and persistent attempts to make a child change from left- to right-hand writing, sometimes produce serious speech and mental disorders.

In an *orderly* mind, not only do words mean nearly the same as they do to other people, but they are associated with some words much more closely than with others. Extreme mental disorder is indicated clearly by the use of disconnected words and phrases, as well as by sentences expressing unrelated thoughts. Psychologists have developed a series of association tests which reveal less marked instances of mental disorder by variations from the usual. The subject responds to a stimulus word by the first word possible. If he responds to " flower " by " rose ", " violet ", " lily ", his minds works in that particular as it has been found to do in a large proportion of minds. The same is true if he responds to " tool " by " hammer " or " saw ". If, however, he responds to " tool " with " rose ", and to " flower " with " hammer ", serious mental disorder would be indicated. To respond to " flower " by the name of a rare variety, or by a Latin or German name would be unusual and individual, but not necessarily abnormal. To give the same response to many different stimulus words is an indication of undue prominence of some mental attitude— called technically a " mental complex ", and is a sure indication of more or less serious disturbance of mental balance.

By recording the response to a hundred standard words, the usual responses to which are known, the per cent of " individual " responses may be found, and if this is high, a disordered mentality is indicated. From this it is clear that mental hygiene is promoted by common experiences that one has learned to indicate by the same word and sentence forms as are used by companions. Good language training and mental hygiene are, therefore, closely related.

Logical thinking is also related to a well-balanced mentality. The self responses must also be limited by the responses of others. When one's facts or conclusions are disputed by several persons who have had an equal chance to know, one must not refuse to give weight to their testimony. If one does, there is no effective check upon the development of all

P

sorts of individual illusions of the senses, and mistakes in reasoning.

(3) A *normal balance* between *situations* and *responses* is a condition closely associated with mental hygiene. An individual who makes little or no response to a situation ordinarily calling forth fear, anger, grief, or sympathy, or who becomes terrorized, wildly hysterical or maudlin in his responses is at least temporarily more or less abnormal. The same is true of one who jumps at sounds which merely cause a turning of the head by most persons ; or who is irritated by small happenings which are little noticed or matters of amusement to most people ; or the person who laughs loudly at things that cause no more than a slight smile in most persons ; or who is in despair because of slightly unfavourable news. Fatigue, indigestion, or a recent disagreeable experience may render some responses excessive, and some individuals are habitually more responsive than others, but persons who fail to mitigate their excessive reactions are likely to become less well balanced and healthy in their mentality.

(4) It is in accordance with the nature of human beings to respond not only to the stimulus of real situations now confronting one, but to memories of past ones, and to plan responses to those pictured as occurring in the future. A *proper balance between the real and the imagined needs to be maintained.* One who acts only in the present is only temporarily adjustive, one who depends chiefly upon memory fails to respond to significant differences in situations being met, while the one who pictures the future only may fail to act as is fitting to the present situation. It is the here and now that demands the response, but to be of the right character the wisdom of past experiences and the hopes of a better future must help direct the efforts being made. The one who acts chiefly in response to his present perceptions may make many mistakes, yet not be troubled by mental disorders. It is the person who lives a great deal in the past or future, continually saying " If so and so . . . I would . . .," either acts not at all, or fails when he acts to adjust to things as they are. Such a condition once started is likely to grow worse

as the individual makes mistakes, especially in his reactions toward other people. Some dreaming of dreams and seeing of visions, is a valuable human trait, but if not balanced by adjusted responses to things as they exist, healthy, vigorous mental activity is not likely to continue.

(5) One of the most important factors in normalizing and harmonizing individual behaviour is human association. Individuals of normal mentality often become queer and many of them insane when placed in solitary confinement, though some through reading and imagination are able to keep in harmony with other human minds. The person who fails to adjust to people or who withdraws from friends and relatives is already showing signs of unhealthful mental functioning which is likely to grow worse the more he avoids companions whose attitudes and behaviour will help restore normality. It is also hard to maintain complete normality if association is with one sex only. A person who as a child was a member of a family of more than one child, and who later married and had children, is, in general, less subject to mental disorders than an only child, or than one from a broken home, or one who forms no home of his own.

(6) Physically and mentally there is need for the maintenance of a proper balance between *work* and *play*, between the necessary carefully made adjustments involved in securing the necessities of life, and the care-free enjoyment of living. Work narrows life interests and leaves many of the essentials of human life—love, beauty, humour—without exercise ; while play may leave unsatisfied the pleasures of achieving useful ends. These two types of activity naturally supplement each other, sometimes being combined in complex activities but more often alternating one with the other. Both physical and mental health are favoured by *daily* rhythms devoted to work, alternating with play. Balance may be maintained by long periods of one then the other, or by some mingling of the two ; but most persons are surer of mental health if they spend a portion of *every day* in some necessary directed effort, and another portion in freely chosen relaxing activity of plays or sports, or of rest and amusement. A complete vacation

period in a new environment is a valuable corrective to extreme mind sets, but not an adequate substitute for daily recreation.

(7) The last and absolute essential in maintaining a healthy personality is success. Just as the bodily organism must adjust to the environment with a considerable degree of success in order to survive, so the personality which is a group of organized behaviour habits and tendencies is dependent for its continued and effective existence upon the making of successful behaviour adjustments, especially to persons. Success is the securing of the results expected and desired, by efforts of some kind ; or in other words, it is the changing of images into realities. The baby who images a bright object that he sees, as touching his lips, has success when he can grasp it and bring it to his mouth. Every voluntary act that brings the expected result, whether it be a simple movement or a complex series directed toward some end for days or years, is an instance of success. A considerable portion of every person's directed activities must bring success if vigorous mental health is to be maintained.

EVIDENCES OF SUCCESS

Objective success in controlling one's muscles in dealing with objects and in altering their relations, comes early, and is always healthful. Many cures of nerve troubles of adults are now effected by occupational therapy.

The human element, however, nearly always enters into such success and modifies the harmonizing results. If companions are much more successful in producing such changes than one's self, the success is minimized. Renewed effort and improvement is of advantage, but is not wholly satisfactory unless achievement seems to be the equal in some respects, of at least some of one's companions. It is not at all necessary that this shall be the case in every undertaking, but in order to maintain normal self-respect one must achieve what seems to him success equal or superior to that of someone else, in *some* field of effort. To the young child and to the feeble-minded, as well as to the average person and the genius, such objective success is equally necessary. In one sanatorium where there are many wealthy men, some of them are greatly helped by the experience of constructing a material object which is so good that someone will buy it.

Praise is an addition to, and sometimes a substitute for objective achievement. Either to purchase or use what has been made, or to employ the maker, gives more convincing evidence of success than mere praise. Everyone craves the appreciation of others as evidence of personal significance. In a good institution for feeble-minded, in a good family, school, community or state, every individual has a task that he can perform well enough so that he will be recognized by his fellows as useful. Without this assurance, normal mentality is scarcely attainable. Elderly people wish to remain useful, and are only partly satisfied by memories of past successes, even though they are exaggerated.

To be able to attract the attention of others is a form of success very stimulating to some individuals. It shows personal distinctiveness and power, and many notoriety seekers are quite satisfied with such success, even though it brings disapproval and punishment. Boys in school who have not succeeded in other ways sometimes become adepts in annoying the teacher. School and society should give opportunity for all to achieve more healthful and useful types of success.

IDEALS AID FEELINGS OF SUCCESS

In some lines, especially artistic and literary, the evidences of success are not certain, and a genius may for long lack objective and social evidence of his success, while a person having a few fond, foolish relations and friends, but no ability, may achieve what seems to him like immediate successes.

The subjective evidences of success in society and art are not closely correlated with objective success. To an individual, success is measured by the approximation of the result to the idea or ideal of results previously formed. To a child or to an adult of little ability, a crude creation or simple act may equal or exceed his expectations, while to a genius a work of superb merit may seem crude compared with his ideal of what should be done. It is for this reason that gifted persons are not unfrequently less confident than are those inferior in mentality. Kipling threw his " Recessional " into the waste basket, from which it was rescued to be proclaimed a great achievement.

The natural tendency of most persons is to overestimate his own achievement and personality. This tendency in the average person in the usual surroundings of living with persons whose abilities and standards are about the same as their own, is checked and balanced by objective results and expressed opinions of companions.

Persons who are all the time with inferiors may get a superiority complex, while those surrounded by superiors may get an inferiority complex. Persons of low mentality are more likely to obey the natural instinct trend and believe themselves superior, as was recently shown by questioning such people in an institution. The gifted person, because of his ability to form higher ideals and to see how far achievements fall below them, often underestimates himself. A person superior in one line but inferior in general intelligence often overestimates himself.

Normal balance for most persons is assured by association with equals and also with those who are superior, and with those inferior ; by experiences of acting as leader of others in some lines and as followers in others ; or by being with a different group. This normal relation to companions should be sought by young people as a preventative of inferiority and of superiority complexes unfavourable to mental health and development of a normal personality.

Everyone needs the corrective of the opinions of others on their work. Some need approval to keep them trying to achieve, while others need some criticism to lead them to more careful work and higher ideals. Mental hygiene is the result of a proper balance between the self-judgment of the individual and the criticism, favourable and unfavourable, of companions and authorities. To rely wholly on self-judgments, or wholly on the opinions of others, may lead to extreme divergences from normal mentality.

The greater the effort required to secure success, the more it means to the person attaining it. Luck, which singles one out in the eyes of others, is, however, regarded as in some way a success of self. To have an unusual object, an unusual experience, even an unusual disease, marks one as distinguished among his fellows, and may serve as a rather poor substitute for success attained by well-directed effort.

UNHYGIENIC WAYS OF SEEKING SUCCESS

A large proportion of abnormal mentality grows out of either avoiding any comparison of ideals and achievements as viewed by self and others, or by failure to adjust one to the other. In the first case the individual refuses to do anything that he does not expect will be judged favourably, and rationalizes or convinces himself that he can, or has, or is going to attain wonderful success " when . . .", or " if . . .", or he " would have done so if . . .". Such persons find many excuses and avoid acts in which exact comparisons are easily made by observing or measuring, such as athletic contests. Such demonstrations prevent them from fleeing from reality and living in an imaginary world in which great successes are attained by self with little effort. Persons who are introverts, interested in what is happening to self rather than in objective events, are especially liable to abnormal developments of this type.

The extrovert individual is in less danger, as he keeps trying one thing after another until he develops ability to do what he attempts. He is not greatly troubled by what people think, but is interested in objectively comparing achievements of self and others, and in improving his own work.

The normal person is by turns an extrovert and an introvert, a realist and an idealist, a practical man and a theorist, and thus he maintains a balanced growing personality. The extreme introvert is likely to avoid all correctives while the extreme extrovert finds them continually in the objective environment, and needs only to have that rich and varied, in order to preserve normality.

Another common cause of mental abnormality is failure to adjust satisfactorily to many slight but often recurring situations in daily life. One is irritated by the creaking of a door, or the lack of order in a companion's habits, and each time it recurs is again irritated, but without any attempt to correct the objective situation, or to subjectively react to it in a more satisfactory way. Irritation is not a successful response, and he who is frequently irritated by the same situation is lacking in success, and is on the way to an abnormal state. One must change his objective responses or his subjective attitude, or continue to fail in meeting the situation successfully. Sometimes it is best to do one, and sometimes the other. The one who tries to change everything may accomplish much, but is sure of many failures, while the one who adjusts himself so as not to be disturbed by anything is often of little use in the world. When it is a person who irritates, it is especially difficult to get a satisfactory adjustment, because the attempt to change the other person is likely to arouse his opposition, while enduring all his obnoxious behaviour may lead to its continuance and increase. Often the difficulty cannot be met without a change in both physical and human environment. One way, therefore, of preserving normality is to avoid objects, tasks, situations and people to whom one cannot react successfully. A man must, however, himself learn to do some adjusting of his own conduct and attitudes, or he will continually have to change his occupations and companions to avoid irritating failures, and this in the end will show him up as a life failure. A change in environment does, however, give a chance to adjust without being so much hampered by previous failure.

Scolding, fretting and worrying are all indications of lack of adjustment. If people would realize that to do these things in response to the same situations again and again is a thoroughly stupid performance, they might be stimulated to change their behaviour. Hamilton's studies of two hundred persons with nervous disorders show that such non-adjustive, irritating responses to situations were the most frequent cause of the difficulties.

There is another way of attaining seeming success which in a moderate degree is healthful. This is by identifying self with a relative, friend, hero or society that is successful, and associating one's own activities in some way with the person or organization. The one who cheers with the crowd may get as much of a success thrill as the chief performers. In modern life this form of success is possible to very humble members of school, church and state, and with a variety of organizations. With specialization in industries, and in organizations where an individual has only a small part in the ends accomplished, it is worth while to emphasize this substitute for evidences of individual success now so scarce in factory life.

Bragging, bluffing, indifference, or showing off in another field are compensatory ways of trying to secure success in the eyes of others, and of partially concealing from self one's deficiencies. This is a false or pseudo success, not quite healthful and never yielding the permanent, peaceful satisfaction of real success won by appropriate effort.

LIFE AS A STRIVING AND ACHIEVING

The impulse to achieve is so strong that it is striven for in countless ways that bring no other reward to the one making the effort. The time and energy spent in solving puzzles of all sorts with no reward save the satisfaction of success, is one strong evidence of this. Most games are interesting partly for the same reason. The rewards of the scientist, the inventor, the artist, the explorer, the reformer, and even of many men in the commercial field, and of women in social affairs, is often chiefly, and sometimes wholly, the satisfaction of the success attained. This ideal may sustain one for years of non-realization and make one think the effort worth while, even if success is never attained.

SELECTED RESEARCHES

'TWINS AND ORPHANS." By A. H. WINGFIELD and PETER SANDIFORD, University of Toronto. From *Journal of Educational Psychology*, September 1928. *Quoted by Permission.*

The twin subjects comprised one hundred and two pairs selected at random from the public schools of Toronto and Hamilton. The orphans were twenty-nine pupils in a fraternal orphanage. . . .

Thirteen tests in all were given—the best that could be chosen. . . .

Summary. 1. There is no significant difference in the amount of mental resemblance in mental traits between younger and older twins.

2. Twins are no more alike in those traits upon which the school has concentrated its training than in general intelligence. . . .

6. There are two distinct types of twins because :

(*a*) The like-sex group which must partly consist of a number of the uni-ovular, or identical pairs, shows a higher degree of mental resemblance than the unlike-sex group.

(*b*) Physically identical pairs show a higher degree of resemblance than fraternal pairs.

(*c*) The degree of resemblance of siblings in mental traits is nearer to that of unlike-sex pairs than to that of the like-sex pairs. This bears out the contention that unlike-sex pairs are, from the genetic standpoint, really siblings that are born at the same time.

(*d*) Members of fraternal pairs of twins show, on the whole, greater diversity in school grades than members of physically identical pairs. This latter group is probably composed largely of uni-ovular twins.

7. Orphan children who have been reared together for a considerable portion of their lives, are no more alike than unrelated children paired at random, either in general intelligence or other intellectual traits. . . .

10. The amount of resemblance in general intelligence varies from $r = 0$ for unrelated individuals to a maximum of $r = \cdot 90$ for physically identical twins. Intermediate values are found in accordance with the genetic relationship of the individuals. Therefore, there is an increasing degree of resemblance in general

intelligence among human beings with an increasing degree of blood relationship among them. *Ergo*, general intelligence is an inherited trait.

CASE STUDIES—JUDGE BAKER FOUNDATION
Boston, September 1922

CASE STUDY, No. 2
Quoted by Permission

WINTHROP STANDEN, Jr., 15 yrs. 8 mos. ; of New England ancestry on both sides.

Introductory Statement

Mr. and Mrs. Winthrop Standen, evidently thoroughly right-minded people, came for advice concerning their son. To them he is a baffling puzzle. Except for him, every member of their families that they have heard of has had high standards of integrity and citizenship. For two years Winthrop has caused them anxiety through school misdemeanours and through repeated and serious dishonesty which began earlier in small ways.

Family

A careful, detailed account of the family as learned through Winthrop's intelligent and much concerned parents may be summarized :

Father : 48, large, fine physique, bears the appearance of the good habits which he is said to have always had. Member of a successful business firm. Had two years of college life and then financial circumstances led him into business. A reader and student along the lines of his own vocation. A hard worker, but outside of working hours very companionable with his children. Evidently an admirable father.

Father's Family : Rural New England people earlier ; in the father's generation living in small towns ; ambitious for education and recently prospering. Substantial people, free from nervous and mental diseases and anything like criminalism.

Mother : Healthy, even-tempered, a good housekeeper, devoted to her children. Graduated from high school.

Mother's Family : Steady and industrious people, mostly living in country districts. Not ambitious for higher education, but there has been no exception to the family reputation for integrity and sound mentality.

Siblings : Four sisters, all younger than Winthrop. All healthy and normal in every way.

Developmental History

Parents healthy at time of conception. Normal pregnancy ; full term and normal delivery ; 8 lb. at birth. Breast fed. No illness during infancy. Walked and talked first at about 1 year. Some disturbance at 2½ years, followed by a period of poor general condition. Some diseases common to childhood very mildly. Tonsils and adenoids removed at 5 years. No illnesses since. All along very large for age.

Home and Neighbourhood Conditions and Influences

Winthrop has been brought up in a very sensible home, where there has been plenty, but no luxury, where there has been no friction and where his parents have endeavoured to give him the best that an intelligent American household affords in pleasant suburban surroundings. There has been good reading, outdoor sports, social life, contact with church, and a very reasonable attitude towards his needs as far as realized. The father has given all of his time outside of his work to companionship with his children.

Companions

In connection with the Boy Scouts and in his own neighbourhood, Winthrop has found some very desirable friends, whom he has retained. But he has also formed a very influential comradeship with one young fellow, somewhat older than himself, who is a notorious scamp, but who has succeeded in avoiding punishment because of the political influence of his family. Through this fellow Winthrop has formed casual acquaintance with an undesirable crowd of older fellows. His association with girls has been very normal and wholesome.

Habits

Winthrop's eating and sleeping habits have always been quite normal. He has not been allowed tea or coffee and has never been in the habit of smoking. He has had almost no experience with bad sex habits, has not been immoral with girls.

Interests

The only two keen interests which Winthrop displays are in connection with his companionship and in things mechanical. His father claims that at the age of eight Winthrop could name and put together all the parts of an automobile. He has now grown quite expert in making repairs and is perfectly happy if he is going over a motor and its parts.

His gregariousness has led to his forming some undesirable friendships as well as some good ones, as mentioned before, and as these ties have been formed it has been difficult for him to break away.

Beyond this, Winthrop is moderately interested in sports, especially swimming ; but he has never taken much part in competitive games. He is a first-class Scout and has been much interested in Scout activities. Earlier he was much of a reader of boys' books, the only kind he reads now occasionally. He was interested in church affairs and in the activities of a social club. But the outstanding point that his father makes is that Winthrop doesn't show much lasting enthusiasm about any of his interests except mechanical.

In school, Winthrop showed a fair amount of interest, at least he never truanted, until he entered high school. Since then he has become very indifferent towards his studies.

School and Work History

Winthrop attended two private schools and one public school as his parents moved about. He was a moderately good student and offered no conduct problem until, at the age of 13 he entered the high school in the town where he now lives. Truancy soon began there and in a few months Winthrop withdrew. In each of the two succeeding years this has been repeated, so that he has never completed one entire year. His grades in the high school have been uniformly poor and the school principal has expressed the opinion that Winthrop is subnormal. His course has consisted entirely of languages and mathematics. Most of the time he has taken three languages and algebra. He had neither shop nor laboratory work.

During the periods when Winthrop was out of school, he worked in several places. His father has tried to prevent what he thought was harmful employment; Winthrop wanted to work in a garage but his father would not allow this because he has been fearful of the association with an inferior class of men. For a short time the boy was employed by his father's firm, although he did not work directly under his father. In nearly every position before he has been long at it, he has taken a day or two off, without permission, and of course his employer in each case has discharged him because of his evident lack of interest.

Delinquencies

Winthrop was first known to steal at 10 years. He took small sums of money from home, and occasionally larger amounts, which he spent in boyish fashion, sometimes hiding the money to spend later on. After his stealing was discovered, Winthrop was neither severely scolded nor punished, because the parents felt that they were largely to blame through their own carelessness in leaving money about. Later, when he was 12, he stole three times, five dollars and ten dollars at a time, from a neighbour at whose house he went to play with a boy. And this was done in spite of severe whippings which followed the discovery of his first thieving. Finally they thought that he had learned a lesson when he was made to pay the whole sum back from his spending money. No repetition of his delinquency was known until a year before we saw him, when with a bad companion, he was implicated in a burglary and petty stealing—a ridiculous affair because it was so petty—for which he was taken to court and placed on probation under suspended sentence. Later it was discovered that he had been repeatedly misappropriating automobiles with this same companion, driving the automobiles away from private garages in the night-time, but returning them. When finally trapped at this he made a melodramatic escape, but was, of course, caught. He was allowed to stay in jail for a week ; then the case was appealed to a higher court, his parents not wishing him to be sent to correctional school. But even after this Winthrop showed no deep concern about making good. He did not hold jobs, and his father asserted he " could not believe him on oath " now.

During the last two years he had also been in school difficulties, mainly truancy, elsewhere mentioned.

Physical

Winthrop makes a decidedly good impression ; he is clean-looking, well-dressed, manly in appearance. His head is well shaped ; he has a very light complexion ; his features are somewhat heavy, with comparatively weak mouth and chin. His expression is pleasant and responsive ; his posture is strong and upright ; his manners are good.

Weight, 155 lb. Height, 5 ft. 9 in. Strength very unusual for age. Particularly large arms and legs. Adult voice. In development of primary sex characteristics almost adult type. Teeth and throat in good condition. Vision and hearing normal. Physical examination otherwise quite negative.

Mental

According to age-level tests, grades as supernormal. Intelligence Quotient 116.

On the auditory memory test (immediate recall of digits) he achieved a superior adult performance. Language ability, very good except for rather meagre vocabulary. Apperceptive ability, with language very good ; with pictorial representations, very good—an adult performance. Speed and accuracy of hand movements, slightly above average. Speed of mental response, very rapid. Ability to carry in mind and mentally work with visual representations, exceedingly good. Ability to handle constructive simple problems with concrete material, very good ; perceptions of relationship of form, rapid. Mechanical ability, very good. Generalizing ability for abstract ideas, very good. Learning ability, exceedingly good for rote visual and rote auditory materials and for ideas.

Mental Balance

From observation and on test results there were no signs whatever of poor mental balance. Winthrop has good control of mental powers, is well oriented and coherent.

Personality Traits

Winthrop is described by his parents as essentially a group boy and as very popular among his companions. He is just one of the crowd, not standing out against influences either good or bad. Indeed, he himself says he is socially suggestible. The traits which have been outstanding in the last two or three years are his easy-going love of pleasure, his restless changeableness, his resentfulness of criticism from his family, and his self-assertive and argumentative attitude. Also, he has grown to have a lack of feeling toward his misconduct; he doesn't seem to mind worrying his parents or to feel disgraced even when arrested. Towards his father he has grown extremely reserved. He assumes an air of manliness in wanting to manage family affairs, but is really boyish and unformed. He is not without some shrewdness, and a sense of humour. In the last year seems to have made very little effort toward doing better, and there has been much lying.

Winthrop has always seemed unusually refined and clean-minded. Many of his relatives have remarked about this.

As a little boy he was very affectionate and nice to the younger children, but somewhat jealous of them. He has always been impulsive rather than deliberate. He has never appeared to have a particularly sensitive nature. He is quite even-tempered, never moody.

His school principal reports him in no way vicious, not insolent or bad-tempered, but apparently thoroughly indifferent to his success, both in regard to his work and his conduct. His employers say that he starts in as " a regular whirlwind ", but soon slacks up, and after a little while becomes worthless.

Boy's Own Story

In talking to us, Winthrop seems sincere, although evidently he lacks energy at all commensurate with his size and strength.

He says it was foolish of him to let anybody get him into things that were wrong. Since he entered high school he has been in with a bad crowd right along. His stealing and truancy have been under the influence particularly of one young fellow who is " the biggest all-round crook " he ever heard of, and who yet gets out of everything because of political influence of his family. The fellow's father is dead and his mother allows him to do as he pleases, and the old friends of the father at the city hall let him off all the time. In answer to the question: "Why do you go with him?" he says, " I don't understand that myself. Everything seriously wrong I have ever done has been his idea."

His earlier stealing was simply taking money from his relatives, and he doesn't feel that was anything of consequence. Come to think of it, he did hear boys talk about stealing—older boys—when he was a little fellow, but he doesn't remember distinctly anything about their influence in starting him.

Concerning his lying, he says, " It is part of the same trouble. Going with this crowd and lying about things makes it seem as if I had a weak will that way."

He takes things as they come, never worries about them. He

doesn't plan his stealing ahead and denies any special impulse or temptation to steal.

It is because he doesn't like the high school that he has been truant. These fellows come around and want him, so he goes out with them ; but anyway, he has had a general dislike for school lately. He has been taking a general course ; he has had no shop work, and that is what he likes. He has always been interested in mechanical things. He wanted to do repair work in a garage, but his father wouldn't let him. He is not old enough to get into a regular factory. Says he has never had any job he liked. At present he is simply working as assistant soda clerk in a drug store.

Although Bill, the boy with whom he goes, smokes heavily and drinks, and although the whole crowd gamble, Winthrop denies that he has done any of these things. He maintains that the crowd is very little interested in girls and that there is no bad sex talk and no bad pictures. " They don't go in for that sort of thing." He learned when he was in the sixth grade about bad sex habits from a older boy, but he soon stopped. " I never had that inclination."

He wants to leave school. Bill and this crowd are there and it would only mean trouble if he stayed on. " There is no use hanging around my town anyway ; I would just be sure to see these fellows." What he particularly wants to do is to study air-plane construction and mechanics. He would soon understand the engines because he knows so much about automobile engines. He thinks it is wonderful that the air-planes are able to carry their own weight up in the air. He knows about the army air-plane fields, but is afraid that he can't get in because he is so young.

Summary of Staff Conference

PROBLEM : Delinquency :—Stealing occasionally for years. Truancy. Court record for petty burglary. Misappropriation of automobiles.

PHYSICAL : Considerable over-development. Unusual strength. Premature sex development.

MENTAL : 1. Abilities ; somewhat supernormal in general ability. Good memory powers. Good learning ability. Very good mechanical ability. No marked defect or disability. Inadequate interests in comparison to capacities. 2. Mental Balance ; Psychiatric examination negative. 3. Personality ; Assumes manliness, but really is unformed.· Pleasure-loving. Socially suggestible.

BACKGROUND : (a) Heredity : Negative in thoroughly reliable account. Family of rather strong characters and standards. (b) Developmental : Practically negative. (c) Home Conditions ; Unusually good physically and in attempts at companionship. (d) Habits : Negative.

POSSIBLE DIRECT CAUSATIONS : (1) Physical over-development and sex prematurity which is not in accord with (2) Adolescent traits. And possibly (3) Personality traits, particularly suggestibility. (4) Bad companion ; very marked influence. Peculiar situation because this other boy is able to avoid arrest, although really the leader. (5) Educational and vocational situation not in keeping with either general or special abilities. (6) Development of a poor standard of values concerning property rights through defective training in otherwise good home.

PROGNOSIS AND RECOMMENDATIONS : The outlook is distinctly bad under present conditions ; the boy is unlikely to get away from the influence of his old companions. His school and work situations, too, are difficult to adjust satisfactorily. His social suggestibility bespeaks his response to good conditions as well as to bad influences.

Any plan for his future should include his removal from his home town. He needs activity suitable to his large size and strength, and if possible in connection with further education along lines of his special interests. Being in some ways practically adult he should have association largely with men rather than only with boys of his age.

Just where suitable conditions may be found can be discussed in detail with parents. We can at once think of the army and navy technical training schools or camps, but he cannot legally enter yet. In the meantime work at air-plane fields or at a commercial factory or flying field might be considered if someone could have special friendly oversight. Or for a tiding-over period until he is old enough for the above plans to be carried out, he might work on a western ranch.

In the light of our experience with boys associating with bad companions, it is strongly advised that Winthrop go away even while his case is pending in court.

SUBSEQUENT HISTORY

Winthrop was at once sent to stay with relatives in the country until his case was heard in court, when he was placed on probation. In the meantime his father was making efforts to locate a suitable place in the West for him. But Winthrop went to New York one day and there enlisted in the army for training in the air-plane field service. giving his age as 19. His parents decided it was best to make no objections, and very shortly he was sent to a training field in the South-West. He has remained in this service with various transfers and promotions during the last three years. He has stood high in his examinations and has had a splendid record for conduct. His parents tell us that when he came home last time on a furlough he was (at barely 18) almost 6 feet and weighed 175 pounds. They were very well pleased at his success. His father now says, " He is a son to be proud of."

Q

SUGGESTED READINGS

The mental testing movement initiated by Alfred Binet of France, introduced into this country by Goddard, and promoted by Terman and others, has proved of great value in the study of normal individuals; while William Healy has been a leader in studying the individuality of youthful delinquents. General works on mental hygiene and personality are:

BURNHAM, W. H., *The Normal Mind*, 1924.
HOLLINGWORTH, H. L., *Vocational Psychology and Character Analysis*, 1929.
JASTROW, JOSEPH J., *Keeping Mentally Fit*, 1928.
MYERSON, ABRAHAM, *Foundations of Personality*, 1923.
WELLS, F. L., *Mental Adjustments*, 1920.

The following are valuable case studies:

BENEDICT, AGNES E., *Children at the Crossroads. Commonwealth Fund*, 1930.
BURT, C., *The Young Delinquent*, 1925.
COX, CATHERINE, *Early Mental Traits of 300 Geniuses*, 1926.
GOODENOUGH, F. L., and LEAHY, ALICE, *The Effects of Family Relationship upon the Development of Personality*.
HARTWELL, S. W., *Fifty-five " Bad " Boys*, 1931.
HEALY, WILLIAM T., and others, *Reconstructing Behaviour in Youth : A Study of Problem Children in Foster Families*, 1929.
HEALY, WILLIAM T., *The Individual Delinquent*, 1915.
Judge Baker Foundation Case Studies. Series 1, Numbers 1–20, Boston, 1922–23.
MATEER, FLORENCE, *The Unstable Child*, 1924.
PRINCE, MORTON, *Clinical and Experimental Studies of Personality*, 1929.
SAYLES, MARY B., *The Problem Child in School. Commonwealth Fund*, 1925.
SHAW, E. S., *The Delinquent Boy's Own Story*, 1930.
SLAWSON, J., " Marital Relation of Parents and Juvenile Delinquency " : *Journal of Delinquency*, page 78, Sept.-Nov., 1921.
SOUTHARD, E. E., and GARRETT, MARY C., *The Kingdom of Evils*, 1922.
THOMAS, W. I., and THOMAS, DOROTHY, *The Child in America*, 1928.
THORNDIKE, E. L., *The Measurement of Twins : Archives of Philosophy, Psychology and Scientific Method*, No. 1.

TJADEN, J. C., *The Tjaden Analytical Interviews for the Study of Individual Delinquency and Problem Cases*, 1929.

ZACHRY, CAROLINE B., *Personality Adjustments of School Children*, 1929.

A method of studying children by means of exact records of words and sentences has been developed by PIAGET, JEAN, *The Language and Thought of the Child*, 1926 ; and in others of his publications.

CHAPTER X

BEHAVIOUR IN RELATION TO OTHERS, OR SOCIAL PSYCHOLOGY

THE NEED FOR A SOCIAL PSYCHOLOGY

THE concept of general psychology is of an organism reacting to the physical environment, and improving in doing so by practice. Individual psychology not only recognizes differences in human organisms but emphasizes the truth that, in reacting in his special way, each individual builds a self whose parts are so organized that what is done in response to a situation is not wholly determined by either the situation or the sense and motor apparatus responding, but by the personality of the actor. Social psychology shows that there is also a social determiner of conduct. It no longer assumes a general " social mind " of which each individual mind is a part, but emphasizes the truth that the individual is directed and moulded by companions and by the customs and institutions of the group of which he is a part. These influences are shown to have more to do with determining behaviour than bodily structure or physical environment. Realization of the importance of personal and cultural influences in human behaviour has led to the present deep interest in social psychology, which is concerned with these interrelations.

THE EFFECTS OF THE BEHAVIOUR OF ONE UPON ANOTHER

A hungry individual animal or man, when food is perceived, responds to the situation in a positive and active way. Another individual, also hungry, observes the response perhaps before he has observed the food, and is then influenced by the two stimuli to more vigorous action than the first one, who had the food stimulus only. As the second approaches and begins taking food, both become more active in getting it than would be the case if each was alone, especially if the amount is limited. If one interferes with the other's attempt to get a portion the natural reaction is one of anger, which usually calls forth a similar response with further interference of each with the other, and increase in vigour of struggle. For a time, perhaps, the food is neglected while each tries to match the aggressive behaviour of the other by more effective responses of a similar kind.

In another situation, a strange stimulus or object is reacted to by signs of fear and the attention of a companion is thus attracted who, either with or without seeing the disturbing object, acts much as if he saw it. Any increase in fear behaviour of one individual stimulates similar behaviour on the part of others, and this often has much more to do with the panic that may ensue than the original stimulus. Again, one individual notes an unusual, amusing or beautiful object, approaches it and watches it. A companion noting this behaviour, approaches and looks as long as the two stimuli hold his attention. In all these cases we see that the behaviour of one not only directs the attention of his companions to the same stimulus and increases its significance, but often leads to a situation in which responses are made more to the individual's reaction than to the stimulating objects. In general, each individual is stimulated to do what the other does, and then does it more vigorously than if alone.

If several persons are present acting in a certain way, instead of only one, and another joins the group, his behaviour is almost completely determined by what they are doing. It will readily be seen, therefore, that man who is much of the time in the presence of others, has his attention to things in the environment directed, not always by stimuli that are strongest in themselves, but by those made strong by the actions of others. What he notices in his environment and whether it attracts or repels him, depends not entirely upon its nature, but upon the actions of the people with whom he associates. Enjoyment of bird songs, or of mountain colours are imitated and increased by companions' expression of pleasure in them. Aversion to bugs, worms, and serpents, is due less to their appearance and one's own experiences of their harmful nature, than to the way in which others behave toward them.

Such attitudes are not limited to action while others are present, but the person is often conditioned for life, so that he always reacts to situations as his early companions reacted. What things are to be eaten and what are unclean or dangerous; what is beautiful or desirable or of no account and detestable; what acts are approved; what clothes are becoming; and what one's reactions to all sorts of religious and national symbols are to be, are determined for the individual almost wholly by his companions, especially where all behave in much the same way. No human being sees the objective world with his natural eyes, but chiefly through the glasses provided for him by those among whom he lives; and to an even greater degree his judgments of human behaviour are coloured by the prevailing attitudes of his companions.

Instead of being imitated, a peculiar individual differing in appearance or behaviour from his companions, is often teased or bullied by them, and is thus driven to conform as nearly as possible in dress and behaviour to customs of the group. When fights result from teasing or other causes, or from competitions of any kind, accepted ways of fighting or of playing usually develop, to which all are expected to conform. Individuals who do not act as expected are made uncomfortable until they do. What an individual pleases to do thus tends to become what the group is pleased to have him do.

When there is conflict between two individuals resulting in one or more complete victories for one of them, the defeated individual soon ceases to try to match the behaviour of the other by similar acts. Instead he is likely to wait his turn, take what is left, or he may snatch something and run away. If such a situation occurs frequently between two animals or two persons, it is not long before the prestige of one over the other is established, and often the habits of domination are carried over into various relations between the two.

Between the young and their parents the helplessness of the young and the care-taking instinct of the parents give to the young a more or less dominating control in early infancy. As they become able to act independently, the greater strength and experience of the adults transfers prestige to them in all these relations. If well established, this prestige may continue after the parents have become old and feeble.

Something of the same condition is found in the relations among animals in the poultry and cattle yards, and among dogs. The author once painted the leading cock of the yard, who was promptly attacked by one of the young ones, and was defeated. The victor began to assume leadership, but when the disguise was removed from the former boss all attempts at leadership and fighting by the younger one were abandoned, and he ran away as he had formerly done, whenever the older one threatened him. Summarizing, we find that the behaviour of one stimulates and modifies the acts of a companion. In general, the act of the second is similar to, or matches that of the first. In the case of equals each change in the behaviour of one produces changes in that of the other. Where they are unequal, the weaker makes most of the adjustments and relations of dominance and subordination are established. In either case, adjustments are made that become comparatively satisfactory to both parties, and habits of acting in those ways are established. Individuals joining a group, especially if they are young or weak, are dominated by the customs already established and are almost completely controlled by them. These truths are fundamental in the science of social psychology.

The influence of others is often increased by praise and reward on the one hand, and by disapproval and punishment on the other. Power, position and honour are given individuals who secure general approval ; while those exciting disapproval are deprived of opportunities and are sometimes punished or executed.

The most important stimulators and regulators of individual conduct in every phase of social living, from eating to religious worship, are desires and ambitions on the one hand, and repressions and rules on the other.   One of the most important problems of social psychology is to determine the comparative effectiveness of praise and reward, of blame and punishment. There is a growing tendency which scientific investigations justify, for all sorts of societies to depend less upon punishment in managing their affairs.   Even conservative governments now recognize that increase in opportunities for all is a means of diminishing crime, which may be more effective than repressive laws and penalties.

SPECTATORS AND BEHAVIOUR

At any time after infancy, one rarely behaves in the presence of spectators just as he behaves when alone under the same circumstances.   Young children look for signs of approval or disapproval, partly, at least, because of previous experience in seeing such signs in adults before something pleasing or hindering was done.   In the presence of strangers one or two opposite, yet related, forms of behaviour are often prominent : shyness or showing off.   Some children are cautious about doing anything lest it be not approved ; while others perform all sorts of acts to get notice and favour.   The same tendencies are shown by adults, either in the presence of strangers or of others who may be critical.   Few persons, as experiments show, are not stimulated or inhibited by an audience.   What others think or are likely to think of one's behaviour is an important factor in stimulating and directing conduct in every-day affairs.   We accept as true what is so regarded by others ; judge of our success in every field by evidence of approval, avoid acts condemned as wrong or out of place.   What is known and believed or acted upon is thus determined largely by social surroundings.

PAST SOCIAL INFLUENCES AND BEHAVIOUR

After having associated with certain individuals, a person in new surroundings naturally behaves towards people and objects as his former companions did.   Such action is likely to be checked by noting the way in which present companions are behaving, and their responses to his acts. In the case of equals not greatly different in habits, the change may be so gradual that the individual is unaware of it until he returns to his former surroundings and it is remarked upon, as is frequently the case when a youth has been away to school. Two children, one eighteen and the other four, were taken with their parents for a year, from the Atlantic coast to live on the borders of the Pacific. At the end of the time the four-year-old pronounced his words like the people of the West, being especially effective in sounding "r's"; the pronunciation of the eighteen-year-old had changed only slightly; while that of the parents changed not at all. Foreigners coming here as adults keep their foreign accents and many behaviour attitudes, while their children are often almost indistinguishable by pronunciation and manners from natives, although the transformation is slowed down by being with the parents. If the family is alone among natives, the change from the old to the new social habits and attitudes is rapid; but if among their own nationality it is slow, and may require more than one generation, *e.g.* the Pennsylvania "Dutch".

If the new language is learned and there is much mingling with natives in school and other places, the principle of prestige is likely to have a good deal of influence. The natives are able to teach and direct the new-comer in many ways, while he can help them but little in practical affairs. The foreign child adopts native ways, while the native child is only mildly amused by the peculiarities of the foreigner. The child acquires the new language and learns the new ways before his parents do, and often thus gains a prestige that seriously conflicts with the former prestige of his parents in maintaining their social habits and ideals. It is because of these facts that our language and social habits and ideals have been only slightly changed by immigrants.

When a single individual joins a group having well-established customs, attitudes and beliefs, either as a new-comer or upon return from association with another group, the pressure to conform is usually irresistible unless the individual, because of personal prowess or superior culture attainments, is able to gain prestige, in which case he may bring about important changes in the practices and beliefs of the group. Even after years of training in the culture of the white man, Indians, as a rule, are gradually but surely forced back into the ways of their fathers upon returning to their own people. Adult missionaries, on the other hand, with a background of superior culture, may produce marked changes in a savage tribe.

What phase of culture shall survive when brought into competition with that of another group depends largely upon the worth of one compared with its competitor, as determined by utility or attractiveness ; but in all cases its acceptance is greatly influenced by the ability and prestige of the persons who introduce it to a group, or who favour its adoption. What and how much of the new is accepted and incorporated into the culture of the group depends upon how readily it can be adjusted to the culture patterns too strong to be given up.

INFLUENCE OF PERSONS NOT PRESENT

The persons with whom we associate have been influenced by the behaviour of their companions, and these by persons they have met ; thus some of our behaviour is partly determined by ancestors, near and remote, and by persons of other climes and ages.

Human beings are also influenced not only by personal contact with others, but by means of word descriptions of their conduct. From early times, folk-lore, tales, and traditional heroes have had important effects upon the attitude and behaviour of children even though companions do not behave in the ways described. When written language was developed, and especially after the invention of printing, it became possible to associate mentally with a greater variety of people by reading histories of the behaviour of important people in the past. Great novelists and playwrights also present pictures of imaginary characters and their behaviour so vividly, that their influence rivals, and sometimes surpasses, that of persons present and known.

With the development of the telegraph, telephone, and wireless, and the great facilities for printing and distributing newspapers and books, we can now learn of the recent behaviour of individuals and groups in all parts of the world and be influenced by them.   In addition to this we may witness in the theatre, or hear over the radio all sorts of performances of people we have never met.   Also we may confer directly with friends and strangers at a distance by telephone and otherwise, and have our behaviour modified or directed.

As a result of modern conditions we are more frequently and continually influenced by the actions of persons at a distance than those near at hand.   The change is not so much in amount of influence, as in variety.   Under the old conditions the conduct of the members of the family and of the community was almost the sole director of our attention and behaviour, while now the number and variety of people who modify our behaviour and attitudes is almost unlimited.   This makes for greater variety of interests and activities, but not for greater firmness and consistency of conduct.   Facilities for travel, bringing us into the presence of a variety of people, are also factors working in the same direction.

ORIGIN AND PERSISTENCE OF CUSTOMS

If an individual changed his companions and wandered from one group to another, he would form some personal habits, but they would not be identical with any particular set of customs.   On the other hand, whenever several families are associated with each other, there are not only individual and family habits formed, but customs to which all the families conform more or less closely.   The longer the same families and their descendants are in companionship, the more definite and firmly established do the customs become. In this, as in the influence of individuals upon each other, the customs developed depend upon the equality or lack of equality in the power and prestige of the families. Both classes will practise their special customs, but some customs will always be dominated by the superior group. The lowest class may be slaves, yet rarely are they entirely controlled by personal whims, without regard to customs concerning relations of master and servant. The good master, conforming to the habits and traditions of his families, and the good slave, to those of his companions, may both recognize the laws governing their relations of dominance and subservience between the groups, and of equality between members of the same group.

When there are several distinct classes, but no slaves, as in England, there may be equality in certain fundamentals of right and duty whatever the class to which the individuals belong. In America, prestige is more temporary, more limited in scope, and more individual, depending not so much upon family as upon office held, position in a corporation or an institution, wealth or personal achievement in some field. In every case the position held carries with it obligations to conform to the customs or rules of the group represented, or to which one belongs.

Customs once formed by a group and its different classes, are likely to be accepted and practised by descendants and successors in office or position. Under a static condition of society, customs continue with little change for ages. Those dependent upon personal achievement are more changeable ; yet the successor of a strong ruler, though himself a weakling, inherits prestige from his predecessor.

A strong individual having acquired prestige by his ability and achievement may succeed in changing customs in many lines, and for people of various classes. Such leaders, and some contacts with people of different culture and customs, are the most important factors in changing social customs and the social status of various classes. In order that such influence may be effective, the difference in the culture of the two groups in contact, or of the leader and his followers, must not be too great. In many of the contacts between savage and highly civilized people the fundamental customs of the lower group are often continued, while the tribe is being weakened by the unequal competition.

When an able, original individual within a group undertakes to change fundamental customs, he, rather than the customs, is likely to be destroyed, unless he grafts the new customs on to the old, instead of trying to uproot the old. To destroy religious practices is difficult, especially if force is used to substitute new gods, but it is not impossible if the familiar ritual forms are not too much changed. It is also most sure when changes are promoted, not so much by quick intensive action, as by making conditions favourable for spontaneous growth in the new direction.

When new products, new machines, new offices, new organization, and new knowledge, are being used for old ends, it is easier to change individual prestige and social customs, than when the attempt is to make old tools, old organization, etc., more efficient. Proving that twice as many motions as were necessary were made in laying a brick, brought about little change in the use of the trowel by masons ; but the method of mixing mortar and conveying it to the mason has been completely changed by the invention and use of mixing and hoisting machinery. It is easy to start new practices in a new industry, school or institution of any kind, but exceedingly difficult or impossible to effect changes in old ones.

INSTITUTIONS AND SOCIAL BEHAVIOUR

The term institution implies fundamental ways of acting of a group, such as its language, religion, types of accepted social behaviour. In a more special sense it is used to indicate organizations, with their traditions and rules of procedure. It is in the latter sense that the word is generally used in this chapter.

Institutions behave in much the same way as individuals. Some of the workings of all groups are automatic, like instincts and habits in persons ; while others are directed by conscious purposes of managers and members. The stimulating effects of the behaviour of one organization on others, are the same as for individuals. Prestige and relations of dominance and subservience also characterize the relations of organizations to each other. Just as one individual whose behaviour has been modified by a companion has a different effect upon other individuals, so institutions are changed by the institutions with which they come into contact.

The oldest and most universal type of institution is the *Family*. It is also the one which grows most directly out of original human nature, and whose organization is least planned. Typically, it consists of an adult male and female, and one or more children. If there is more than one husband or wife in most families of a given population, it is usually because of a more or less temporary condition of excess of one or the other sex.

Children do not all come at once, nor remain for life when they do come, so they are not always essential to the existence of the family. If both parents die, a family may consist of children only. Again, several families may live as one. In general, a family is unified by common economic and other interests that keep them in more intimate association with each other than with outsiders.

In practically all families there are relations of dominance of parents over children, and often of older children over the younger ones. In the case of the husband and wife there is rarely complete dominance of one over the other in all things, nor of complete equality. In tribes where the husband lives with the wife's people, she is often dominant; but in most other tribes the man, because of his superior strength and aggressiveness is likely to be the head of the family. There is everywhere less rivalry between adults of the opposite, than between those of the same sex. In the family there is little rivalry between husband and wife, nor are the children nearly equal enough when young, to bring about the same sort of equilibrium as is usually gained when persons of the same age associate with those of their own grade of ability outside of the home. There is indeed rivalry among children for good things, including parental favours, but the older child or the parent is usually powerful in determining what behaviour is supported.

Temporary dominance by the weak is a condition found in the family *more than* in any other institution or human relation. The youngest child by his helplessness, may direct the behaviour of the whole family. So, also, a chronic invalid in a family may dominate it more completely than more powerful members can possibly do. With diversities of age, sex, experience, and the appeal of helplessness or of love, and with relations disturbed by new births and the changes of maturing, it is not strange that in many families there is never a settled adjustment of all members to each other. A well-adjusted family prepares its members for successful individual and social living. The lack, if any, is in the experience of adjusting to equals. This is obtained outside the family, where there is more association with equals who are not obligated or compelled by relationship or authority to act in certain ways, and where choice of leaders and companions may be freely made.

There is no other institution which exerts so intimate and permanent an influence, and none so intimately connecting generations with those of the past and the future. The family not only perpetuates human life physically, but culturally.

Social failures are more frequently found among families that have been broken by death or separation, and among adults who are without family connections. Psychiatrists and social workers are impressed with the great influence of well-adjusted home life upon normal living and social adjustment. Their views are supported by statistics showing that foster homes bring quick and permanent improvement in about three-fourths of the children placed in them. This method of dealing with problem children is now generally admitted to be more effective than that of sending children to institutions such as orphan asylums or truant schools.

To a considerable extent a family group is always an economic and industrial unit co-operating and specializing according to sex and age, in providing necessities and sharing equally and unequally in the advantages gained. Property rights to lands and personal possessions are largely family rights, and names, titles and prestige are passed on to individuals of succeeding generations of the family counting the descent in one or both lines of parentage. Families are important influences in community life. Usually families related by descent constitute genes or patriarchal groups where inheritance is counted in the male line, or clans when counted in the female line. Not unfrequently these clans or genes are distinguished by some common symbol such as the name of an animal. Marriage regulations are often founded on actual or supposed blood relationship, or lack of it. Certain rituals and beliefs are usually characteristic of each of the genes or clans. Political institutions are determined partly ·by local association and partly by real or imputed relationships. In most groups, savage and civilized, there are voluntary societies partly independent of family life. As civilization develops these increase in number, and rival the family in their influence over individuals.

The *School* is now organized and consciously directed as an institution supplementing the family, and acting as a partial substitute for it. The teacher dominates instead of the parents ; but the children are here more influenced by others near their own age than in the home. In so far as this takes place without the teacher's interference the individuals make their own adjustments to each other as comparatively equal competitors, and the customs which become established on the playground, and to a less extent elsewhere, are often quite different from those formed where parents or other adults dominate. In thickly settled regions, children of the same age seek each other outside of school also, and form gangs that are still more independent of any dominating direction by their elders. As a result, before children reach their teens the customs and attitudes developed from associations with equals are often more powerful than those developed under the dominance of elders, either in the home, school or elsewhere.

The school, though beginning its influence later than the family, thus supplies more opportunity for development on an equality basis than the home. The behaviour of each child in school is a stimulus to similar behaviour on the part of others. In the home, with fewer individuals and these of varying age and experience, it is difficult to get the stimulus of uniform behaviour within the group. The teacher has not only the prestige of age and knowledge, but that of a representative of a system of schools consistently directed and supported by society; while parents are strong or weak in their own personalities and often do not have the support of other parents behaving in the same way. Indeed children often find reason for contrary action in observing what their chums' parents do or do not require. For these reasons the relative prestige of school and home is sometimes reversed. Instead of teachers appealing to parents to support them in controlling children in school, parents not infrequently ask teachers to help in controlling the children in the home. Sometimes teachers who have been very successful in directing children in school with the indirect assistance of other teachers, and the habits of pupils developed by other teachers, find the situation entirely different when they try to deal with their own children unaided by the conduct of other mothers and children.

When husband and wife do not support each other in directing the behaviour of children, there is little chance of success by punishment and fear of punishment. On the other hand, the personalities of parents in constant association with children without the concealing protection of school forms and customs, through which the teacher as a person is only partly revealed, are sure to mould the personalities of their children permanently. In many instances, the attempt to maintain authority diminishes the beneficent influence of a loving parent. Parents often accomplish far more by merely being what they are, than by making conscious attempts to make the child what they think he should be.

In both school and home there is growing recognition of the fundamental equality of all human beings of all sorts and ages. Both are slowly becoming less autocratic and more democratic; or in other words, are conducted on more of an equality

R

basis than on the former one of dominance and subordination.

The *Church* as an institution has, in every land and in all
ages, exerted a powerful influence in directing behaviour.   In
many ways its direct influence has decreased, while the indirect
has increased.   It can no longer coerce as formerly.   Attendance
at its services and the observance of religious forms in the
homes and at public meetings have decreased ; and while
religious doctrines excite little interest, the church has
organized numerous societies for various purposes and for
persons of all ages.   By means of these, more people are
brought into contact with each other than by almost any
other institution except the school.   Representatives of the
church, holding to her ideals, are prominent in all sorts of
societies, and many political questions are settled by the
sentiments of church members.   No other institution receives
so much voluntary financial support or has so many helpers
in carrying on the various activities of associated societies.

The institutions of *Government*, local, state and national,
not only forcefully direct human conduct but are important
means of control in other ways.   This influence is most
directly exercised in the support and control of schools, in
bureaus for research and the distribution of information to
the people.   It is concerned in many affairs of common interest
to large numbers of people, and is a medium for registering
and executing their will.   How things are done by the government influences every sort of society, from the village club
up to the largest national organizations ; *e.g.* a constitution
slightly resembling that of the United States, is usually
adopted, and the " rules of order " of Congress are followed
in transacting business.

A common American citizen has a certain prestige which
is increased if he becomes an official of city, state or nation.
Every official in any department of government must conform
to government regulations, and in so doing has power in a
limited field, and something more than personal influence
outside that field.

Industrial and *Financial Institutions* function much as

individuals do. The articles of incorporation are analogous
to the native endowment of the individual ; the way in which
it is managed, to his character. *Esprit de corps* and *morale* in
an institution are as important as ambition and reliability
in the individual. Every one connected with an institution
has his actions directed and his companionships determined
by it. Every official from the office clerk up, answers questions
and approves and disapproves of what is brought to his
attention in accordance with the customs and rules of the
institution and the directions of the manager, rather than
in accordance with his individual wish or opinion. A well-
managed industrial or financial institution also influences the
conduct of employees outside of working hours. The best-
managed institutions are as careful to preserve their reputations
as individuals are to preserve their personal honour.

Voluntary Organizations for fellowship, benevolence, etc.,
many of them national in scope with branches in every
community, are important features of social life today. Just
as machines have taken the place of tools, so organizations
have taken the place of individuals as cultural forces. Their
facilities and support are necessary in every attempt to bring
about social changes.

Institutions have many advantages over persons ; their
life is usually long and may even be everlasting ; their rules,
customs, and policies have been tried out in many situations.
They combine the abilities of many, and wield influence based
on the prestige of past achievements.

COMMUNICATION

The most primitive of institutions, the *family*, is the least
affected within itself by modern facilities of communication,
since most of the association of its members, is face to face.
In local communities, various organizations bring people
together, but telephones and the local newspapers greatly
facilitate a common community life. *Schools* are known to
the public through children, parent-teacher associations, items
of news in papers, public events, and school reports. Schools

communicate with and influence each other by means of visits of teachers, public educational meetings, local and national, by state and national reports, and by means of special journals and books. Courses of study and methods of teaching and managing are similar in all the forty-eight states, not at all because of national regulations, and only to a limited degree because of state laws, but principally because one school copies from others. A new method of teaching spreads among schools nearly as rapidly as a new game or a new style of hat among individuals. Every school-board, superintendent and teacher is influenced in all that is done by knowledge of what is being done elsewhere. Schools imitate and compete just as people do, although they may be thousands of miles apart. The use of scientific tests and measurements, along with greater facilities for publicity, has increased the tendencies to common standard practices. Schools and school-rooms sometimes gain prestige by inventions and innovations, but the larger number imitate and compete in the same types of activities, and thus become more standardized.

Churches are more like families than schools, the denominations corresponding to races, and the local church to a family. The local church members are brought into association partly by the regular services, but more by the various church societies concerned in activities not distinctly religious. Churches of some denominations keep in touch with others of their denomination by general assemblies and the help of travelling officials, but especially by denominational journals. The most effective means of preserving denominational unity are the denominational creeds, hymns and rituals, and the common training of pastors. The old, more ritualistic churches, of course, preserve much greater uniformity than the non-ritualistic churches where individuality of ministers is shown in the church services and management.

There is some competition and imitation among churches of the same denomination, and between the different denominations in the same neighbourhood ; but not a great deal because rarely do the several churches have many of the same people at their services. Most persons go only to the church of their parents, or to the one nearest or the one attended by their friends, and a few " shop around ", but these latter usually do so for only a short time. The churches compete for new-comers ; the wealthy ones using fine music and other incidental attractions, rather than inducements along distinctly religious lines. As a result, changes in churches come not so much from the influence of one church on another as from changes in the home and other institutions which modify incidental and supplementary activities of the churches.

The social influence of the church in the nation is great, because every Sunday the idealistic attitude on all sorts of questions is presented by the ministers to people who during the rest of the time are observers of more selfish and realistic behaviour. The attitude of churches on disputed moral questions such as slavery and temperance, has always been a strong force in national life. The idealistic programmes, however, often originate outside of the churches ; but the church is an important medium for getting them to the people and making them powerful by giving them the prestige of church sanction. This explains why churches may be instruments for stirring men to " holy war ", or leading them to give aid to the needy regardless of nationality.

Industrial and Business Institutions in which success is frequently measurable and expressible in figures, are subject to the greatest stimulus by similar and associated institutions. In no other type is the stimulus to efficiency so great as in manufacturing and merchandizing establishments where success is obtained by the extensive use of modern means of communication.

Commercial institutions not only imitate and compete with each other more intensely than any other type in improving their organization, management and personnel, but even more in their attempts to gain prestige by advertising and all sorts of publicity methods. No social climber or ambitious politician ever put forth such intense effort to make himself prominent during long periods of time, as is put forth by many big industrial and mercantile corporations. In doing this they use printing in all forms and places, pictures, motion pictures, coloured lights, airplanes, telegraph, telephone and radio. Many companies and their products are better known in every home than the personalities of our greatest men. In a variety of situations they outrival teachers and preachers in giving advice and direction. Every science and art is called upon to aid in getting the attention of people and inducing them to save, use, adorn, enjoy, protect, etc., by means of some object or service. No one above a few years of age is free from the influence of such propaganda for scarcely an hour of their waking life.

Voluntary Institutions, amusement, literary, fraternal, artistic, scientific, humanitarian, social, political organizations small and large, old and new, make extensive use of means of communication. Many persons are thus brought in closer touch with strangers thousands of miles away, and are more influenced by them than by near neighbours. A large part of the public speaking done now is done under the auspices of some such organization. Legislation at the national capital and in the state capitals is influenced more by speakers, letters, petitions, and telegrams initiated by institutions, than by ballots on election day.

With the numerous organizations now existent and the possibility of leaders getting in communication with members by means of circulars, newspapers, letters, telegrams and radio it is now possible to arouse and assemble (mentally) a crowd, and organize and direct them as if they were armies, while they remain widely separated in space. Emotions are not quite so readily aroused by these means as by personal presence, gestures, and tones of voice—hence they are not so likely to excite the furious mob to violence ; but considerable emotion may be aroused by pictures and vivid descriptions, and thought is effectively directed toward a definite line of action in the future.

With a free press and not too much limitation as to the sources from which communications are received by most people, there is opportunity for different courses of action to be presented to all, before action takes place. This is the best safeguard against dangerous propaganda. It must be admitted, however, that if a group of writers have enough means and are sufficiently skilful in their methods of propaganda, almost any idea may be made to prevail, just as the best orator formerly carried the crowd with him.

NEWSPAPERS AS A SOCIAL INFLUENCE

The most important means of influencing behaviour of people by ideas is the newspaper. Leaving out of account those that are continually and intentionally used to further partisan and other special causes, there is still much possibility that newspapers may serve not merely for presentation of news of acts and ideas of people everywhere, but to give information and produce attitudes, favourable and unfavourable, toward certain persons, organizations, laws, and conduct. In general, the American newspapers are primarily mediums for communicating news. The Associated Press and other press organizations for the gathering of news items, are largely drawn upon for other than local news. The chief standard of selection by the agencies is that of interest. This means that new or unusual happenings are presented, such as sudden deaths, crimes, disasters, etc., and new facts regarding persons, countries, activities, events, in which there is already some interest due to previous knowledge. The newspapers, more than any other agency, present the world with all its activities to the individual, and thus have a broadening effect not given by special journals. However, each person reads chiefly about that in which he is already most interested, and consequently is not as broadly influenced as would be the case if he read the whole paper.

Newspapers are almost as distinctive in the way in which they present the world's events to their readers, as are persons in their particular type of individual reactions. This is shown not so much in what is presented as in the amount of space given an item, and above all in the wording and size of the head-lines. Head-lines force themselves upon the attention and are read by at least ten times as many as read the details under the headings. Editorials were formerly regarded as important directors of opinions and conduct, but now they are probably insignificant in comparison with head-lines. A shrewd editor who devoted his abilities to influencing the people by means of head-lines could probably prove as effective as several editors devoting all their abilities to editorials.

BROADENING OF SOCIAL INFLUENCES

There has been great change in the manner in which human beings are influenced by other persons. Formerly this influence came directly from companions and indirectly from their ancestors and others associated with them. The prestige of family and tribal customs was great, and each new generation was strongly impelled to behave in accordance with the habits and customs of the older. Now, after early childhood, institutions of many varieties direct the behaviour of every person. Parents are with their children less of the time, and are themselves less influenced by their immediate neighbours and by local traditions than formerly. The behaviour and customs of people everywhere and in all ages are brought to the child's attention by modern means of communication, and often come to be stronger influences than those gained from personal contacts.

The psychology of the development of culture and social control is always and everywhere the same, but the special culture of every group is being modified by that of other groups, and it is almost inevitable as facilities of travel, transportation and communication increase, that a common world culture will rapidly develop.

SELECTED RESEARCHES

".THE EFFECT OF A SMALL AUDIENCE UPON EYE-HAND
   CO-ORDINATION." By Lee Edward Travis, State
   University of Iowa. From *Journal of Abnormal and Social
   Psychology*, July 1925. *Quoted by Permission.*

Does a person play better or worse before an audience ?   Or
what satisfaction will the football coach obtain when he applies
for information regarding the effect of the spectators upon his
team ?
This study bears specifically upon these two problems which
have to do with neuro-muscular co-ordination.   The test used was
the eye-hand co-ordination test of Koerth.   Briefly, the test is to
hold a flexible pointer on a revolving target.   The target is on a
disc which revolves at the rate of one revolution per second.
The disc is electrically wired so that if the pointer is held continually on the target for one complete revolution of the disc,
a counter will indicate 10.   Twenty revolutions or seconds constitute a trial and a perfect score is 200.
Twenty freshman boys, one sophomore boy and one junior boy,
acted as observers.   The small audience consisted of from four
to eight upper classmen and graduate students.   There was
always an approximately equal number of men and women in
the group.   The subjects were not acquainted with any members
of the audience.
Each observer practised in the presence of the experimenter
twenty trials a day.   His learning curve was plotted each day,
and when for two consecutive days there was no general rise
in the curve it was considered that O* was about as expert as
he would ever be.   This is probably an accurate criterion of
complete mastery of the task as the learning of eye-hand co-
ordination is very rapid, the learning curve showing an abrupt
ascension.   When it thus seemed that O had obtained his
maximum efficiency, the audience was admitted.   But on the day
that O performed before his audience, he was required to do
five trials under the usual experimental conditions, just prior to
the introduction of spectators.
The audience was essentially a passive one.   Its members
seated themselves in a semicircle in front of O, who was standing
at his accustomed place for the carrying out of the experiment.
O was told that here was a number of individuals who wished

* O =subject observed.

to observe him follow the target. Unknown to O, the spectators had been asked to intently watch him but not to make a sufficient distraction by means of noises, laughing, or talking to forcibly draw his attention from the experiment. Nearly every observer displayed various signs of confusion and uneasiness, but no attempt was made to study these. Ten trials were done in the presence of the onlookers.

In this study there are several ways to make comparisons between the performance in the presence of spectators and that when working alone. It would have been permissible to compare the average of the forty scores of the last two days plus the five attained just before the introduction of the audience with the average of the ten scores received in the presence of the audience. Or a legitimate comparison would have been between the average of the five trials just before the appearance of onlookers and the average of the ten during the presence of onlookers. A third way to compare the observer's performance under the social situation with that under the non-social is to compare the average of the highest ten consecutive scores received while working alone with the average of the ten scores received while working in the presence of spectators. This latter method is the one adopted because it comes more nearly comparing the maximum ability under a non-social environment with actual performance under social pressure. On the other hand, it is a rather strict comparison and the one that will put the results in the worst possible light, because each observer has several chances to make his best ten consecutive scores when working alone as compared with only one chance to do his best in the social situation. That is to say, the average score given the subject under the social conditions is probably representative of his mean ability under these conditions while the average score given O while working alone is more representative of his greatest ability under non-social conditions.

Another check on the comparative performance is to compare the highest score of the non-social situation with the highest score of the social situation.

Here it is seen that 18 of the 22 individuals or 81·8 per cent had a higher average for the ten scores in the presence of an audience than for the highest ten consecutive scores when working alone. Sixteen or 72·7 per cent obtained their highest scores while working in the presence of the audience ; 3 or 13·6 per cent had scores during the performance in the presence of the audience that were equal to the highest obtained when working alone ; and 3 or 13·6 per cent had scores in the presence of spectators which were below the highest attained when working alone.

" THE EFFECT OF ENCOURAGEMENT AND OF DISCOUR-
AGEMENT UPON PERFORMANCE." By Georgina
Strickland Gates and Louise I. Rissland, Barnard
College, Columbia University. From *The Journal of Educa-
tional Psychology*, January 1923. *Quoted by Permission.*

. . . In the present experiment an attempt has been made to
investigate further the effect of the experimenter's comments on
two very simple performances. The subjects used were 74 college
students who were given individually, after a preliminary exercise,
two trials of the motor co-ordination (Three Hole) and two of the
colour-naming test. After taking the first co-ordination test, the
first subject was told, " That is really splendid ! Do you always
make such good scores ? In a curve of distribution your score
would be way up here (indicating a position at the top of the
curve). Your score was so good that I wonder if you would
mind repeating the test ? " After taking the test again and after
performing the first test of colour-naming, she was encouraged
similarly with words and inflections which had been previously
standardized. To the next individual who took the co-ordination
test, the experimenter said, " O dear, that is really a very poor
score. I am afraid that you would fall at the bottom of the curve
of distribution," etc. Expressions of disappointment and sympathy
were similarly offered at the completion of the first colour-naming
test. To one-third of the group no comment concerning their performance was made ; they were simply asked to repeat the test.

Certain obvious precautions were observed. The subjects
promised not to tell any other persons about the experiment.
They were asked to write down what they believed the purpose
of the test to be. Only two suspected the object. . . .

The results of this study seemed to show, then, a very slight
difference in average improvement or even in percentage of
individuals who improve in the three groups. In this, the facts
found are similar to those observed in experiments on fatigue,
lack of fresh air, sleep or food ; the external factors seem to
be of relatively little importance in determining the score. Such
difference as there is seems to be in favour of encouragement
or discouragement rather than mere repetition. We might say
then (with the usual realization of the inadequacy of the data),
that it is better to make some comment about the score than to
make none ; that it is a little better to make an encouraging
than a discouraging remark ; that relatively poor individuals
are more likely to be unfavourably affected by discouragement
than are relatively proficient persons ; that the effect of these
incentives does not seem to be constant for the two tests. The
desirability of performing such an experiment on more susceptible
subjects, as children, using more complex, and more reliably
measured functions, is obvious.

Note.—Children tested by the author in a similar way, with few exceptions did much better after being praised, and fell far short of their first
performance when told that their work had been poor.—E. A. K.

Quoted by Permission

E. W. BURGESS in *Am. Journal of Sociology*, July 1928, presents in detail the increase in means of communication. Some of the most significant figures are :

	1900	1927
Passengers carried . . .	576,831,251	841,463,000
Registration of passenger automobiles	8,000	20,230,429

	1902	1922
Number of telegraph messages .	90,834,789	181,518,774
,, ,, telephone calls .	5,070,554,553	26,645,000,000

	1921	1927
Home radio sets . . .	60,000	7,500,000

	1909	1925
Copies of books and pamphlets published	161,361,844	433,211,253

	1899	1925
Copies of daily newspapers circulated	15,100,000	38,000,000

He says :

But the process of civilization, now as always mediated by the prevailing modes of transportation and communication, does not operate uniformly for all the countries of the world, nor for all regions within the United States . . . in moulding a social order. . . . It should be possible to measure for any country, region, or community, not only the rapidity of social change, but the process of civilization and the resulting stage of social organization, by the construction of an index number of communication. . . .

SUGGESTED READINGS

The idea of a vague general group mind was dissipated by :

ALLPORT, FLLOYD H., *Social Psychology*, 1924.

Since then books in this field have been appearing rapidly :

BERNARD, L. L., *Introduction to Social Psychology*, 1926.
DUNLAP, KNIGHT, *Social Psychology*, 1925.
FOLSOM, JOSEPH K., *Social Psychology*, 1931.
KRUEGER, E. T., and RECKLESS, W. C., *Social Psychology*, 1931.
MURCHISON, CARL, *Social Psychology : The Psychology of Political Domination*, 1929.
MURPHY, GARDNER, and MURPHY, LOIS B., *Experimental Social Psychology*, 1931.
YOUNG, KIMBALL, *Social Psychology*, 1930.
JUDD, CHARLES H., *Psychology of Social Institutions*, 1927, shows the significance of language and other institutions in mental development.

Other books on special phases of Social Psychology are :

HERTZLER, JOYCE O., *Social Institutions*, 1929.
LASKER, BRUNO, *Race Attitudes in Children*, 1929.
LIPPMAN, WALTER, *Public Opinion*, 1922.
STERN, BERNHARD J., *Social Factors in Medical Progress*, 1927.
THRASHER, FREDERIC W., *The Gang*, 1927.
THURSTONE, L. L., and CHAVE, E. J., *The Measurement of Attitude*, 1929.
WATSON, G. B., " The Measurement of Fair-mindedness," *Teachers College Contributions to Education*, No. 176.

A list of articles follows, indicating how Social Psychology is becoming an experimental science, the possibilities of which are extensively pointed out in the one by HULL :

ALLPORT, FLLOYD H., " Influence of the Group upon Association and Thought," *Journal of Experimental Psychology*, vol. 3, No. 3, June 1920.
BERNAYS, EDWARD L., " Manipulating Public Opinion : the Why and the How," *American Journal of Sociology*, May 1928.
BOGARDUS, E. S., " Measuring Social Distance," *Journal of Applied Sociology*, page 299, 1925.
BOWDEN, A. O., " Study of Personality of Student Leaders," *Journal of Abnormal and Social Psychology*, page 149, 1926.

CHAPIN, F. S., " Measuring the Value of Social Stimuli," *Social Forces*, March 1926.

DAVIS, JEROME, " Testing the Social Attitude of Children in the Government Schools of Russia," *American Journal of Sociology*, May 1927.

HULL, CLARK L., " Quantitative Methods of Investigating Waking Suggestions," *Journal of Abnormal and Social Psychology*, Sept. 1929.

HURLOCK, E. B., " Value of Praise and Reproof," *Archives of Psychology*, vol. 11, No. 71.

LAIRD, D. A., " Changes in Motor Control and Individual Variations under the Influence of Razzing," *Journal of Experimental Psychology*, page 236, 1923.

STRICKLAND, G., " An Experimental Study of the Growth of Social Perception," *Journal of Educational Psychology*, Nov. 1923.

WARNER, M. L., " Influence of Mental Level in the Formation of Boys' Gangs," *Journal of Applied Psychology*, page 224, 1923.

CHAPTER XI

ORGANIZED GROUP LIVING, OR SOCIOLOGY

THE SCOPE OF SOCIOLOGY

EVERY science, whatever its scope, has difficulty at the outset in determining the limits of its field. Each makes use of truths learned from older sciences and in turn contributes to them facts and general principles gained from its own specialized investigations. The complexity of man's nature, his intimate relation to earth forces and to all living things; and especially his reactions to his fellow-man and the influence of his past history upon present life, make all studies concerning him particularly difficult.

In no field of human knowledge is it harder to select, classify and organize into a system the facts to be considered, than in Sociology. Scarcely a fact dealing with this science can be named which has not already been observed and used by some other science. This partially justifies the claim that sociology has no distinct field, but is merely a collection of facts and truths from other sciences; yet to make too broad a claim of this kind would not be correct. Other sciences may be compared with sociology in this respect—providing one is careful not to make improper use of analogies. Physiology, for instance, draws heavily upon the sciences of physics, chemistry and biology for most of its facts and truths, and also takes some account of psychological and sociological truths. The special problem of physiology is to discover how certain types of organization of cells and organs function under the more usual environments so as to continue to live as a unit. As a pure science it studies the effects of changes in environment, and in its applied forms of Hygiene and Medicine, seeks to show how functioning may be preserved and increased

271

in vigour, and how, when it has declined, it may be restored.

Sociology is not concerned primarily with isolated persons but with groups living in some sort of organized relationship. To maintain such organization there must be balanced action and reaction of individuals and institutions analogous to the balances found in the functioning of cells and organs within the animal body. Sociology as a pure science is concerned with the study of functions and relationships of individuals and institutions in all groups that are able to continue to maintain a separate existence.

Since some truths are common to animals and men, sociology must give some consideration to biological facts. The problems of anthropology and sociology are similar, but the former deals chiefly with what is called savage society, while the latter confines itself mainly to the study of civilized societies. Any society that has existed for a long while having little contact with others, is sure to have special types of organization and functioning, just as species of animals separate into varieties in different environments.

In order that a society may continue to exist it must contain individuals of both sexes and produce children to replace the older generation. The individuals composing this society are continually changing. The chief ground for regarding any group of human beings as the same as the centuries pass, is that the fundamental traits, patterns and complexes remain nearly the same. These are so related as to conserve organized group life.

METHODS OF SOCIOLOGY

Truths of human biology, physiology and psychology serve as a necessary background for the science of sociology. Special researches by economists and students of history and law, the study of various institutions such as the family and the church, all researches of anthropologists upon races of men, relation of environment to behaviour, and relationships of cultures, give important data. All branches of psychology must be largely drawn upon in studying sociological phenomena.

Such a background gives a good basis for theoretical sociology, but it also demands a more thorough study of how all these factors work in civilized societies over a long period of time. Changes in the life of a group take place so slowly that no sociologist lives long enough to observe the various stages of the development of a people. The memories of older persons and the historical records upon which sociologists have to rely, are usually incomplete and inexact. Societies also differ so much in racial stock, environment, tradition and cultural contacts, that it is hard to classify facts so as to show the comparative importance of the various factors upon which vigorous group life depends. For example, there is little agreement as to the chief factors in the rise and fall of Greek and Roman civilizations.

A single group must be studied in all phases of living for as long a time as possible to determine how various factors combine and balance others. This is now being done by anthropologists more than ever before. Sociologists, too, study minutely a period of history, carefully trace the development of an institution or custom, or survey a town, city, or industry.

The sociologist, like the astronomer, cannot experiment readily, but must study sociological phenomena as it is found. But he may select problems and materials for observation admitting of reliable measurements and comparisons. In gathering data, single events or actions of single individuals, are of little use. He must get many facts of the same type under nearly the same conditions but varying in degree, and treat them statistically before he can say what is true of a county, city or institution.

As reports of all sorts, especially census reports, become more complete and accurate, the data will become more useful for the sociologist. He can then measure some of the causes which are working in the direction of increased expenditure for amusements, decreased church attendance, increase in crime, decrease in death-rates, or increase in accidents due to machinery. He must make many comparisons between the places where one or several possible factors are

s

most prominent, and others where these same factors are of least prominence. He must continually try to distinguish between things which incidentally occur together and those that are related as cause and effect.

Exact and reliable methods of obtaining facts, and more perfect statistical methods, are not enough. Sociologists must cultivate an impersonal and scientific attitude in studying social problems if sociology is to be a real science. How difficult it is to do this without being influenced by one's own beliefs is shown by the use made of statistics by some of our most careful sociologists, according as they were believers or disbelievers in tariff or prohibition, or had opposite opinions regarding population increase.

It is because of this tendency to personal bias in sociological research that the more careful sociologists are making more use of objective facts. If subjective states are involved, they seek to measure them indirectly, by random selection of associated indications. For example, increase or decrease in interest in amusement, religion and education are tested statistically by attendance in movies, churches and colleges ; by amounts expended for these various purposes, or by other significant facts. To insure this freedom from bias, great care is necessary in choosing the objective data to be considered, and in interpreting the figures obtained in the light of truths previously established.

SOCIOLOGICAL AVERAGES OR NORMS

A society, like the human body, is in good working condition in proportion as all processes are harmoniously adjusted so as to maintain the balance necessary to vigorous functioning of all of them. Norms are useful not primarily as permanent guides or ideals to which approximation is sought, but to facilitate comparison, and to determine what are the usual and healthful ratios of one function to others. In civilized countries where there are reliable public records and census reports, it is becoming possible to compare different cities and countries with each other in important particulars, such as health conditions or amounts expended for various purposes. Where the records have been kept for many years, changes can also be measured over a term of years. General trends of development may be discovered : *e.g.* the sociological effects of increased use of machinery ; change from rural to urban life in the United States ; and the increase of products per man.

All kinds of institutions, from churches to banks, issue reports from which standards or norms may be computed and comparisons made of one year with another, or one city, state, or industry, with others. These norms may be used, too, for comparisons with other corporations in the same field. Norms of all sorts may be constructed showing whether any or all churches, urban or rural, are growing more or less rapidly than formerly, and whether religion is gaining or losing in numbers and financial support.

In similar ways it is possible to get evidences of differences in the sociological trends of nations and states at different periods. Financiers construct indexes of prosperity in each industry and in the country as a whole, and on that basis give advice on the probable future demand and prices for materials, labour and securities. Norms of public expenditures per person for libraries, schools, health, playgrounds, police and fire protection, etc., are made, by means of which the sociological condition of cities, states and nations may be compared over a given period.

Norms of this type are much more convenient and reliable for scientific and practical uses in sociology when expressed on *per capita* basis, than when gross figures only are given. Great care is necessary, however, in constructing and using these ratios, or serious errors will be made. General averages need to be corrected for various reasons. Library, school, and other figures, for example, are usually more valuable when compiled separately for cities or towns of like size. Allowances always have to be made for other marked differences, such as for a city that is dominantly industrial and another that is mainly residential. A wealthy residential town in Massachusetts, paying high average salaries to teachers, and spending large amounts per pupil, spends fewer dollars per thousand of its *taxable property* than a small town paying low salaries ; the latter, however, spends more in proportion to its wealth and a larger part of its total expenditures for schools, than the town first named. Statistics show that families living on a small income spend a far greater proportion of it on food and rent than those having larger resources ; and that this ratio becomes smaller in families with larger and larger incomes. The per cent of incomes spent on books, arts, amusements and luxuries, on the other hand, increases with the size of income. Standard budgets for various incomes are thus constructed by which families of similar financial status may check up their own expenditures.

The use of statistical norms has been greatly increased by surveys of all sorts. Whether a community will support another movie, needs another playground, another church or more doctors, is decided in part by considering population and other data in relation to averages derived from studying many similar communities. The trends of development in various lines are also indicated by the change in general norms and figures in a given community, from what they were in a previous survey or census. Every carefully made survey in a town, city, state, nation, industry or institution, adds to the data which may be used by sociologists in studying the normal functioning of social groups. As in the case of physiology there are no absolute standards, but merely averages, mediums, or norms based upon data from as many similars as possible which serve as standards for comparison but not as goals to be reached.

The individual variation is greater from mental norms, as we have seen in studying individuals, than from the physical norms. The extremes in sociological data are even greater. One community, for example, may have ten or even twenty times as much taxable property per person as another. This means not only great individual and community differences in purchasing power for anything except the bare necessities of life, but that the amount of money to be used for public expenditures, such as roads, public health, schools, libraries, police and fire protection, etc., are in one case limited to absolute necessities of community existence, and in the other are ample for these and other purposes, without as high a tax rate as in the poorer community.

Considerations such as these were forcibly brought to the attention of sociologists by the report of representatives of a philanthropic board on how to help education in certain states. This report showed that from the standpoint of sociology, it was not wise to use the old-time method of such organizations, *i.e.* giving directly for school purposes, but to proceed by methods that would bring about such economic improvements as would make it possible for the communities to support their own schools. One of the most important means of doing this proved to be through an organization concerned with getting the boys and girls interested in better farming and better food-preserving methods. This ultimately led to general improvement in the economic activities of the people of those states.

It is becoming more and more possible for a sociologist to survey a community, determine its degree of social health, and prescribe treatment, much as the hygienist or doctor gives an individual an examination and advises as to health conditions and their maintenance, or recommends the best ways of curing ills.

POPULATION PHENOMENA

The more or less accurate and comparable records of population, deaths and births in all civilized countries, have been kept by the same methods for a sufficient time to furnish a measure of the changes taking place in five- or ten-year periods. Our census reports show population increases by decades with considerable accuracy. The sources of these increases are shown, but less reliably, by statistics of immigration, births and deaths. Not all immigrants have been registered, and many have emigrated, so that the net increase due to additions from without is a little uncertain. Only a few of our states have kept accurate records of births and deaths from the beginning, and many have only just begun keeping these records in the way prescribed by the census bureau.

For the registration area of the United States there has been progressive decrease in birth-rates during the last half century, as has also been the case in most civilized countries. This seems to be true not only of native born, but of foreign born after the first generation here. The rate for foreign born of the first generation is now near that of the native born a century ago.

Birth-rate alone is not significant as to population increase. Countries like India and China with a high birth-rate, are almost stationary in population, while England, with only a little more than half the birth-rate, and little immigration, is increasing its population.

Statistics show that in most countries birth- and death-rates are in inverse ratio. This is partly due to the fact that the death-rate is always greater during the first year of life. Another important reason is that because of improvements in hygiene and medicine, death-rate is decreased, especially for infants in countries where birth control is known and practised.

It is not entirely correct, however, to say that all the improvement is due to physiological and medical discoveries. Better economic conditions bring about better living conditions even without new discoveries as to how health may be promoted. Discoveries also have little effect on death-rate until by education, or the force of law, changes in health practices have been effected among a large proportion of the inhabitants. Cheaper or more easily obtainable foods, better food-preservation methods, or improved transportation facilities, sometimes produce improvements indirectly. Better health activities promoted by athletics, styles of clothing, and ideals of beauty, may also have an influence. It is easier to ascertain facts regarding increase or decrease of population than it is to measure the direct and indirect, near and remote, causes of the changes and the results that follow.

Whatever the causes, it is important to know the facts as to changes in a nation's population. The life of the nation is threatened by continued decrease. No change, or an increase, may or may not be desirable, according to conditions. Increase is to be welcomed so long as the nation's resources can be utilized by the larger population to a corresponding extent, or so as to admit of raising the standards of living ; but it is usually to be deplored in a country where increase of production cannot be made to equal the increase in population (unless there are places for the excess population to go and colonize).

Population problems have many other aspects than that of mere numbers. In all countries the number of males and females are usually nearly equal, and any marked change in their proportion is likely to complicate economic and social problems. In every country also, there are industrial, social, racial and intellectual classes whose birth- and death-rates usually vary considerably from the average of the whole population. Which are increasing and which are decreasing, is often of great sociological significance, as has been indicated in the chapter on Eugenics.

From special studies of birth- and death-rates in industrial and professional classes, it is possible to determine which classes are increasing most, *e.g.* families of college grade or those not able to fully support themselves ; also the intelligence and birth-rates of occupational groups may be compared.

SOCIOLOGICAL HEALTH

The death-rate per thousand of population over a term of years, in any community established long enough to allow time for the various factors concerned to become effective, is the best indicator of its sociological health. Rate for one year only might not be significant because of some special cause of death, such as an earthquake or a new disease. Some allowance may need to be made in comparing population groups in different climates, but in general, a people after living in a given locality for a century, is sociologically inefficient, if it has not studied the effects of climate and used effective means for keeping the death-rate low. It may seem impossible to become thus efficient, because population in relation to resources which are being used is, in some communities, excessive, so that the best health conditions cannot be provided. However, this situation is sociologically preventable, either by better use of resources, or by decrease of population through birth control or emigration.

A stock farmer with a small death-rate in the stock born on his farm, is more successful than one with a large death-rate. Similarly, a nation with a low death-rate is likely to be superior in its sociological functioning to one with a high death-rate. There is one difference, however, which is not easily overcome. If the farmer has an inferior strain of horses or hogs, he can rather easily change to a better strain ; but for a nation to make such a change is a long process, and although not quite so impossible, it is somewhat like lifting one's self by pulling at one's own boot straps.

In a new country with population small in proportion to resources, a high birth-rate (if death-rate is medium or low) is a sign not only of general individual health but of sociological conditions that are normal, *i.e.* balanced, and tending toward continued balance. In a country with large population in relation to resources and no emigration outlet, a low birth-rate with a very low death-rate, is a sign favourable to continued balance and sociological health.

Average life expectancy is merely another way of expressing nearly the same conditions as death-rate. Figures showing the reduced rates of death from diseases which in the light of present knowledge are theoretically entirely preventable, such as typhoid, are indications of the effectiveness of the various social agencies and methods concerned in using means of prevention. The increase of twelve years in the life expectancy of every child born in this country in a half century, is due : (1) to better feeding, care and treatment of infants, as influenced by economic conditions, medical knowledge, and training of mothers ; (2) to decreased deaths due to preventable diseases by increase in medical knowledge, public health measures such as quarantine and public education ; (3) to improvement in hygienic living of adults by various means such as larger incomes, better sanitation, and hygienic teaching.

At present, the figures indicate an increase rather than a decrease in cancer, heart disease, and old-age maladies such as hardening of the arteries. This may be due in part to a larger population over sixty years of age than formerly. In any case it shows the lack of sufficient knowledge and use of means to materially reduce deaths by certain causes. It may turn out that control of such diseases is impossible, but it is probable that some improvement, either by better hygienic practices, medical treatment, or eugenic means of decreasing susceptibility to such diseases may be made.

A very important factor in social health is the economic condition as indicated by wealth and income per person, *e.g.* death-rate of infants is inversely correlated with income of parents.

The purchasing power of a dollar or other money unit, and the standard of living in terms of cost, may be much less in one country than in another without a corresponding difference in well-balanced living activities of all sorts.

A people with little wealth may have freedom and leisure for art, literature, social intercourse, religion, and amusement, nearly equal to that of a more wealthy people. If the proportion of the average working and leisure time of the people of two countries could be secured, it would be a pretty good indication of social health, although differences in intensity and specialization of work, and in the modes of using leisure would modify the conclusions to be drawn. Where work is intense and specialized, more leisure is necessary to health and to the higher forms of living, than where it is less vigorous, less specialized, and less fatiguing.

The wealth and income ratio to population must be interpreted in the light of other figures than the averages. The *distribution* of wealth and income is of great significance. If a few men have more than they can use and many others have not enough to maintain physical life on an efficient basis, the group as a whole will not be vigorous. In general, the more evenly distributed the income, the better (allowance being made for getting people suited to do the various forms of work and for the efficiency that abundance of capital makes possible). Wealthy individuals or corporations, however, are of advantage only when they increase the average income of the people generally.

One of the best single indications of *mental* vigour in civilized countries is the percentage of literacy, or the number of persons of ten years or more who can read and write with a standard degree of facility. In a country where conditions have been stabilized for a few generations, this is as significant of many influences acting in this direction as is the death-rate. Some of the conditions and results of factors concerned are, the average number of days of schooling per person ; the number of books, magazines and newspapers published and the circulation of these ; the variety of general industrial, literary, scientific, artistic and social publications ; and the number of organized societies concerned in the development and spread of different phases of culture.

The surest indications of social inadequacy are the statistics of famines, accidents, contagious diseases, poor relief, crime, insanity, and physical and mental deficiencies such as blindness and feeble-mindedness. Statistics in this field are, however, generally incomplete and difficult of interpretation. What is classed as crime is often a matter of legislation ; yet a country with many crimes shows inefficiency, whether in its legislation or in its administration of laws. Laws that become a " dead letter " or that show increase in acts classified as crimes after they have been on the statute-books for a generation, are out of harmony with other social influences.

Statistics regarding deficient and dependent classes are often based on number of persons found in public institutions only, and so may imply conditions the opposite of those supposed to be indicated. For example, a state having all of its insane in institutions or under institutional supervision, will appear to have a larger percentage of population of that class than a state that makes meagre provision for such persons. Again, certain classes of people may provide philanthropic institutions for their own people, and send only a few to public institutions

—as is true to a considerable extent of Jews in this country. Properly checked and interpreted, however, such statistics are most significant indications of sociological trends and of degrees of social efficiency of different communities or nations.

The best indication of the complexity of the civilization of a people is in the number, variety and functioning of its organizations of all sorts. The group that has the activities of the individuals of its population correlated by means of public and private institutions that are well balanced as to equality or dominance and efficient in functioning is more vigorous than one where the people are not thus fully organized for co-ordinated, competitive and co-operative activities.

As a broad generalization regarding balance of institutional activities, it is safe to say that wherever action is to be controlled by force, the government should be supreme. Whenever the church has assumed such authority, not only the nation but the church has usually been the loser. Religion is most effective when it uses persuasion rather than force. The church, like other institutions and individuals, may appeal to the government to protect it from injury from without, but not to enforce its decrees on its own members. For the state to dictate as to church officials, doctrines, or policies, is equally as undesirable in America, as for the church to choose government officials and control government action. A government official, as such, should have no more power in the church than a humble citizen ; and a church official should have no more influence in state affairs than a citizen having no church affiliations. Each, because of his position and following, is likely to have prestige, but this should not be increased by legal recognition.

The school as an institution has claimed and exercised a good deal of authority in its own right or as a representative of the state or the church. Both church and state properly engage in the education of their present and future constituency. Even when the schools are separate in support and management, much of the education given is likely to be the same ; in the portion that is different, the state should not dictate as to religious and church teaching, nor the church as to what the state deems necessary to citizenship. In education needed for citizenship the state should have control, both in state schools and in church schools ; in that needed for church membership, the church should have control in its own schools, but not in the public schools.

The officials of the schools should select the materials and exercises they deem suitable and effective to accomplish the ends desired. The less either state or church interferes in the detailed processes of education, the better. Every teacher should have some part in determining the general policy and management as well as considerable freedom in administering details. These rather dogmatic statements are in harmony with investigations made as to the most efficient types of control, especially in education.

The best relation of government to industrial institutions is difficult to define. It is, of course, supreme in its authority to prevent individuals or corporations from injuring others, and may make regulations in the interest of the people, and of fair competition between institutions. How far it should go in regulation, and whether it should own and control economic means of production, transportation, etc., other than those concerned directly in government, is still in dispute. There is now no objection to government management of the mail service, and in many places it operates public utilities such as light, gas, and water ; in some cities the government owns and manages or supervises parks, playgrounds, art galleries, hospitals and clinics. It regulates, usually without managing, every means of transportation and communication, banking, insurance, factories and stores. Government control is more likely to be justified by the results when it is limited, leaving room for initiative and private gain, than when each individual is merely a cog in a machine.

The developments of Civil Service management instead of political management has greatly improved the post office and other governmental undertakings, and partly obliterated

conflicts between "good economics" and "good politics";
but it is difficult to get as strong an incentive to individual
effort in government service as in affairs managed by individuals and corporations. Instances can be cited, however,
of superior work under government management, as well as
of inferior work under private management. There is still
much to learn about the best relations of government to
industrial activities, and the subject is now being studied by
the Civil Service and other bureaus.

What has been said of industrial affairs applies to a considerable extent to voluntary associations of all sorts. It is
clearly necessary for government to regulate these in some
of their activities, *e.g.* insurance features of fraternal organizations which at first were so unwisely planned. Social welfare
institutions may do some forms of work much better than
they can be done by a governmental institution. Private
organizations have been especially useful in showing the value
of playgrounds, clinics, etc., and in developing methods of
conducting them which may be used when their management
is taken over by some unit of government. The Red Cross
is a notable example of an institution that is voluntary and
public, combining community, national, and international
co-operation.

GAUGES OF SOCIAL PROGRESS

Progress from the standpoint of sociological science cannot
be measured by opinions as to what is a good or a bad change.
To radicals and progressives, nearly all changes are evidences
of progress; while to conservatives and reactionaries they are
evidences of sociological disturbances and diseases. The
sociologist as a man of science, is chiefly concerned with a
study of phenomena of social *change*, regardless of its character;
but in applying the science he must try to determine the
effects of any changes taking place upon the social health
of the group concerned. He must look to past history and to
special sciences before deciding what changes, and correlations
of changes, are likely to add to the health and vigour of the

life of a people as a co-operating group. He will consider the effects on certain norms, such as death-rates, literacy, dependency, deficiencies, and upon dominating institutions and their functioning.

Many of the questions of greatest sociological significance are now connected with the family. This is to be the starting-point of the Yale Foundation research on Human Relations. There is no question that divorces are increasing, and that many functions formerly performed by the family are being taken over by the school and other institutions. Both the size and the dominating influence of the family is decreasing, except possibly in isolated regions. What influence such changes will have upon fundamental social norms in twenty, fifty or a hundred years is not easy to say. Some investigations have shown that children in town schools are larger, stronger, more healthy, and make higher scores in educational tests than rural children in the same state. General health statistics, however, show less sickness in rural than in urban populations, except in the case of diseases caused by defective water and milk supplies, of which there is little public inspection in most rural sections.

Not enough studies of this kind have been made to settle the matter, but it is probable that children of parents of the same type and income, living in well-managed cities with the advantages offered by schools and voluntary societies of various sorts, are in a more favourable situation for physical and mental development than those in rural regions, where such institutions are few and inefficient, and most of the facilities for development are supplied by the family. As to morals, statistics show that juvenile crime in cities is greater than in the country, less in residential and business sections than in intermediate areas, and still less in the vicinity of playgrounds.

Children spend less time with their families in cities, and are less continuously under their influence, but much of the time are under the influence of institutions and companions which direct their behaviour almost irresistibly. The conditions favourable to gang life in cities are favourable also for the development of clubs of all sorts. The real question is, are the valuable influences of the family life which are declining as urban population gains over rural being replaced by equally effective influences of other institutions ? Perhaps Scout law and rules are more efficient social implements than parental commands and precepts. There are reasons for believing that the two kinds of influence bring better sociological health than either one alone. The important thing is not to try to do in the home what can be more efficiently performed by organizations outside the home. Many delinquencies are traced to bad home or community conditions ; and many youths are restored to normal behaviour by changes in both, and some by changes in only one.

The possibilities of studying and improving the organizations most directly affecting social welfare are almost unlimited ; but many phases of family life are not readily observed or improved. The study of families is more like the study of individuals, where statistical generalizations are not easily applied to particular situations. To deplore divorce and poor family life accomplishes nothing. Divorce shows that something in the family life is not working well, but throws no light on causes or remedies. It is true there are statistics showing the causes named to the courts, but it is well known that these are only slightly indicative of real causes. Legal causes for divorce are prescribed variously by state laws, and parties seeking separation select the cause that makes it easiest and least objectionable to procure the divorce.

The laws governing divorce and marriage are obviously inefficient and inconsistent if they are supposed to be made in the interest of the family as an institution for producing and sharing in the training of future generations. It would not be in the interest of an efficient government postal department to permit any person applying to enter the service, but to allow no one to leave it without giving certain definite excuses for doing so ; but our present laws allow almost any person who chooses to marry, almost regardless of fitness to produce healthy children and to care for them properly, and then compels them to run this family institution no matter how inefficient they may be in performing the task, unless they offer one of a few reasons for quitting. It is obvious that there should be more research on what is needed in order that the family as an institution shall function well in the case of each marriage ; and that means, probably educational rather than legal, shall be provided to prepare individuals for establishing and successfully conducting institutions of this type.

Social changes are indicated by the raising and lowering of important norms, and most persons will agree that decrease in rates of death, sickness, unemployment, crime, number of defectives ; and increase in income, in leisure time, in literacy, in expenditure for the arts, among a large proportion of the people, would be indications of progress. In general, the numerous changes of the last fifty years have brought these results ; hence, however unfortunate some of the changes may seem to some who are conditioned to the former ways, there is scientific ground, as indicated by these significant sociological statistics, for believing that civilization has progressed rather than regressed.

SOCIAL CHANGE

That social changes occur in cycles and in accordance with certain general laws has long been believed. The attempt is now being made to state such theories in a form that will admit of their being tested by scientific methods. The problems are much the same as those of evolution in biology : one kind concerned with the origin or traits, and the other with their survival and development, or decline.

It has already been pointed out that any type of culture a group has developed after many years of existence in the same environment, is likely to persist. The greatest changes are usually initiated by emigration to new surroundings, or by contacts with other people and their culture, practices and attitudes. But some changes, usually more gradual, take place without outside stimulus ; *e.g.* changes in population and economic conditions and standards of living which involve many readjustments.

When new situations are met, new machines, new ideas or modes of co-operation are introduced, then the changes are likely to take place in a way similar to that in which an individual learns. Old attitudes and ways of acting persist, followed by more or less trial attempts to adjust to the new, during which time other activities are modified. The third phase is the standardization and continuance of the new as an essential feature of cultural living.

When the steam-engine was invented it met with resistance everywhere, and old modes of transportation by land and water were continued. The form of the early locomotive cars was similar to wagons, but as the railways came into favour, numerous changes were made. Now, locomotives and cars are of the few standardized types found most efficient, and are changing very slowly. Bicycles and autos have had a similar history. Chapin has shown that the development of the commission form of government has been similar. At the time when a large number of cities were adopting it, it was being most modified. Now that it is gaining slowly, changes in details are unusual. The development of departments in city and state governments has also followed a similar course.

When it comes to the problems of the effects of a new invention and other culture traits the matter becomes quite complex. The auto, for example, has gone into the third stage of general use and standardization, but the changes that it is producing on other culture traits are still going on. How much it may yet influence the relations of city and country, and modify moral standards by decreasing home and community association and restraint, and by bringing individuals into new and varied material and social surroundings, cannot now be predicted with any certainty.

On the other hand, the invention and adoption of the auto was itself dependent upon other trait developments. Previous mechanical inventions, scientific knowledge and cultural attitudes rendered such an invention inevitable. A history of inventions and discoveries shows that they are likely to

T

originate independently in the mind of more than one person. It is also found that most inventions are made, not by any type of individual, but by those prepared for the new idea by previous training and specialization. In other words, inventing is a result of culture development and not wholly the product of an individual genius.

These considerations lead to the thought that in societies, as in biological life, every new trait must engage in a struggle for continued existence in which other traits are active, and each is helping or hindering others to survive. Biological traits are subject chiefly to selection by physical surroundings and the helping and hindering activities of other species. Social traits are subject to the same biological selection, and in addition to societal selection. Culture traits whether originating within or outside the group are subject to such selection, survival depending on the environment in which they appear. Democratic ideals and organizations were generally short-lived and weak until about the time our government was formed. World conditions were favourable at that time, and the American colonists, with many democratic traditions, were better prepared to organize and carry on democratic political institutions than any other people. The governments of states and cities were patterned after the national government, with an executive head, two legislative bodies and a judicial department. Nearly all voluntary societies in America adopted the democratic ideal, and also the rules of procedure of the national legislative bodies (Roberts Rules of Order). Business and manufacturing companies at first largely ignored the democratic ideal, and continued until recent times to be conducted by a head man much as kingdoms were formerly ruled. Now stockholders have a voice in controlling policies, as the people have in the government. In some industries the employees are also being given a share in the management. Schools remained autocratic rather than democratic until recently. Now teachers are having a part in making courses of study and pupils are beginning to exercise self-governing functions. In the home there is as yet little attempt to recognize democratic ideals.

This slowness of a new trait to be accepted and adopted is sometimes called " cultural lag ". In reality it is merely an example of more or less favourable conditions in certain groups and types of activities for the development of the new trait. The " lag " may be due largely to custom and attitude inertia.

If the advantages of the new traits are based on usefulness, then those that are clearly most efficient under the circumstances are likely to survive unless there are artistic, social, religious or other cultural traits actively opposed to their adoption. The more complete the scientific knowledge of the world and of human nature becomes, the better chance will all useful traits have of surviving. As will be shown in a later chapter science is becoming the chief selector of what culture traits are to survive except in fields where the emotions play a large part, such as in art.

In applied sociology, partially successful attempts are being made to predict the curve of development in many lines of business, government, and politics. There are many corporations using these predictions as partial guides in deciding what the general business conditions will be during the coming year, or the increase in special lines, *e.g.* building materials used, or automobiles bought. Politicians seek to know how fast certain ideas are spreading, and to determine the effects on elections to be held during the year. As the science of sociology develops it will be possible to predict with considerable accuracy when conditions will be favourable for initiating a certain type of change and to draw a curve showing the probable progress of the new trait and to indicate other changes that will follow from it. Sociology will never attain the certainty and accuracy now possible in astronomy, physics, and other natural sciences, but we may look toward a future in which the prophecies of sociologists will be given a good deal of weight by practical men in sociological as well as in economic affairs.

SELECTED RESEARCHES

"FACTORS AFFECTING THE MARITAL CONDITION OF THE POPULATION." By WILLIAM FIELDING OGBURN, Columbia University. From *Publications of the American Sociological Society*, vol. 18, 1923. *Quoted by Permission.*

AGE

The percentage of population who are married is dependent on the age distribution of the population. For instance there are smaller percentages of persons married under thirty years of age than over thirty (see Table I.). So a population with a larger percentage of middle-aged persons will have a larger percentage married than will a population with a large percentage of young persons under thirty years old. For instance, in 1920, 59·5 per cent of the population of the United States fifteen years old and over were married, while in 1890 only 54·3 per cent were married. There has thus been an increase in thirty years of 4·6 per cent of the population married. But this increase may be due to the fact that there are smaller percentages of young persons in 1920 than there were in 1890. For in 1890, 41·1 per cent of the population fifteen years old and over were under thirty years old, while in 1920 there were only 38·5 per cent. In fact, if, in 1920, there had been the same age distribution that existed in 1890, only 56·8 per cent would have been married instead of the 59·9 per cent, other factors being as they were in 1920. Thus the increase in age of the population from 1890 to 1920 accounts for 3·1 per cent increase of the 4·6 per cent increase in percentages married during this period. The age of the population is therefore a very important factor in determining the percentages married. . . .

THE RACIAL AND NATIVITY FACTOR

The percentage of the population married depends also upon the composition of the population as to racial and cultural groups. . . .

The percentage married among the native stock is 59·7 per cent, and is about the same for the United States as a whole as the percentage married among the negroes, 60·0 per cent. The immigrants have a much larger percentage married, 68·6 per cent. This high percentage is due largely to the fact that there are such small percentages of very young persons among them.

But, of course, in studying the effect of immigration on the percentage married, the age distribution of the immigrant is irrelevant. On the other hand the percentage married among the children of immigrants is small, 52·4 per cent. This tendency not to marry among the American-born offspring of immigrants is not due to age, nor to urban and rural influences, nor to locality. If therefore a state or city has a large percentage of immigrants, for this reason the percentage married tends to be high. But if there is also a large percentage of the children of immigrants, the percentage married tends to be small. In many states and cities these two influences offset each other in about equal degrees. . . .

TABLE I.

Age Group	Percentage of each Age Group who are Married in U.S. 1920.
15–19	7·3
20–24	40·6
25–29	66·0
30–34	76·5
35–44	80·0
45–54	77·8
55–64	70·1
65	49·4

" THE MIGRATION TO TOWNS AND CITIES," II. By CARLE C. ZIMMERMAN, University of Minnesota. From *Am. Journal of Sociology*, July 1927. *Quoted by Permission.*

In a recent issue of this Journal I gave some preliminary figures concerning migration to cities and to different occupations by children of Minnesota farmers. Since that time I have gathered more information and material for an analysis of the quality of the families which furnish recruits from towns and cities. The purpose of this paper is to present the conclusions drawn from this first-hand material.

The material consists of data on migration from 694 farm families in Minnesota. These resided in thirteen communities and were selected by random sampling so as to represent the farm population of the state. They represented all types of farming, from cheese-producing areas to the wheat regions on the one hand, and from the cut-over country to the corn-belt on the other. Farms varied from 10 to 640 acres in size, and gross cash incomes from $125 to $15,000. The sample is typical of the state. These data were secured by personal interviews during 1925 and 1926.

From 494 of these families information as to cash receipts was secured. Subsequent studies have shown that these incomes form a fair index of the living conditions and the quality of the farm population. For purposes of qualitative analysis of migration, the farmers were divided into five groups according to the amounts of cash receipts. Table I shows this distribution and the number and present location of all living children eighteen years of age or over.

TABLE I

SOME OF THE MATERIALS OF THE STUDY

Income Groups (Dollars).	Number of Families.	Number of Children 18 Years or Older.	Number on Home Farms.	Other Farms.	Villages or Towns (under 10,000).	Cities (over 10,000)
Under 1,400 .	106	181	46	52	25	58
1,401–2,600 .	175	270	109	75	42	44
2,601–3,800 .	119	179	76	40	27	36
3,801–5,000 .	44	65	36	14	10	5
More than 5,000	50	86	44	31	9	2
Total .	494	781	311	212	113	145

The $1,400 to $2,600 group included the modal number as well as those with mean incomes ($2,500). Fifty-seven per cent had incomes below $2,600. This asymmetrical distribution is typical of most economic phenomena. Those still on the home farms numbered 311, and those who had migrated numbered 470. These 470 were divided into 195, or 41 per cent, who were on other farms, and 375, or 59 per cent, who had entered urban life. These 494 farmers had 781 children eighteen years of age or more (at which time migration begins).

These data were analysed to find if towns or cities selected a larger proportion of children from any one economic class than from another; if the large cities selected similar proportions of each class; if the children from each group rose at a similar rate of speed to the non-wage-earning classes; and finally, if selection affected both sexes alike.

. . . The group with incomes under $1,400 had 23·2 per cent of all 781 children. If the selection affected all classes alike, we should expect to find that this class furnished about 23·2 per cent of all urban migrants and the same proportion of all migrants to large cities. However, an examination of Tables III and IV shows that this is not true. The group with incomes under $1,400 furnished 30·9 per cent of all urban migrants, 40·0 of all migrants to large cities, 18·7 of all farmers, 39·0 of all wage-earners, and 14·4 of all non-wage-earners. On the other hand, the upper group (incomes of $5,000 or above), which had 11 per cent of all children eighteen years or older, furnished 4·0 per cent of all urban migrants, 1·4 of all migrants to large cities, 14·3 of all farmers, 2·7 of all wage-earners, and 6·7 of all non-wage-earners. These differences might have arisen through errors of sampling ; but as a matter of fact, the major portion of the variance may be attributed to differences in selectivity of the population groups and occupations. The proof of this lies in the size and consistency of the differences. They have been tested by comparison with the standard errors.

By making similar analyses, but in greater detail than in the tables given, and by separating the sexes, I have been able to establish some tentative conclusions. For the sake of brevity I am not presenting the detailed figures. These conclusions are :

1. Children of the successful farm families stay on the farms more often than those of the less successful.

2. These children, when they do migrate to urban areas, rise more rapidly than those from the lower-income families.

3. Large industrial cities are greater agencies for non-proportional selection than are towns and villages.

These conclusions must be qualified with the following statements. The sample is small and includes only Minnesota farm families. However, judging from all statistical tests of sampling which we have been able to make, we feel that this one is truly representative of Minnesota. These data may not apply to areas in the east, which in some cases have suffered large net losses in farm population. Families which migrate as units are not included. We have no data on the types of selection affecting the reverse migration from towns and cities to farms. In addition, some of the children are still young and may migrate again or rise to higher social classes. And, finally, we do not know whether or not selection within economic groups or within families is normal. Perhaps the brightest children within each family migrate to urban occupations. However, this last consideration may not be of great biological importance.

" THE PROLIFICACY OF DEPENDENT FAMILIES." By H. JEANETTE HALVERSON, University of Wisconsin. From *Am. Journal of Sociology*, Nov. 1923. *Quoted by Permission.*

For two years the University of Wisconsin has been carrying on an investigation through Prof. E. A. Ross and Dr. R. E. Baber to determine the change in size of American families in one generation and the relation between the decrease in size of family and such factors as education, occupation, and nationality. . . .

The dependent families studied were selected because they

were complete and of American stock. We termed families American if the husband, the wife and the husband's father were all born in this country. There were three conditions under which the family was judged complete : (1) if the wife was forty-five or over ; (2) if the wife was between forty and forty-five and had not borne a child for at least eight years ; (3) if the wife was known to be sterile because of a surgical operation or venereal disease. Families were deemed dependent if they had been regular recipients of relief from private or public agencies over a period of several years. No figures were recorded for families in which there were children by more than one marriage.

In order to find 100 families of this type, it was necessary to go to several communities. Thirty were found in Madison, Wisconsin, 31 in Kalamazoo, Michigan, 26 in Bloomington, Illinois, 5 in Omaha, Nebraska, and 8 in Des Moines, Iowa. Information regarding the past generation was available only when the family was visited, as they were in Madison. There was no selection of cases except on the bases mentioned. . . .

Although every case-record was carefully studied to ascertain the total number of births in the family, it is possible that some births were not mentioned in the records. This may account for the fact that the average number of children returned for the families living in Madison was somewhat larger than the average from the records in other cities.

In the 100 families described, 649 children were born, giving an average of 6·49 children per family. The births ranged from 1 to 13 per family with 8 the most frequent size, occurring 19 times. In 20 families there were fewer than 5 children, in 61, from 5 to 8 children, and in 19 more than 8 children.

The data obtained by interviewing 28 families in Madison showed that their parents, representing 55 families in the past generation, had 429 children, an average of 7·8 per family. In this generation the range was from 1 to 16 births per family with 8 again recurring frequently.

The figures stated are startling when compared with the average for self-supporting families, obtained in the central study of this department. In the present generation, 1,895 filled fertile families were found to have an average of 3·35 children. When the infertile families were included in the calculation, the average fell to 2·80. The parents of these men and women, representing 671 families of the past generation, had an average of 5·44 children. According to these figures, *dependent American families of today are almost twice the size of self-supporting families in which there are children ;* they are one child per family greater than the self-supporting families of the past generation.

SUGGESTED READINGS

It is difficult to select from the immense volume of sociological writings. The following are standard texts :

DAVIS, J., and BARNES, H. E., *An Introduction to Sociology*, 1927.
HANKINS, F. H., *Introduction to the Study of Society*, 1928.
HAYES, E. C., *Sociology*, 2nd ed., 1930.
LUMLEY, F. E., *Principles of Sociology*, 1928.
PARK, R. E., and BURGESS, E. W., *Introduction to the Science of Sociology*, 1921.
SOROKIN, P., *Contemporary Sociological Theories*, 1928.
SOROKIN, P., *Social Mobility*, 1927.

The latter two volumes give a good idea of all significant theories, facts and books.

Methods in Sociology are described in :

LUNDBURG, GEORGE A., *Social Research*, 1929.
ODUM, H. N., and JOCHER, KATHERINE, *An Introduction to Social Research*, 1929.

Books of the survey and case study type are :

BRUNNER, EDMUND De S., and others, *American Villages*, 1927. (140 villages studied.)
KIRKPATRICK, E. L., " Farmer's Standard of Living," 1929.
LYND, R. S., and LYND, HELEN, *Middletown*, 1929.
SHAW, C. R., *Delinquency Areas*, 1930.
STEINER, JESSE F., *The American Community in Action ; Case Studies of American Communities*, 1928.
THOMAS, W. I., and ZNANICKI, F., *The Polish Peasant in Europe and America*, 2 vols., 1927.

Good books on the family are :

GOODSELL, WILLYSTINE, *Problems of the Family*, 1928.
GROVES, E. R., and OGBURN, W. F., *American Marriage and Family Relationships*, 1928.
REUTER, E. B., and RUNNER, J. R., *Family ; Source Materials for the Study of Family and Personality*, 1931.

The following are concerned with population problems :

DROCHSLER, JULIUS, *Intermarriage in New York City ; Studies in Economic and Public Law*, edited by the Faculty of Political Science, Columbia University, vol. 44, 1921.
EAST, EDWARD M., *Mankind at the Crossroads*, 1923.

OGBURN, W. F., and TIBBETTS, CLARK, " Birth-Rates in Social Classes," *Social Forces*, September 1929.

PEARL, RAYMOND, *The Biology of Population Growth*, 1925.

PHILLYS, J. C., " A Study of the Birth-Rate in Harvard and Yale Graduates," *Harvard Graduate Magazine*, 1916.

REUTER, E. B., *Population Problems*, 1923.

ROSS, EDWARD A., " Standing Room Only," 1927.

THOMPSON, WARREN S., *Population Problems*, 1931.

The following are significant discussions of social change and adjustment :

CHAPIN, F. S., " Cultural Change," 1929.

CHASE, STUART, *Men and Machines*, 1929.

DEXTER, ROBERT C., *Social Adjustment*, 1927.

HERTZLER, J. O., " Social Progress," 1928.

RANDALL, JOHN H., *Our Changing Civilization*, 1929.

Standard works on social pathology are :

HAYNES, F. E., *Criminology*, 1930.

QUEEN, STEWART A., and MAN, DELBERT M., *Social Pathology*, 1925.

SUTHERLAND, E. H., *Criminology*, 1924.

CHAPTER XII

CHANGING HUMAN BEINGS, OR EDUCATION

POSSIBILITIES OF CHANGE

PREVIOUS to the development of modern science, ideas of human nature that took little account of the original nature of man were common. According to one theory, nothing could be accomplished since everything was supposed to be predetermined. This idea, originally set forth both by theologians and philosophers, has been supported in part by some scientists who believe in the theory of hereditary determinism ; but it has almost never been a guide in practical life. The attempt to educate anyone implies a practical belief that the person will be different because of the educational practices used. This accords with scientific conceptions as well as with common sense.

The other theory which made consideration of original nature almost unnecessary is that man is like a white sheet of paper upon which you may write what you will. On this supposition there is little need to consider the nature of the creature being educated, but only to know how to do the writing. A modern form of this theory conceives of man as having a complex structure and a few simple native ways of acting which may be dealt with so as to make all men exactly alike, or each different from the others in any desired way. This theory of Watson's demands some knowledge of the nature of the organism and of the most effective means of changing it into some specific type, such as a physician, musician, mathematician, engineer, mechanic, etc.

Neither of these two modern views of nature as everything, or nurture as the only factor to consider, are in their extreme forms in accordance with all the facts known to science ; but there is some truth in both, justifying further study of the original nature of man and of the changes that may be effected by educational means.

All studies of plant and animal life show that each individual specimen is constructed in general as are others of its species and variety, though differing in detail. Man cannot survive without certain essentials in the environment, but with these present, individuals show marked variations when placed in a new and different environment. The effects that various elements in the environment have upon development of traits desired, as well as the original nature of each species and sometimes of each individual, must be known in order that a desired type of plant or animal may be produced.

Man is a living organism of a distinct species and becomes what he is in maturity by the influence of the environment on his original nature. The kind and degree of change that environment, including education, can make upon original nature is limited. Individuals differ so greatly in their capacity for general and special development that the results of a given amount of training upon different persons are far from equal. Some at ten years of age are in advance of others at twenty in nearly all mental activities that can at present be measured with any accuracy; while many are superior or inferior in special achievements such as music or mathematics. The science of education must, therefore, recognize the truth that the same surroundings do not have the same degree of effect on individuals of different capacities, and sometimes not even the same kinds of effect.

EDUCATIONAL IDEALS

Ideals of what men should be vary with every age and people, and often undergo rapid changes. The church desires men of a certain type of religious belief and practice; the state desires obedient subjects or resourceful citizens, as the case may be; while moralists put forth all sorts of ideals as to what man should become. Science as such, cannot *directly* decide which ideals are the best. It may, however, modify them in important particulars. It may show that some ideals are impossible of attainment for any man or for certain types of men ; and that others demand the development of traits that cannot exist in the same individual at the same time, *e.g.* a strictly 'obedient individual, showing great initiative. It may show also that it is a waste of time to try to develop certain traits in every one to the degree indicated by the ideal ; or to try to make the new generation quite different from the older under whose influence they are growing up by pointing out the results of dishonesty and inefficiency ; or to try to make all alike or all different in certain ways. In many particulars common sense and scientific study may thus modify and reconstruct purposed ideals of what education should attempt to do in the way of making men different from what they would be, if no definite type of education were given them.

In this country some of the ideals and practices of education are under the more immediate direction of the home, others of the church, and still others of the industrial and other institutions to which an individual may belong ; but the chief social organizations for realizing ideals are the public schools.

FUNCTION OF THE PUBLIC SCHOOLS

In a very general way the function of the public school is to change the children from what they are as the result of heredity, the incidental influence of their surroundings, and the intentional influence of the home and other institutions, into men and women of a type fitted to live in civilized society as it exists, and to maintain, and perhaps improve upon the culture of the present generation. Since the state supports and controls the schools, it prescribes the main ideals of what they shall do ; but scientific educators are to a considerable extent in control of the means to be used in preparing for citizenship the general type and variety of individuals desired by the state. The solution of the scientific as well as the practical problems of how to attain these ends devolves largely upon schools. Educators take what they can from researches of physiologists, psychologists, and sociologists as partial guides, and make special researches as to how truths in those fields work under school-room conditions as they are, or may be. In this way courses of study and types of methods are determined, then as great efficiency as possible is sought in carrying on the work of instruction.

Though only recently begun, educators' use of scientific methods is rapidly being extended. The broadening of the courses of study in recent times has been due partly to an effort to find more effective means of education ·for all, and partly to meet the needs of special types of persons. Another important source of addition to the studies offered is the recognition of the fact that institutions other than schools are not doing their part efficiently. As a result not only has the elementary curriculum been changed and broadened, but public education is being provided for older children in high schools, junior colleges, and colleges, and for those under six years in kindergarten and nursery schools. The limits that may be set to the functions of the public schools are not as yet definitely settled. Evening classes, vocational instruction, Americanization classes for adults, and playground facilities for all ages, are in many places also a part of the school system.

SCIENCE AIDS IN SELECTING WHAT SHALL BE TAUGHT

From the beginning of the public schools it has been admitted that every one should know something of the three R's. Considerable research has been devoted to determining what parts and how much of these subjects are needed in present-day life. It is impossible to teach the spelling of all the half-million words in the English language, and few persons have occasion to spell more than a small per cent of them. Extensive studies were made showing what words are used in ordinary business and social correspondence, in newspapers, books, and by children in their written work in the various grades, and what ones appeared most frequently. From these a list of about four thousand of the words most frequently used are now usually selected for teaching in the grades. It is, therefore, likely to be worth one's while to learn to spell every word in the modern spelling-book since, if one knows these he can, with occasional aid from a dictionary, spell all the words he has occasion to write.

Similar studies have been made of the mathematical knowledge and facility needed in daily life and in common occupations, and the new arithmetics are based on these studies.

As most persons now read silently ten times as much as they read aloud, more time is given to developing silent reading efficiency than to oral reading, and by means of reading tests it is possible to measure the ability to read with sufficient speed and understanding for the purposes of the average citizen.

The invention of the typewriter has made rapid and perfect writing less useful than formerly, and research has produced measuring scales and has established standards of average efficiency to be approximated by all pupils.

Since people do more talking than writing, the schools are wisely giving much attention to training in oral expression. A number of researches have also been made to determine what teaching and training will give greatest facility and accuracy in oral and written English. The results are not as consistent and definite as in spelling, but have justified less teaching of grammar and rules of speech, and more study and practice of good usage. Subjects such as Latin, formerly supposed to help in learning English, have in part been replaced by direct study of English.

 Other additions and subtractions from the curriculum have been made as the result of investigations as to their usability. The former belief that mental discipline was gained from studies that gave little or no knowledge or skill of a kind likely to be needed at any future time, has been largely dissipated by the researches of psychologists and educators. Consequently junior high school, high school, and college courses of study are undergoing changes in the direction of including work of proved practical value.

A most important development has been in the realization that only a few of the many subjects offered in these schools should be taken by all, and that special needs, interests, and capacities may be served by óptional courses or subjects. This opportunity for election and specialization, which began in the college and extended down through the high school into the junior high school, is having some recognition in the grades, although it is generally agreed that most of what is given in the first grades is, and should be, almost equally useful to all persons.

RESEARCH AS TO THE NATURE OF THOSE TAUGHT

Biology, physiology, and psychology have in recent years been much concerned with the genesis of function and behaviour. These studies bearing on the nature of children and the processes by which they mature have been supplemented by the researches of educators. From the social point of view, what the future citizens shall be taught is the important thing ; but from the educators' point of view it is still more important to know the nature of the creature being taught and the effects the subjects and exercises chosen as means for changing him, have upon him. They have been especially concerned not only with selecting what will be most useful from the immense mass of culture, but with presenting the materials in a form and at a time best calculated to effectively produce the changes desired. They have given some weight to what children as individuals wish to become, partly because of their belief that each child should have a chance for developing his individual possibilities, and partly because they know that educating him into what the state desires him to be can best be accomplished by knowing what he is and what he desires for himself.

Many experiments have been made in special schools and some in public schools, of postponing the formal teaching of the three R's, and of introducing material formerly used only in upper grades or high schools. Few, if any, of these experiments have been conducted in rigidly scientific ways, but they have aided in reaching intelligent, common-sense conclusions. Tests show that the best experimental schools which are guided chiefly by what interests the children, give as much of the knowledge and skill usually sought as is gained in the schools having regular courses of study. Much more experimenting, observing, and testing will be necessary before the double advantage of an ordered arrangement of the materials of instruction can be secured, while utilizing the advantages of having children freely doing things that their natural and acquired interests impel them to do.

The order in which things are learned is closely connected with method. For example : to teach geometry in the first grade by the method of logical deductive reasoning would be absurd, while a high school student would not gain much by the purely observational study of geometrical figures which is so valuable to younger children. Almost any subject may be taught in any grade if the method is sufficiently and suitably modified. It is not clear whether it is better to fix the place of a subject in the curriculum, then adapt the method to it, as is usually being done in the public schools, or to determine the methods best suited to the different ages, then choose material suitable to those methods, as is more often done in progressive and experimental schools.

Final conclusions as to which procedures are demonstrably the most efficient are difficult, because all the results of a given type of procedure do not show themselves at the end of a year, or two years, nor even at the end of schooling, but only in the subsequent lives of those educated in the different ways.

SCIENTIFIC STUDIES OF METHODS

Children engaged in interesting work and play of all sorts may learn incidentally, without conscious effort, colours, shapes, materials ; how to construct, count, draw, read, write, spell, etc. ; or they may devote themselves to the definite tasks of learning and practising one after another of the elements of these subjects. The first method is used to a greater or lesser extent in what is generally known as the project method. This indirect, unsystematic method of learning works well in some cases, especially with young

U

children, but is not necessarily the most efficient method to be used at all times.

One of the chief differences between the project method and the direct study of elements in their logical or psychological order, is in the interest excited. The project method involves varied activities in which ends desired and things learned and done are closely related, while the direct study and practice of elements is more monotonous and more distantly related to objectives. To learn to hold a pen and make the various writing movements, and to drill on number combinations, is far removed from the end of being a book-keeper ; but writing labels on an exhibit and calculating how many things will be required to make several rows of things, is more immediately interesting. On the other hand, it is necessary at times all through life to give attention to monotonous acts in order to secure distant ends.

It is largely because of children's natural lack of interest in means to remote ends, that resort has been made to artificial rewards, punishments, and marks, in order to produce more immediate interest in school work. In well-chosen project work none of these are necessary, which means a great saving of time and energy of both teachers and pupils. The advantages of the project method are, of course, nearly all lost if pupils are not interested in the ends involved.

All researches upon the psychology of learning furnish truths that are being used to an increasing extent in all schools. Some of the more important of these are given in the chapter on General Psychology, especially in the section on Economy in Learning.

A number of experimental studies of methods have been made in which pupils of equal intelligence and school advantages are placed in two or more groups and each group taught the same subject by a different method for a certain time, then tested, care being taken to keep all other conditions the same for all the groups. Reliable tests of achievement in various school subjects now make it possible to test various procedures in causing children to attain knowledge and skill in every school subject.

Changes in emotional and volitional attitudes are not so easily tested as are subject achievements. Progress is being made, however, in developing tests, and there is reason to expect that effects of teaching and training on personality traits such as honesty may be tested and evaluated with considerable accuracy.

ADAPTING EDUCATION TO INDIVIDUALS

A good deal of progress toward scientific direction of education has been made by co-operation between psychologists and educators. Before much scientific work had been done teachers were making many common-sense adjustments to individual pupils ; and superintendents were doing such sensible things as providing seats of a proper size, and arranging separate classes for children who were exceptional in a marked degree.

With the development of intelligence tests, changes in the grading of children have been made. It is found that nearly all children who are of a mental age of six years can do the usual first-grade work in one year, that most of those under that mental age fail, while those of a year or two greater mental age can do the work of grade I and a part or all of grade II in one year. In the average school, in Detroit and other cities, it has been found that about sixty per cent are of about the mental age of six years when they enter. These are placed together and given the usual work. The twenty per cent under that mental age are given exercises suited to their capacity until ready for regular grade work. The remaining twenty per cent are given the first-year's work in a shorter time, or with extra work. This procedure eliminates wasteful repetition, and gives all pupils the mentally hygienic advantage of success in what he undertakes.

In some experimental schools, and especially at Winnetka, Illinois, the adaptation has been carried farther. Very definite outlines and tests of what is to be learned in the grades are prepared, and each pupil spends whatever time he needs in mastering them. He then either goes on to the next piece of work, or more often devotes his extra time to projects and group exercises. In some schools it is found that the essentials of the principal elementary subjects may be mastered completely by the majority of pupils in about half the day, leaving the rest of the time for specialities and for group exercises. The pupils thus get the advantages of both direct and indirect methods, and of individual and co-operative project work. Definite aim and complete success in the subjects studied make for efficient study, and relieve the teacher of the necessity for supplying artificial motives.

Some experiments have been made to find whether the method best suited to children testing low in intelligence is also best for those testing high. It is found that there are considerable differences. The former need, and are interested in drill repetitions to a greater extent than the latter. It also appears that there is not a large gain from arranging class groups according to intelligence, unless the amount of work required and the methods of working, are varied for the different groups.

VOCATIONAL EDUCATION AND GUIDANCE

The problem of determining the most efficient means of giving the knowledge and training that will best prepare for success in the various occupations is not a general one to be solved by public schools, but is composed of many special ones to be solved by educators and representatives of the special occupations. The first six grades of the public schools are, however, expected to give the training suited to the needs of all citizens of every occupation, while the junior high schools, high schools, and colleges give the additional general and special training required by leaders and those engaged in the more technical and professional vocations.

An important function that the public schools may perform is to give information and direction that will help individuals to choose and prepare for the occupations for which they are naturally fitted. It is a great waste of time and energy if those unable to deal with symbols with facility continue that sort of training, and try to prepare for the higher occupations ; and it is a waste of talent if those having such facility are not kept from engaging in vocations requiring only mechanical work with things. It is now possible to discover by tests who will be likely to fail in an abstract subject like algebra, and it will probably not be long before prophecies of individual success or failure in many subjects may be made with considerable assurance. This will make it possible to arrange that children, especially in high schools, shall take only subjects in which they can succeed, and which will prepare for occupations in which they will be efficient workers. Tremendous economy would thus result.

Traditions of secondary and higher education are strongly against such adjustments to individual abilities and needs. Even where the schools are ready to do their part, the parents often insist on their children taking the traditional course which was originally designed chiefly for the professional classes. Teachers would not need to waste so much time and energy in inducing the children to study efficiently, and what they learned would be more beneficial if all children were doing work suited to their abilities and interests.

At present educational and vocational guidance in a scientific way is possible only in the way of determining what subjects and occupations are open to children on the basis of abilities shown by tests, and these are not yet sufficiently perfect to be complete guides. What subjects and occupations shall be followed within the limits set by physical and mental ability, vary greatly with interest of pupils, with untestable personality traits, and with all sorts of practical considerations. Notwithstanding this lack of a complete scientific basis for educational and vocational direction of youths, there is justification for the growing practice of public schools, in providing advisers for pupils.

These advisers are differentiated into two types—an expert on vocations knowing the abilities, traits, and training needed in each industry, the conditions of supply and demand now and in the future, various details of choosing and securing employment, working conditions, pay, etc. ; the other an expert in individual psychology who can test children, aid them in finding that for which they are fitted, and help them in personal problems. In the nature of the case, advisers, though helped by every advance of scientific knowledge in their field, will always have to be guided to a considerable extent by sympathy, insight, and common sense. To be successful they must continually maintain the faith that success is possible for the person advised in some field of activity, and must help the children to have a proper faith in themselves.

ORGANIZATION AND SEQUENCE IN EDUCATION

Until recent years educational systems have developed from the top downward. The higher institutions deemed it necessary that the professional classes demand a certain type of secondary preparation, and that secondary schools, in turn, demand uniform elementary schools. In response to this demand, each year of study must prepare for the next, and thus the graded system was developed. Subjects and topics were arranged to follow each other in an order dictated by tradition and logic. The aim in every grade was to teach these things in a way that would give a good foundation for the education to be given in the next year. Colleges were particularly insistent that high schools should make it their chief purpose to prepare for college, and some high-school men became almost as insistent that elementary schools should prepare for high school. This has emphasized the marking system as a means of determining what subjects are mastered to the degree assumed to be necessary to assure success the next year or in the next higher school. This assumption was not supported by experiments or justified by general truths regarding mental processes used in the various subjects.

The elective system in colleges changed practices and awakened doubt of the assumption that a college education must consist of certain subjects pursued in a certain order. Entrance requirements, however, were, and still are, made to some extent on the presumption that only by taking certain subjects in high school can students be prepared for successful college work. Slowly the scientific attitude of determining the truth as to what preparation is needed in order that one may be able to study any subject effectively is gaining ground and being put into practice.

Extensive studies have recently been made of the types of students who succeed or fail in college work. Below a certain standard set by intelligence tests few or none succeed, but the *degree of success* is not closely correlated with intelligence score nor with success in special subjects, but is correlated with previous general success in high school. This is understood to mean that those having the mental ability and other traits that bring success in high school have what is necessary for success in college, rather than that taking certain subjects made possible the success attained in college. Some colleges now frankly recognize this and admit all who have been successful in high school whatever subjects they may have taken, but many still name at least a considerable proportion of subjects that must have been pursued, although they have little or no scientific evidence that these subjects are any better preparation for success in college than others.

Theoretically it seems to educators that some subjects are more valuable as foundations than others, but experience with individuals in the same classes variously prepared throws doubt on all presumptions that have been made, and demands that requirements as to what shall be learned before passing to another grade or school or phase of a subject shall be tested by research as soon as possible.

There can be no question that in preparing for a very specific occupation or type of scholarship, economy would be furthered by a certain kind of training given in sequence, but for general personality development it is of doubtful desirability. This truth must be recognized in the general organization of a system of schools. The old type of German education subordinated the individual to his vocation, while the less carefully planned American system allowed a choice of any occupation without a carefully worked-out system of training preparatory to it. After about ten years of age, education in Germany became different according to the occupations to be followed. It was not easy after that to pass from folk schools to gymnasia, or from one type of gymnasia to engineering schools, or from the other type to the university. In this country it is not usually made difficult for a child to take one special course in junior high school, another in high school, and still a different type in college, and even then the graduate is not greatly limited as to choice of occupation.

The demand that there shall be special training in order to get into any of the higher vocations is growing, but it is not at all certain that on the whole it is best for the schools to be so organized and conducted that they shall be devoted largely to preparing for *technical* training to be given later. More should be known about the value of such preparation and about its effect on producing broad, well-balanced personal development before allowing lower schools to be so conducted as to give vocational training, rather than general advantages to the individual and society.

It will be seen from the brief summary given above that education is beginning to be put on a scientific basis, yet in choosing materials and exercises to be used in general education for all, in preparation for each vocation, and in deciding on the most efficient method to be used, education is in many respects an art rather than a science. It is provided for individuals and administered by differing personalities ; hence, in many respects it must adjust to individuals and special circumstances, while conforming to general principles scientifically established.

SELECTED RESEARCHES

" THE CONTRIBUTION OF TEN CHRONICLES - OF -
AMERICA PHOTOPLAYS TO SEVENTH-GRADE HIS-
TORY TEACHING." By J. W. Tilton and David C.
Knowlton, Yale University. From *Journal of Social
Psychology*, February 1930. *Quoted by Permission.*

The photoplays used are historical dramas setting forth a
number of important developments in American History very
much as the playwright unfolds his plot by dialogue, change of
scene and action. The length of the photoplays, 3 reels, is fixed
by school practice which makes it almost imperative that the
story be unfolded, if it is to be presented in its entirety, within
a period of from 40 to 45 minutes. Accuracy of portrayal is
vouched for by specialists in the phases of history portrayed.
The dramatic structure of the photoplays has been carefully
supervised by Professor George Pierce Baker of the Drama
Department of Yale University. Of the 15 photoplays already
produced, 10 were used in the experiment. . . .

The purpose of this experiment was to measure the contribution
of the photoplays to enrichment, retention, and the creation of
an interest. . . .

This plan was carried out in Grade 7 of the Troupe Junior
High School of New Haven, Connecticut. The grade was composed of 521 pupils divided into 15 sections of approximately
35 pupils each. The pupils had been sectioned, within the
limitations of administrative necessity, on the basis of Otis
Classification Test quotients and teachers' judgments. The
15 sections were designated by letters in alphabetical order
from A, the highest, to O, the lowest. The 15 sections were
taught by 6 teachers, A, F, and K, by one ; B and L, by another ;
C and H, by a third ; D, I, and N, by a fourth ; E, J, and O,
by a fifth ; and G and M, by a sixth. For the whole grade the
median mental age was 12 years and 11 months, and the median
intelligence quotient was 105. For reasons stated later, sections
F, H, I, J, L, and M were chosen to constitute the experimental
group, and B, C, G, K, N, and O were chosen to constitute the
control group.

The course of study pursued by the experimental group differed
from that of the control group in only one respect, viz. that it
included the use of the photoplay in addition to the textbook
and such other class-room equipment as was common to all

seventh-grade history and social study classes. No other visual material was introduced into the classroom except that which was already in use there, such as wall and blackboard maps. Teachers were at liberty to make such use of the pictures and maps in the textbooks as might commend themselves, provided they used such materials in control and experimental groups alike. . . .

. . . The Van Wagenen Information Scale C–2 was given at the beginning and end of the experiment to 9 of the 15 sections. The nine were fairly representative of the whole grade in that, of the 6 omitted sections, 2 were bright, 2 average, and 2 dull. The 9 sections made an average gain of 14·4 points. Allowing for the effect of the experimental factor and for practice effect, this improvement made in 6 months is equal to the improvement normally made in both the sixth and seventh grades in the Minnesota cities from which the norms were obtained. The period covered by the experiment was therefore one of real progress, as measured by the use of this standardized scale. . . .

. . . The experiment was conducted under unusually good experimental conditions. All study was directed and supervised in the classroom ; books were not taken home. . . . Experimental work had been conducted in the school before, and the teachers knew the necessity for control. They exercised it carefully and conscientiously. In the case of two teachers the extent to which they were consistent in their teaching from section to section was measured. Alongside of each of the 395 questions in the test, record was made of the number of pupils who learned to answer it correctly in the course of the experimental instruction. This is a good measure of the extent to which the same things were taught in different sections. Control sections D and N were taught by one teacher, and control sections E and O were taught by another teacher. We combined the measures for D and O and for E and N. The coefficient of correlation between the combined measures is ·76, and for all six teachers it may be estimated to be ·91. If many pupils learned to answer a certain question in one section, then many learned it in the other control section taught by the same teacher. From the number of pupils in one section who learned to answer a certain question, there could be predicted with a probable error of two pupils, the number who would learn to answer the same question in another section taught by the same teacher.

In every way the teacher's influence was held constant as possible, and whatever was done in one section was done in all sections taught by that teacher. . . .

No particular effort was made to keep conditions constant from one teacher to another, for all comparisons have been made between control and experimental groups upon which each teacher had an equal influence.

. . . The grouping of the pupils into homogeneous ability sections, all different, afforded a good opportunity to evaluate the photoplays in terms of the ability handicaps which they enabled the experimental group to overcome and afforded an opportunity for testing the precision of experimental control by comparing two control groups taught by the same teacher. On the other hand, this plan of homogeneous grouping made it necessary to match control and experimental groups as a whole, without matching within each teacher's influence. This method is inferior to matching by individuals, other things being equal.

The objection to the method of matching used lies in the possibility of a teacher being a better bright-section teacher than she is a dull-section teacher, or vice versa. The mental ages of four control sections taught by two of the teachers are such as to permit a determination of the extent to which that factor invalidates comparison in the case of these two teachers. D and N are bright and dull sections taught by one teacher ; E and O are bright and dull sections taught by another teacher. The average of 300 measures of gain for sections D and O is $11 \cdot 8 \pm 5$. The average of 297 measures for sections E and N is $11 \cdot 2 \pm 5$. The difference is $\cdot 6 \pm \cdot 7$. Being less than its probable error, the difference is a statistically insignificant one. . . .

SUMMARY STATEMENT OF RESULTS AND CONCLUSIONS

On the Knowlton tests, designed to measure enrichment of a worth-while sort, the experimental group gain exceeded the control group gain by 19 per cent. . . .

The greater gain of the experimental group consisted of learning about, in descending order, causal relationships, persons and places. The experimental group gained less of worth-while time knowledge, but learned twice as many worth-while *causal* relationships not frequently known by history teachers. . . .

Retention, over periods varying from 3 to 7 months, was measured in two ways which we call relative and absolute, relative being the percentage retained of what was gained, and absolute being the retained gain or net gain after forgetting.

The experimental group retained more, relatively, of knowledge of relationships, to the learning of which the photoplays also contributed most. Of person and place knowledge, the experimental group retained relatively about the same or a little less. Of time knowledge the experimental group clearly retained relatively less. Of all combined they also retained relatively less.

In the so-called absolute units, even though the experimental group forgot more, they retained more of relation, person and place knowledge. Of time knowledge they retained less. Of all combined they retained more. Compared with the 19 per cent contribution on full gains, the contributions based on net gains is about 12 per cent. The loss was due chiefly to the forgetting of time knowledge. . . .

The control and experimental groups were compared as to the reading of history in the school library and outside of school, as to their liking for history as compared with their liking for six other subjects studied, and as to information contributed in class and obtained outside. In none of these measures did the experimental group average exceed the control group average.

However, more weight should be attached to the findings in the classroom, since they were obtained under controlled conditions. In the classroom discussion the experimental group participated more to the extent of about 10 per cent and showed more desire to participate. This was especially true of the more voluntary participations. . . .

"THE RELATIVE INFLUENCE OF TWO TYPES OF MOTIVATION ON IMPROVEMENT." By VERNER MARTIN SIMS, Louisiana Polytechnic Institute, Ruston, La. From *Journal of Educational Psychology*, October 1928. *Quoted by Permission.*

The experiments here reported are attempts to evaluate the influence upon improvement of two different types of motivation : in the first type, which we have called individual-motivation, the individual competes against his own record and against that of other individuals of like ability ; in the second type, which we have called group-motivation, the individual as a member of a group, competes against another group. Two experiments are reported, the first using substitution as the function to be improved, the second using rate of reading.

The method of conducting the experiment in substitution and the results of the experiment are as follows :

An initial practice period of three minutes at substituting digits for letters was given to 126 college sophomores and juniors, and on the basis of the number of substitutions made per minute, three sections of twelve each were equated by selecting trios the members of which made the same initial score, one member of the trio going into each of the three sections. This manner of selection made the sections equal in range as well as in central tendency.

These three sections practised at substitution three times a week for a total of twelve practice periods, using the same as that used in the initial period, but with varying forms. The practice periods after the initial one were two minutes in length.

The three sections were motivated as follows :

Section I. The Control Section.—No motivation other than that which came incidentally from seeing their own progress and that of their neighbours was used. The blanks were collected immediately after the practice, no attempt was made to prevent them from watching their progress or to encourage them to improve. They perhaps knew approximately what their score was ; and they left the room in a body immediately after the practice, perhaps discussing it to a slight extent.

Section II. The Group-motivated Section.—The section was divided into two groups, whose total initial score was approximately equal, and they were competed against each other. Before beginning practice the average score of each group for the preceding practice period was read to the section, the amount of improvement for each group was given, and a graph showing the total progress of each group was presented. They were then encouraged to put forth their best efforts to make their respective groups win. After the practice the blanks were collected and the group dismissed.

Section III. The Individually-motivated Section.—The section was divided into pairs, the two members of a pair having approximately equal initial ability. Before beginning practice each individual score was called out, and as they were called each member entered on a graph his own score and that of his particular competitor. In addition, the names of the three persons who showed the greatest improvement with the three that made the least improvement and the names of the three persons who made the highest scores with those three that made the lowest scores on the previous day's practice were reported to the class with the praise or blame which the record deserved. All were encouraged to surpass their previous records and if possible to defeat their respective competitors. Immediately after the practice the blanks were collected and the groups dismissed.

Using the average of the last two practice periods as the final ability we find that:

Section I improved from 36 substitutions per minute to 72·8 substitutions per minute, or 102·2 per cent.

Section II improved from 36·1 substitutions per minute, to 75·8 substitutions per minute, or 109·9 per cent.

Section III improved from 36·2 substitutions per minute, to 93·3 substitutions per minute, or 157·7 per cent.

Similar experiments on rate of reading gave the following results:

TABLE II

INITIAL AND FINAL RATE OF READING FOR
THREE SECTIONS

	Initial Rate (Words per Minute).	Final Rate (Words per Minute).	Per Cent Improvement.
Section I .	167·3	181·9	8·7
Section II	167·5	191·9	14·5
Section III	167·7	226·0	34·7

To summarize, with these two types of material, rate of reading and rate of substituting, and with the groups here used, individual-motivation is vastly superior to group-motivation and group-motivation is but slightly superior to no motivation other than that which comes incidentally in learning. To the extent that reading and substitution are typical of learning in general, one may say that for the groups here concerned individual-motivation is the superior form of motivation. To the extent that these students are typical of students in general, one may say that for improving the rate of substituting and the rate of reading individual-motivation is superior to group-motivation.

From the standpoint of efficiency in learning, there is urgent need for a repetition of these experiments using different functions for improvement and different age groups as subjects. More than this, it is essential that the groups be tested after periods of no practice in order that the permanency of the improvement may be ascertained. The superiority of the individually-motivated group may represent a " forced growth " which in time will disappear. And finally, before any practical educational value can be derived from such information, we must know that a function thus improved will show general improvement in the various situations where it may be used, *i.e.* that an increased rate of reading under drill conditions such as those here outlined will mean an increased rate in other situations involving reading.

SUGGESTED READINGS

Of the countless publications on Education none are concerned with a body of knowledge which may be called purely scientific. Nevertheless, education is utilizing the results of scientific research in choosing and in gaining its objectives. These are so numerous and so mingled with the arts, that it is not easy to name outstanding books that are dominantly scientific. Those concerned with the use of intelligence and achievement tests are most distinctive. Goddard, Terman, Thorndike, Courtis, Thurstone, are prominent leaders in developing reliable tests and in showing how they may be used as aids in educational research; but the actual uses of tests in schools are being tried out by the common-sense observation of teachers, principals, supervisors and superintendents, aided by psychological experts.

Good accounts of tests and their use in schools are found in such books as :

FREEMAN, FRANK N., *Mental Tests, their History, Principles and Application*, 1926.

GILLILAND, A. R., and JORDAN, R. H., " Educational Measurements and the Classroom Teacher," 1924.

PINTNER, R., *Intelligence-testing Methods and Results*, 2nd ed., 1931.

Among superintendents using scientific aids in improving schools, Washburne of Winnetka, Illinois, is prominent; while the progressive type of school is set forth in :

COBB, STANWOOD, *Progressive Education and its Effects upon the Child and Society*, 1928.

Most of the researches in education will be found listed and summarized in the Year-books of the Society for the Study of Education, printed by the Public School Publishing Company.

Some of the newer type of educational research are indicated by the following :

CHAMBERS, O. R., " A Method of Measuring the Emotional Maturity of Children," *Pedagogical Seminary*, page 637, 1925.

LINCOLN, EDWARD A., " The Later Performance of Under-aged Children Admitted to School on the Basis of Mental Age," *Journal of Educational Research*, January 1929.

SYMONDS, PERCIVAL M., and CHASE, DORIS H., " Practice *versus* Motivation," *Journal of Educational Psychology*, January 1929.

WINSOR, A. L., " Inhibition and Learning," *Psychological Review*, Sept., 1929.

Chapter XIII

MAN AND THE UNSEEN WORLD, OR RELIGION

CHARACTERISTICS OF RELIGIOUS BEHAVIOUR

THE common objective feature of all religious behaviour is that it is influenced by some sort of existence that cannot be directly perceived by the senses. It has the same basis as the belief that a man is not simply a visible body, but that he has a mind or spirit, which directs his acts in accordance with purposes. In dealing with men this presupposition is justified by experience. One can usually react more satisfactorily to other persons by interpreting and anticipating what they are doing and what they are going to do, than by reacting to the observed objective movements. The higher animals, plants, forces of nature, and sometimes even stones and other animate objects are treated as if they, too, acted with a purpose.

Such attitudes are assumed not only by savages and poets, but under certain conditions are manifested by all sorts of men. If one is hurt by anything with which he is dealing, there is an impulse, not infrequently acted upon, to try to smash the offending object. The weather is commended or condemned every day as if it were a person, and all nature seems to partake of our moods like good friends, or to ignore or jeer at them, like strangers or enemies. This universal human tendency, much disguised in this scientific age, is of the same texture as all behaviour that may be called religious.

All religions involve some sort of a conception of forces, spirits, or persons associated with whatever happens in the objective world, and the practice of a ritual of some kind supposed to be effective in influencing these invisible powers in ways analogous to means that are effective with persons.

All acts of men indicating such beliefs and practices are religious in some degree. In its higher forms religion implies prayer and reverence ; but in its lower forms gods may be beaten like slaves to make them do one's will, may be bribed, cajoled, tricked, or compelled by magic formulas, signs, or rituals to grant favours.

Superstitions and beliefs in luck which have some influence on most civilized men even in this scientific age, have the same basis in human nature as religion. Beliefs of this kind may be denied, but if one refuses to begin a journey on Friday, to eat at a table of thirteen, or does something to change the luck in gaming, he shows an underlying belief in the unseen.

If one has a feeling that his luck is going to be good or bad because of some acts he has recently performed, he is in much the same situation as the religionist who seeks the favour of gods not only by rituals, but by daily conduct which he supposes to be pleasing to his gods. " What have I done to deserve this ? " is one of the most universal cries when sudden calamity comes. The moral expectation derived from human associations of other persons acting toward us much as we act toward them, is applied to the universe. " I have not abused the universe. Why should it treat me thus ? " This belief, that certain kinds of acts are more acceptable to spirits or gods or to the universe than others, is a more or less prominent feature of all religions. In Confucianism and some forms of Christianity it is very important, whilst in some religions all that is regarded as necessary is that rituals shall be observed in proper ways and at suitable times and places, and then one may behave as he pleases the rest of the time.

THE PSYCHOLOGICAL BASIS OF PRAYER

The essentials of a correct answer as to why men pray are embodied in this sentence : " All men have been helpless infants and had their wants supplied by persons of seemingly unlimited power." The child in his helplessness is apparently powerful, for when he wishes or commands it comes to pass.

x

In his earliest conscious experience the feeling of hunger or pain, perhaps accompanied by a cry or gesture brings relief and satisfaction, and there is no need to consider ways by which things are made to happen. Later when difficulties arise he calls for help. The first method of getting things is therefore by prayer, and all through life whenever insurmountable difficulties are encountered there is resort to prayer for help to a being more powerful in some or all respects than self. No matter how strong an adult's beliefs in mechanical causation are, or how long he has acted in accordance with known causes, this attitude of getting the unattainable by appeal to a superior power remains. It is evident, therefore, that religious and prayerful attitudes are the inevitable results of man's nature and of experiences that all persons have, especially in early life.

Thus we see religion in general is the outcome of a subjective view of man and of the world in which one dwells. It is not concerned with physical forces of nature, but with human purposes and powers. All observable phenomena are thus regarded. Religion, and religious attitudes and practices, can be understood only by studying the nature of man as shown in this tendency to view all things subjectively and personally. His nature being what it is, and having a period of helpless infancy, he would probably be religious no matter what sort of world he inhabited.

On the other hand, the ideas of gods and of how they may be propitiated are modified by the objective surroundings, and the culture of the time and place, and are in many respects distinctly local and individual. The great religions of the world with their infinite varieties of belief and ritual are the products of individual imagination and thought. They have survived because of the personal influence of their originators and disciples, their supposed objective usefulness, and their adaptation to subjective needs. Shamans and priests emphasize the usefulness of religion in this life, and usually foster belief in its value to a future life.

SCIENTIFIC AND RELIGIOUS ATTITUDES DIFFER

The scientific attitude also has a basis in human nature, but develops out of a different type of facts. It comes from experiences in which results are gotten not in unknown ways, but by known means. The closer one observes objects and events, and the more accurate his generalization as to what means always accompany a given result, the more scientific does one become. In its earlier, cruder stage it is what is called the common-sense attitude of expecting that objects, and to some extent persons, will behave as we and others have found them to behave when certain acts are performed or certain conditions exist. If a stone drops on one's foot the results are painful whether anyone made it drop or not. Water wets, however it may come to a person or object. Stones sink in water and wood floats in it, regardless of what people do. But human beings actuated by purposes are much more variable. Inanimate objects and tools are usually viewed objectively, while animals and sometimes plants and phenomena of nature, such as day and night and unusual happenings, are often regarded as personal in their behaviour. Some tribes have rituals connected with utensils, weapons, and tools, that are supposed to insure that they will function properly. Planting of seed, births, and deaths are generally occasions for rituals recognizing the subjective, human, and religious attitude toward things that are variable or not well understood in the light of ordinary objective experience.

Science has advanced in proportion as man has taken the objective attitude in looking for causes of changes produced by things, instead of imagining the variable purposes of forces or spirits in things, that determine what shall happen. In the latter case there is no way of checking imagined causes by objective study.

Only within the last two or three centuries has the scientific attitude toward the world in which we live prevailed over the personal, sufficiently to bring a rapid advance in knowledge. When it was believed only a century ago that cream failed to change to butter because it was bewitched, there was no encouragement to study carefully the exact condition of cream when it was being churned. Science has led to so many practical applications in every field of known affairs, especially in mechanical things, that even the uneducated people have been led to acquire something of the mechanistic attitude toward the world, and now view nature as a vast intricate machine acting in accordance with physical laws, rather than controlled by powers resembling human beings. This mechanistic attitude at first asserted for stars and inanimate objects, gradually extended to plants, animals, and to human beings, individually, and in groups. Justification of the view has been found in the increased ability to predict and control changes in nearly all phases of practical life.

Achievements of science have been greatest in the objective world where exact observations and measurements by more than one person are possible. Subjective facts may be observed by one person only, thus the observations of many supposedly similar phenomena cannot be accurately compared. This does not mean that it is impossible to acquire subjective truths, but merely that they cannot be formulated with the same generality or exactness as in the objective world, nor can they be as accurately checked by experience and experiments. It is much more difficult, for example, to find *persons* enough alike and in as nearly the same situation to secure exactly the same results from an experiment, than to get two pieces of iron that are alike, in the same temperature, etc., so that chemical and physical tests will give the same results for each. The objective behaviour of two persons may be compared with some assurance by taking the average of many tests under as nearly the same conditions as possible ; but there is no way of accurately comparing the ideas of emotions of individuals as experienced or described by themselves, since there is no way of knowing how much the conscious states indicated by their words differ. In dealing with human beings the interpretation of behaviour as governed by subjective purposes is practically useful, but accurate scientific study of subjective purposes is impossible except by indirect means. Furthermore, the objective view is analytic, while the subjective is concerned with actions as performed by a person as a whole. The subjective view is much like that of the driver of an automobile who expects it to do his will as he makes various movements, but gives little thought to the parts of the auto and their relation to each other ; while the objective and scientific view is more like that of a mechanic who knows all the parts and their relations, though he may have little skill in driving. The non-mechanical driver of an auto is pleased or irritated by the behaviour of the machine as a whole, much as he would be by the acts of a person. In the typical subjective attitude causes are thought of in terms of human motives and purposes rather than those determined by mechanical laws.

In the objective view the final result is the sum of a series of parts or causes, while in the subjective view the aspect of the whole is something different from the parts. There is ground for the claim that the two views are not of the same phenomena. A machine is not merely the sum of its parts, a word is not merely so many letters, a blue stripe is not the same when seen with red as when it is placed beside yellow. In other words, elements, objects, and forces when combined are not merely so many chemical elements, so many cells, or so many organic parts, but something more than all of them.

As social creatures, a purely scientific description of the parts or traits of a person cannot mean to us what a person is as a whole. The behaviouristic psychologists may describe the impersonation of Lady Macbeth by an actress in terms of attitudes and gestures, and give us exact measurements of movements of eyes, eyebrows, lips, tongue, vocal organs, changes in breathing, heart-beat, and the muscular tensions of all sorts, yet such a report, however accurate, would not correspond at all to the mental states of actor and observer. A trained actor or an expert critic might note some of these details, but both would be more concerned with the general mental states of the actors and the audience. The natural human reaction to the behaviour is to think of a person as thinking and feeling as one's self would under the same circumstances, in accordance with certain emotions and purposes. To consider the physical stimuli and the physiological mechanism involved in the movements made, is quite a different sort of observation.

Long training is necessary in order to take a purely objective attitude toward the behaviour of any person. Even skilled observers disagree as to what happens when actions of human beings are in question.

It is possible by the use of machines to get accurate records of all objective signs and determine which of several reports is most nearly correct. It is not, however, the accuracy of a description or of a moving picture that gives it interest, but the interpretations of those actions in terms of human purposes. Purely objective methods of searching for truth can never tell us what God and man are as subjectively viewed or conceived personalities. Neither can the detailed study of scientists serve as guides to poets and artists in their creative effort. The world as seen by religionists and artists in the light of man's own spirit is of supreme interest and value to man. However far objective and inductive science may extend its researches into the elements and nature of human behaviour, the conduct of persons in the home and in social life will be based on the idea that each is a conscious, purposeful personality. Religion, like common-sense belief, is based on the ideas of subjective personality, and hence its angle of viewing man and nature is different from that of science. The child, the poet, and the artist in all men finds this personal idea more or less satisfying, and so does the religionist. It is a profound truth that " Except ye become as little children ye cannot enter into the Kingdom of Heaven " (*i.e.* the religious attitude). As a way of knowing and using what is true of the world in which we live, science is supreme ; but life seems worth-while largely because of the subjectively viewed personalities with which we naturally people the world.

The childlike impulse to rely on powerful personalities to bring wishes to realization by unknown means, rather than to study painfully the exact and fixed relationship of means and ends, continues in certain fields during the whole life, and is not necessarily contradicted by scientific study. The scientist and the practical man satisfy themselves by discovering and using truths regarding means of insuring objective results, while the religionist uses rituals and prayers and satisfies phases of his nature by wishes that are to a greater or less extent subjectively, if not objectively, realized.

The thoroughgoing scientist having obtained objective success in so many fields, believes that success in every field, however mysterious, may ultimately be gained by scientific study. The religionist, on the other hand, on the basis of subjective realizations is inclined to rely upon wishes to bring results where there is no definitely known means of getting them by objective means. To relieve a toothache one now goes to a dentist instead of resorting to self-examination and prayer as did Cotton Mather ; but an unknown disease or danger drives men to prayer just as a child calls for help when he knows not what to do.

NATURE OF DEITIES

The child's first cry of discomfort which brings relief is not made to any definite portion of the universe ; and the same is true of many of our wishes throughout life. In the child's early experiences the usual fulfiller of his wishes is a person, much more powerful and wise than self. It is natural, therefore, that there should arise the idea of gods who, like persons, fulfil wishes (or sometimes thwart them). In nearly all religions God is personal, with characteristics similar to those of human beings but possessed of superhuman power and perfections. In all religions involving worship (and it is a question whether the word religion should be applied to beliefs and practices which lack that element) God represents what is considered by his worshippers as best in human nature. The Hebrew God was frankly regarded as the friend and helper of his people as long as they obeyed him. He gave them not only spiritual help but also material prosperity, if they loved and served him. The Christian God, as presented by Jesus, is like a loving father who sends rain on the just and the unjust and who does not wait to hear words of repentance from the prodigal son. He is to be trusted as one who clothes the lilies, notes the fall of a sparrow, and views with sympathy all that befalls man. To many persons such a God is a resource and comfort that can be replaced by nothing else.

To the individual who has become obsessed with the idea of a mechanical world where every event is only a link in a series unvaried by chance or personal wish, the idea of a personal cause seems absurd. Such a man may, however, love his auto or sail-boat which responds to every wish, though he knows that it is merely an assembly of parts which work in accordance with mechanical laws ; but whatever one may believe in theory, his son, daughter, mother, or sweetheart are interesting to him as *persons*, rather than as an assembly of chemical substances.

An attitude analogous to that of religion is fostered by modern everyday experiences. When one addresses, stamps, and mails a letter, he expects without considering all the details of how it is done, that " Uncle Sam " will deliver it as desired. When one buys a railroad ticket or sends an express package he trusts the company to care for himself or his valuables, although he knows nothing of the details involved in bringing about the result. Every day our faith in men and corporations is justified by our experience and by that of others. We wish, and there are mechanisms, or persons, or institutions, ready to fulfil our wish when it is properly signified. We can now get our wishes granted with little more knowledge of means than when we were young children. We continually appeal to experts to do for us what we cannot do for ourselves.

To many persons it is natural to believe that there is a God who cares for one when there is need, in the way that parents did in childhood, and that an insurance company does now. This attitude of depending on God " who works in mysterious ways His wonders to perform " is more satisfactory to a large proportion of human beings than the scientific one of expecting everything to happen in accordance with fixed laws, partly known and partly yet to be discovered.

It is not impossible, however, for individuals to alternate

between the two views, or even to combine them. One may conceive of the laws of nature as the uniform and consistent ways of acting of either a Supreme Being who is conscious and personal, or of a non-personal Power or Force. The nature of Deity can never be determined by scientific methods, hence, what God is, is a matter of faith. All religions of large influence have taught faith in a personal God. The more science reveals a universe of law the less God is appealed to for material help and the more he is relied upon for spiritual satisfactions, if appealed to at all. A strong religious faith properly directed may be worth more to some individuals than any truth given by an expert in mental hygiene. The best way of judging of the value of a man's religion to himself, is whether it gives him mental health and peace.

RELIGION IN A SCIENTIFIC AGE

Inductive science in theory, and religion in theology, have opposite methods of obtaining and verifying truths. In all cases where there is difference between them regarding explanations of events in the material world, science has become the more powerful, and religion on its theoretical side, weaker. In the explanations of *human* behaviour, science is gaining but is not yet overwhelmingly powerful. The growing dominance of science is perhaps shown most clearly in the transfer of prophecy from the field of religion to that of science. In all the more advanced fields of science a study of the past and present makes it possible to predict the future with a high degree of certainty and exactness. This is perhaps greatest in astronomy where the exact minute of an eclipse may be foretold a century ahead. In physics, the exact time required for a sound or a beam of light to reach a certain place can be calculated, or the weight necessary to crush a stone can be given. In chemistry, what will happen when a given amount of one substance is added to another under proper conditions may be expressed in exact terms. The action of individuals or of societies under certain conditions is also predictable. As this power of prediction by using the methods of science increases, there is no prospect of a corresponding increase in faith in the prophecies of religion, many of which must wait for a future life for verification.

When we turn from the theoretical differences between science and religion to their place in the minds of the great mass of people in their daily living, there is frequently little realization of conflict. The attitudes involved in the child-parent relationship requiring certain actions toward parents, do not prevent a child from acting toward companions in quite a different way. The study and use of means does not prevent us from wishing with some expectation that things, and especially people, will serve our ends. The attitude of believing what we see, does not prevent us from accepting in full faith statements of other persons regarding things they have experienced. Much of what is known both of scientific truths and of those of religion is not the result of individually acquired knowledge, but of what is learned from others. There is no fundamental difference in attitude between quoting the Bible, or a scientist; or between pressing a button to light the room, and saying a prayer to bring peace of mind. We accept and use the facilities provided by science and religion with only occasional questioning by a few as to the ultimate and justifiable reasons for so doing. With few exceptions the child accepts the religion of his parents nominally if not actively. It is the exception rather than the rule for an adult to inquire into the foundations of religious belief and practice, and as a result to change his church affiliation.

A large number do give up their religion because of their scientific study. This is most likely to occur when facts of the physical world are involved and when religious doctrines seem to be in conflict with the facts and theories of science. When such questions are not raised, most individuals in their daily living are probably not aware of conflict between their attitude toward religion and toward science. To pray for the recovery of a sick friend while ministering to his needs and asking for the help of scientific experts is not at all incongruent. To provide for every comfort of a friend going on a journey is not contradicted, but supplemented, by the *wish* that he may have a pleasant and safe journey. Indeed the consciousness that a friend has expressed the wish, and the idea that he is still wishing or even praying for one, may give a peace and confidence that cannot be supplied by the mere furnishing of every known scientific means of insuring safety and comfort. The satisfactions that come from the thought of the attitude of persons toward us is quite different, and to many much greater than the knowledge that all that science can do has been done to bring the desired result.

The same truth holds in attitudes toward the universe. The view of it as a system of mechanically acting forces is, for many people, less natural and satisfying than one which conceives of it as the embodiment of a personal deity whose attitude is like that of human beings. If the two views of the world are not forced into conflict, the majority of men may continue to maintain both the scientific idea of impersonal cause dominating in the best-known fields, and the idea of spirits or deities in the less known and less controllable events of life and death. In ordinary living the thought of personal approval, human and divine, may mingle with the effort to use every means of science to secure the wished-for result.

Science satisfies the impulse to know and understand, and gives power to do all sorts of things, while religion gives hope and subjective satisfactions. Both are the outgrowth of man's nature and experience. The early experiences of childhood, and of personal associations in later life, foster religious tendencies ; while the later experiences of childhood and adulthood foster the scientific attitude of using known means to gain ends. Complete dominance of the scientific attitude is prevented by personal associations with others, by interest in æsthetic wholes rather than elements and their relations, and by meeting situations where science cannot predict or control, and the only resource is to wish or pray in thought or behaviour for the end desired. Science satisfies the desire for order and consistency, while religion and art satisfy other phases of one's nature. An increasing number may choose scientific satisfactions to the exclusion of religious ones, but many human beings will, more or less successfully, continue to secure religious and subjective satisfactions in an objective and materially ordered world.

There is no possibility that science will prove that there is no God, no future life, and no subjective answers to prayer. Nor is it possible to prove that the scientist is wrong in his presuppositions that this is an ordered world, the truths of which may be discovered by the use of scientific methods. The basis for reasoning in the two cases is different, and men accept whichever is most satisfactory to them. Some find ways of harmonizing the two views ; such as conceiving of a universe whose uniform laws are the will of a deity who made or permeates it, and believing that such a deity's will may be discovered by scientific research. A scientist in his investigations must proceed on the supposition that if there is such a deity his will is uniform in its action. Scientific knowledge would not necessarily be *wholly* impossible if there were rare variations in the form of special " acts of providence ", but expectation of such variations would be a serious damper on scientific research.

The choice of either the scientific or of the religious attitude, or of both as harmonized or in separate compartments, is for the individual to make in the same way in which he classes one work of art as preferable to another. There is little gained and often much lost by trying to show that either view is wholly false. Science may vindicate itself in all objective affairs and religion in subjective, without compelling an individual to carry over conclusions from one field into the other.

Religion, as expressed in a body of theological beliefs regarding the world and man is the natural rival of scientific theories, but religion as a way of feeling, acting, and thinking is not necessarily so. To respond to a person, a poem, a song, a flower, a landscape or to the universe or a god as something to be enjoyed and made a part of living without much thought of why or how, is a natural reaction of the untrained human being. The why and how, so far as they are present in thought, are chiefly of the child, wish, purpose, fulfilment, and artistic types. When an attempt is made to understand the exact nature of deity and how he acts, intellectual activity dominates over the emotional, and some sort of a theology is formulated. The success of science in showing how objects may be changed and disease prevented or cured, has been so far in advance of efforts to get results by prayer or other theological or religious means, that there is no longer much competition in the minds of intelligent people. The same is true of scientific explanations of storms and other physical phenomena, as against the theological explanation of their being the will of God.

In the subjective world the advantages of the scientific as compared with the religious attitude are not so great, partly because psychology is still a new science and partly because the personal attitude is more natural and usable in that field than the impersonal, analytic, objective attitude of science. There is little doubt, however, that long-distance plans for changing the behaviour of human beings may ultimately be carried out more successfully under the guidance of scientific knowledge, than by subjective knowledge of conscious personalities.

Every advance in science and in the scientific attitude of men toward situations that they meet, results inevitably in enlarging the field of activities in which behaviour is directed by science. Religious leaders are unwise who oppose science in objective affairs, where it is strong, and who neglect to seek for the forms of belief and ritual that will enable religion to render its best aid in giving subjective satisfactions.

CO-OPERATION OF SCIENCE AND RELIGION

As previously indicated religion is to a considerable extent based on the experience of early childhood of wishing and getting results in accordance with purposeful acts of superiors, while science is the result of studying the objective means by which results may be reached. On this basis we may expect religion to set before men goals to be attained, and science to provide the means of reaching them. Desire and the study of means naturally increase together. This accords with the facts of history which show that desire to reach goals set up as desirable by religion have exercised a powerful influence over human behaviour. Until recently, however, the means used were also prescribed by religion, sometimes wisely by great leaders who knew human nature, and sometimes unwisely.

With the development of psychology and sociology, the church has begun to rely more upon scientific research to point out the best means of attaining desired ends. Some kinds of religious training have failed, or have produced results contrary to those desired. The results of scientific study of psychology, child nature, and education are being used in Sunday School and in other religious training. Churches are also having church surveys made to determine scientifically what methods are most effective under various conditions.

It is the special function of science to supply knowledge that will help in attaining any end that may be desired by man ; but it can only incidentally indicate what ends to desire. When several ends are desired, science may show how they are related to each other in the way of one helping or hindering in the attainment of others.

By eliminating some of the ends proposed by religion, both common sense and science have been important influences. In most civilized countries the idea that religion must not demand continued action injurious to physical and mental health, or to the disruption of the social life of a people, places considerable limitation upon religious objectives. At one time, any way of securing a better eternal life for human beings was favoured regardless of the immediate effects on individuals and society. Religion now usually considers what is desirable in this life as well as in the life to come. Few forms of religion ignore temporal life or regard its ends as directly opposed to those of eternity. This change is doubtless due in part to the fact that science has provided so many reliable means of securing present ends, and has thus made a future state of less immediate interest. The other-worldly types of Christianity have therefore declined.

It is less easy to point out the direct and indirect influences of religion upon science, and its usefulness in scientific effort. In so far as theologies involved facts and theories of the material world, they were rivals of the scientific theories and often hindered the advance of science. On the other hand, as is true in every line of effort, devotion to scientific research has often been increased by religion as a motive in the mind of the searcher after truth. Men who looked only to sacred books or other authorities for knowledge did not help scientific discovery, but those who studied nature's laws to discover the divine will were more faithful labourers in the field of science because of their religion. The great function of religion is to furnish ideals and motives. It is religion and art that inspire men to rise, while science continually provides more effective means of realizing what has been conceived. The more religion and science limit themselves each to its special function, the fewer errors will be made by each.

RELIGIOUS TOLERANCE AND APPRECIATION

There are several hundred denominations in this country professing the same Christian religion. All are guided more or less by the same Scriptures, and all aim to promote a good life here and hereafter. Most of them originated when theology was a common subject of discussion, and each was formed to emphasize some particular doctrine, ritual, or mode of living. Many are practically alike except in form of church organization. The keen rivalry that once existed between them has now nearly ceased, and they are co-operating in many ways. All the Protestant churches are more democratic in their government than formerly, and the theological differences between denominations is growing less prominent. The difference between Catholic and Protestant is more in ritual, and in the place of the church and its representatives in managing religious affairs, than it is in fundamentals of beliefs and in the ideals of conduct set forth.

Unfortunately both Protestants and Catholics know more of what to them are the objectionable features of the other, than they do of the best features. Every church has much in its history and present practices that could not fail to commend itself to persons of other churches, if they were informed of them.   It may be that in order to bring about the understanding, tolerance and appreciation of all beliefs so desirable in citizens of a common country, the good work of various churches will need to be presented to young people in school.

Assuming that good actions are, in general, such as are approved by the majority of the group to which one belongs, it is clear that all religious observances of a people who have common religious beliefs, are regarded as good.   There is no distinction made between acts that directly bring injury to a neighbour, and those that offend the deity worshipped, and thus may bring injury to the entire group, except that the latter are regarded as much more serious.   Theoretically, there is a clear distinction between classing acts as good or bad (a) because of their results to men, or (b) because of the way in which they are believed to be viewed by a god.   To take part in all religious observances as to sacred days, places, objects, and acts of worship are religious duties ; while to do good to one's neighbours, to refrain from robbing, killing, or injuring them in any way are moral duties.

This distinction is sometimes clearly made by individuals of the same group : one individual carefully conforms to all religious requirements, while another ignores them, but is strictly moral in his dealings with his fellow-men.   In many minds there is no clear distinction as to whether acts are right because of relations to deity, or of relations to one's fellows.   In the form of Christian religion which accepts God as a father and concludes that every man is therefore a brother, the two motives of pleasing the Father and of doing good to the brother, are combined.   The religious minded are concerned with doing the Father's will, and the more socially minded with justice and kindness to the brother-men.   In the past these two motives have sometimes called for opposing types of action.   Among savage people, human beings were often sacrificed as a religious duty, and not many centuries ago it was deemed a religious obligation to punish and torture unbelievers, or those who believed and practised a different religion. At the present time, especially in this country, it is generally agreed that religious beliefs and practices should be left to the individual's own conscience and the discipline of his own church ; while moral practices affecting general welfare are to be regulated in other ways, especially by the state. A few laws such as those relating to Sunday observance and to marriage are still inconsistently based more on religious than on moral grounds.

In general, throughout history there has been a reciprocal influence of religious beliefs on morals, and of customary or moral practices on religious beliefs and practices. This has been especially true in Christian countries except at times when theological and " other-worldly " ideas of Christianity were most prominent. Whenever a change in moral practices has been attempted by reformers, it has been difficult to secure general acceptance and practices of the newer ideals without the assistance of religious leaders. The modern health movement has been greatly furthered by religious endorsement. With the common people, new moral ideals, even if accepted in theory, are often not put into practice unless they are also set forth as being religious duties. The most disagreeable duties may be faithfully observed when strongly sanctioned by religion. Social reforms have been greatly advanced by religious leaders who emphasize social rather than individual salvation.

There are at present an increasing number of persons who live according to their moral beliefs without the direct stimulus of religious beliefs. Whether the great mass of humanity may be brought to a higher plane of moral life without the aid of religion is a disputed question. However that may be, there can be no question that moral advancement will be greater if religionists and moralists can agree in sanctioning the same types of conduct. No matter how clearly science may show the way to human betterment, there is a chance that without the direct and indirect influence of religion, the new way will be followed tardily, if at all, by the masses.

Y

SELECTED RESEARCHES

"EXPERIMENTAL EFFORTS TO TEACH HONESTY."
By HUGH HARTSHORNE and MARK A. MAY. From *Studies in Deceit*, 1928. *Quoted by Permission.*

We have not as yet undertaken any experiment in the teaching of honesty. In several instances, however, we have co-operated with others who wished to do so by furnishing tests in order that they might be able to measure their results. Two such experiments have been reported to us which, though too brief and incomplete to be conclusive, are nevertheless of considerable interest. . . .

The six junior high school groups used for the experiment were selected with a view to equivalence in sex, age, and intelligence. A ninth-grade civics class consisting of both boys and girls, a seventh-grade home room of boys, and an eighth-grade home room of girls were each given fifteen minutes of daily instruction for three weeks in The Honesty Book. The lessons consisted of interesting stories of honest and dishonest behaviour and discussions of the problem of honesty as it appears in various life situations. For such direct teaching the material offered seemed the best available. The other three classes which served as "controls", were another ninth-grade civics class of boys and girls, a seventh-grade class of girls, and an eighth-grade class of boys. To each of these six classes were given the Sims Score Card and the Speed and Co-ordination tests. The deception tests were given just before the three weeks of intensive teaching began and again just after it was completed. It was expected that the effectiveness of the teaching would be shown by comparing the change that had taken place by the end of the three weeks in the experimental groups (those subjected to the teaching) with the change that had taken place in the control groups (those which had *not* had the teaching). . . .

Figure 88 shows that in the case of the Co-ordination tests all groups except the first experimental group were slightly more deceptive after the training than before. The first experimental group changed insignificantly for the better. When combined, the three experimental groups show a slight loss in honesty, and the control groups a somewhat greater loss in honesty.

The facts for the Speed test are somewhat different. Here all experimental groups were less deceptive after three weeks of training. But so also were two of the *control* groups, and the one that was more deceptive at the end of the period was only insignificantly so. . . .

So far as our results go, the particular method of teaching honesty employed in this experiment for fifteen consecutive school periods of fifteen minutes each did not make the pupils concerned less inclined than they already were to falsify their records in order to improve their scores. This does not mean that individual pupils may not have been benefited by the teaching, but that such benefits, if any, were confined to very few or were so restricted in character as to make no difference in the classroom behaviour of most of the children.

The second experiment we shall report was conducted by Dr. J. Maller, a graduate student at Teachers College, Columbia University. His purpose was to find what effect the mention of God in connection with a test would have on the honesty of children. The idea of God was introduced by the statement: God loves an honest man. But the ideas of God and honesty are here used in conjunction, so that it was necessary to determine the effect of the idea of honesty when the idea of God was not associated with it. This was accomplished by using first the statement: Honesty is the best policy.

The Speed tests were used for measuring deceptiveness. As there are six of these, they could be treated in three groups of two each. First of all, the entire six were administered as usual for the two practice trials, which were then collected. Then when the last trial was given, which the pupils were to score, the procedure was as follows:

1. Tests 1 and 2 were given and scored without comment, so that whatever deception occurred was without reference to the two ideas to be introduced.

2. Before beginning test 3 the examiner wrote on the board, " Honesty is the best policy ", and then administered tests 3 and 4, after which he erased the words and left the room.

3. Before the fifth test he wrote, " God loves an honest man ", and then, having given tests 5 and 6, he erased the phrase and left the room. There was thus introduced into the situation not only the stimulus of the words which theoretically would operate to lessen cheating, but also the additional time and the factor of having the examiner leave the room for a moment, which theoretically would operate to increase cheating.

This plan was followed with three groups of children, two of them being classes in Hebrew schools and one being a public school class consisting in part of children attending religious school during the week and in part of children without such training. The facts are summarized in Table LXIX, which gives the mean deception score for each of the three pairs of tests, the SD of the distribution and the SD of unreliability of the mean, and the number of cases

The first row R, is the record for the public school children who have religious instruction. The second row, H1, is for the

Hebrew school giving mild religious instruction, and the last row, H2, for the school giving more careful instruction.

TABLE LXIX

EFFECT ON DECEPTION OF THE MENTION OF DEITY

Group Number.		Tests 1 and 2.			Tests 3 and 4.			Tests 5 and 6.		
		M	SD	σM	M	SD	σM	M	SD	σM
R	25	8·9	5·3	1·06	6·4	4·2	·84	5·5	3·8	·76
NR	15	3·8	1·4	·36	7·8	3·5	·90	10·0	4·6	1·19
H1	29	5·2	4·8	·89	6·1	3·9	·72	6·3	2·4	·45
H2	26	7·8	2·8	·55	6·3	4·3	·84	1·1	4·9	·96

Of the public school class, the children who have religious teaching get progressively more honest as the idea of honesty and then the idea of God in association with the idea of honesty are introduced, whereas the children of the same classroom who do not attend religious school get progressively less honest under the same circumstances. Of the two Hebrew classes, one is not changed by either phrase ; and the other while not responding to the first phrase, is apparently greatly affected when the idea of God is mentioned.

This experiment was only preliminary to a more adequate study, and the number of cases is too small for reliable conclusions. It is reported, however, as suggestive of the kind of experiment that might be easily conducted to discover the values for conduct that inhere in various customary forms of control. The differences between the groups and between the behaviour of the same group under the described conditions are large enough to warrant the feeling that in certain forms of religious training there are potential values for the control of conduct that are far from being realized in the ordinary life of the children concerned. . . .

SUGGESTED READINGS

Since the psychological studies of Religion by STARBUCK, E. D., *The Psychology of Religion*, N.Y., 1900, o.p., and LEUBA, JAMES H. A., *Psychological Study of Religion*, 1912, there has been an increasing tendency to study religion in a factual way by religious workers as well as by sociologists. The Federal Council of Churches maintains a research department, and issues many publications.

The following books present various phases of religion :

AMES, EDWARD S., *Religion*, 1929.

ATHEARN, WALTER S., *Measurements and Standards in Religious Education*, 1924.

BRUNNER, EDMUND De S., and others, *American Agricultural Villages* (analyses the economic, social and religious life of 140 villages), 1927.

CLARK, ELMER T., *The Psychology of Religious Awakening*, 1929.

COE, GEORGE A., *Social Theory of Religious Education*, 1927.

DOUGLASS, H. PAUL, *The Church in the Changing City*, 1927.

DOUGLASS, H. PAUL, *How to Study the City Church*, 1928.

EDDY, SHERWOOD, *New Challenges to Faith*, 1926.

KIRKPATRICK, CLIFFORD, *Religion and Human Affairs*, 1929.

LIVY-BRUHL, *Primitive Mentality*, 1923.

TILLYARD, AELFRIDA, *Spiritual Exercises and their Results ;* an Essay in Comparative Religion, 1927.

WATSON, GOODWIN B., *Experimentation and Measurement in Religious Education*, 1927.

CHAPTER XIV

REGULATION OF HUMAN INTERACTION, OR MORALS

MORAL CODES AND SCIENCE

WHERE a group have lived together for a considerable time, there are certain ways in which individuals and classes react toward each other that are recognized as good. Those most generally approved, constitute what may be called the moral code of the group. This code is usually not only approved, but where all are affected by its observance, is enforced by public disapproval of those not conforming, and usually by punishment. Persons who conform to this code without compulsion and in details that never are enforced, are regarded as genuinely or morally good.

Different peoples have widely varying standards or codes of conduct. Among Arabs hospitality is the supreme virtue, and truth-telling of little account. Moral practice and ideals, like other forms of culture, are exchanged and diffused by the meeting of one people with another, and are usually supported by religious sanctions.

ORIGIN OF MORAL CODES

There is no question that scientific methods may be used in determining the nature, origin and results of all the various moral practices of the human race. Such a study will give a body of knowledge constituting the pure science of ethics, but will not directly aid in determining which of the various approved modes of behaviour of the various groups are the better. As an applied science, however, the knowledge gained may be a help in showing what means can best be used to secure what is desired. As the science of engineering can help a town to choose the type of bridge that will best serve the purposes for which it is constructed, so the science of ethics may help in choosing an ethical code, if the ends to be secured can be agreed upon ; the greatest difference being in the large number of objectives to be gained by an ethical code. In the following pages the help that science may now give in reaching some of these objectives is indicated ; and the hope is held out that it may ultimately help to choose the codes that will be most helpful in attaining all the ends of living sought by man.

Accepted ideas of right have risen and developed into more or less definitely formulated codes of morals chiefly in two ways : (1) by the idealistic thinking of superior persons, and (2) by the practical experience of common people in adjusting their behaviour to each other when living in groups.

1. Religious and humanitarian idealists have been active in forming codes of conduct supposed to be better than those existing and suited to human beings of the highest type. The more socially minded ones have sought for a basis not so much in the original nature of men as individuals, but in the relations of men to each other. The latter, from the time of Plato's *Republic* down to the present time, have been portraying Utopian states where, because of wise regulatory codes, a people may enjoy all the delights of perfect living individually, and as a group. Some of these have been greatly admired and have had a limited influence on conduct ; but for the most part they have never been put completely into practice. Their suitability to such a creature as man has never been adequately tested by adoption and continued use. The practices of only a few persons have ever completely conformed to the ideals of religious and humanitarian leaders.

2. In common law and the ethical attitudes associated with it we have, on the contrary, codes that have developed from the experiences and judgments of ordinary men living together generation after generation. There can be no question, therefore, that as far as they go, such laws are suitable to man's nature and represent modes of conduct which of all that have been tried, work best in the situations

that have arisen. The basis of the common law is in the natural tendency to adjust one's actions so that the responses of others will help rather than hinder in reaching desired ends. When it is the custom for persons meeting to turn to the right, each is justified in expecting that the other will thus turn, and each has an obligation to do so, and when both conform neither is impeded in his journey. This is typical of most codes developing from experiences, except that it is a very simple adjustment involving exactly the same action by both parties. In most situations the acts are not the same, but one is accepted as the equivalent of the other, *e.g.* one constructs a tool and the other supplies him with food.

The tendency for persons to adopt a type of action relatively satisfactory to both after various actions and reactions have been tried, is hastened by the example of those around one, and also by group judgment of approval or disapproval which is often associated with punishment for the one who acts differently.

When there is dispute, and the case not clear as to which of two individuals is in the wrong, someone acts as a judge. His decision as to acts that do or do not conform to the usual approved practices of the group becomes a precedent for deciding other cases similar to it. In this way traditions are established in every group of people living together for several generations, in support of what may be called the accepted code. In England a very complete set of common laws applying to all sorts of situations involving property and personal rights were developed in this way. The whole English constitution has really been formed by an accumulation of accepted practices of government. In America, the English common law serves as a guide to judges in all cases where no statute law has been enacted to cover the case. Engineers and lawyers are now developing professional codes based on the decisions of a committee as to what should be done in cases brought to them for decision.

Every important cultural change makes it necessary to fit the principles of common law to new cases. For example, one question now open is how shall the old rights of protection against trespass be applied to flights over or landings on property by airplanes ?

It has been assumed with good reason that practices which have been found satisfactory for all members of a group during many generations of experience have some claim to be called right or moral since they are the outcome of the best judgment and experience of the people in a variety of situations. Such a set of common precepts, ideals, and laws, having continued for centuries must have had the essential element of being balanced in relation to each other so as to preserve the group under the conditions in which they have been living. The more stable the society behaving according to them, the stronger is the evidence of their being good. It would not follow, however, that any special practice is itself good or would work in another group when associated with different conditions and customs. A curious example of balancing one type of conduct with another is mentioned by Miss Kingsley. In certain African tribes where poisoning is common, the cook, wives, and house slaves of a king or chief are killed if he dies from unknown causes. This crude and seemingly unjust rule has protected leaders and generally curbed poisoning.

Customs and codes are not infrequently founded on false beliefs, especially superstitions, *e.g.* punishing of witches. Laws may also remain long after the conditions justifying them have ceased to exist. The old common law that a workman could not get damages from his employer unless he proved that neither he nor his fellow-worker was the cause of the accident, continued to guide decisions in this country long after there were big establishments using dangerous machines, under conditions which made it impossible for an individual worker to protect himself against the accidents that might occur. Since the employer controlled most of the conditions under which work was done, judges finally decided that he was responsible for injuries to his workman, unless he could prove that the injury was due to the employee's own act, after due precautions had been taken by the employer.

With the development of new conditions and more scientific

knowledge, laws better adapted to work may well be enacted without waiting for customs, common law and judges' decisions to adapt them to newly developed situations. Insurance companies were perfected in this way, in this country, much quicker than in England where regulative customs gradually developed them. Banking institutions are now required to conform to laws founded on business principles and not merely to customs governing individual borrowers and lenders. Science may soon have a larger part in constructing codes, than customs or idealistic thought, yet the worth of a law or code must be tested by actual experience, as in all applied science.

Social changes are now so rapid and customs so variable that the help of science is more than ever before needed in determining what legal and moral codes will work best.

HEALTH AND MORAL CODES

It is not difficult to show on the basis of scientific knowledge of physiology and psychology, that in general more of the ends desired by all men in this life are realized by people who individually and by public regulations act in ways that help maintain physical and mental health. It may be admitted that a few people enjoy being helpless invalids, and that ministering to those in need is satisfying to some persons. These two traits of human nature do not, however, demand ill-health for their realization. Abundant exercise for them may be found in the healthful reactions of children and parents to each other, and of adults who, because of varying experience, ability, and special conditions may give and also receive favours. A learned doctor in a strange city may need the aid of a motor-man in finding his way, but under other circumstances may be the one able to give help. Thus, although all may be in perfect health, there may exist mutual helplessness and helpfulness similar to that which obtains between sick and well, without the handicaps of weakness and the wasted effort of ministering to it.

With this ideal of what may help to realize all the ends desired by man, science may compare moral codes of various people by health tests and statistics and decide which is the best.   The rightness of individual acts is not so readily decided because there are usually special features not covered by the general rule.   For example, by scientific use of statistics it is possible to tell with a good deal of accuracy the comparative death-rates in Boston suburbs and Detroit suburbs next year, but it is not possible to predict whether a given individual will live longer in the Boston suburb where the water-supply is more effectively safeguarded, than if he lived on the river below Detroit.   Science may justify codes that provide for sufficient rest each day and week for every one, but it cannot say in a given case whether it would be right or wrong for an individual to go without rest for twenty hours.   Results to self and others might justify the individual act.   A people, however, who so managed their affairs that twenty hours' work a day was a frequent necessity could easily be proved by health statistics to be conforming to inferior ethical codes.   In a properly organized and regulated society the seeming need for overwork is almost entirely eliminated.   In general, science is becoming increasingly able to decide what regulations of behaviour for most people in the long run promote health, and hence it is becoming more helpful in making ethical codes.   These codes are of some help in determining the rightness of individual acts, but leave much to individual judgment.

In using standards, care must be exercised to take account of indirect and remote consequences of regulations.   The average health condition of one city could be made temporarily better than that of another, by at once destroying all weaklings.   This does not necessarily mean, however, that a people who practised this for many generations would ultimately be more healthy than one that continually studied causes of weakness and sickness to find means of avoiding such deficiencies.   By sufficient study and care, domestic animals have been made more vigorous than they were when nature killed off the weaklings, but did nothing to decrease the sources of sickness and death.   Savage peoples also who do little to maintain health or to cure the sick are not more healthy than civilized people who are partly guided by the sciences of hygiene and medicine.

It is not only the knowledge gained in caring for the sick and in promoting health that is valuable, but the attitude of helping those who need help tends to carry on all sorts of co-operative efforts where the advantage to the individual is indirect or remote. The adoption of quarantine and other health measures where there is an epidemic calls for the same kind of co-operative effort as is needed in providing for a future water-supply or for sanitary tenements. It is quite probable, therefore, that man by studying hygienic conditions and remedies for diseases and modifying his environment and his behaviour in the light of the knowledge gained, becomes more healthy than he would be should he omit such study and kill off all weaklings.

There are, however, some more special problems involving behaviour toward weaklings that are not so easy of solution. What shall be done in cases where it appears to be absolutely certain that no cure or improvement can be effected by any means known to science or likely to be discovered within the possible lifetime of the defective or sick individuals, such as the hopelessly insane and feeble-minded, or those who because of age or disease are in pain with no possibility of relief except by opium or death? The situation allows only (1) of keeping them alive as long as possible either (a) in pain or (b) in an unconscious state; (2) of allowing nature to take its course by doing nothing; or (3) by taking means of quickly ending the useless, burdensome life. In the case of animals the last course is now usually taken by civilized people, as being the more humane. Some savages take the same course with their aged and infirm people. Many civilized persons now say this should be done under carefully regulated conditions with those who have no minds with which to choose, and with those who prefer death to future burdensome suffering.

At present, these cases cannot be positively decided by the standard of ultimate health conditions, although evidence is accumulating that there may be cases to which the law, "thou shalt not kill" should not apply, especially among people who do not follow it in the case of criminals or in war-time.

Few forms of Christianity now favour actions directly opposed to the maintenance of health. Persons whose health would be weakened by fasting or performance of religious duties are temporarily excused by both Catholic and Protestants. In this country there are few who object for religious reasons to health codes.

SELF-SACRIFICE AS AN ETHICAL IDEAL

A code of morals much endorsed by religion has been maintained in a form which sometimes ignores and condemns the health standard in judging moral actions. This is the code which regards self-sacrifice as the highest form of moral action. Popular moral heroes have almost universally been persons who gave up wealth, ease, and often health and life to minister to others. Under some circumstances, such action may temporarily be justified by science, but in a properly ordered society occasions for such action will be made rare, and the value of the ideal much limited. With proper provisions and training there should be few people to be saved from death by drowning, fire, etc., and when there are any, the coast-guard, the firemen or other rescuers should be so trained and equipped that they can do it, usually without injury to self. Storms and earthquakes cannot be wholly guarded against, but when there are insurance companies and organizations such as the Red Cross, having supplies and trained men and women ready to meet such disasters on call, there should be little need for self-sacrifice, or of injury to the health of those giving aid. With increased knowledge of hygiene there is less sickness, and invalids are better cared for by trained nurses working regular hours than by relatives, who destroy their own limited efficiency by overwork. With proper health arrangements in a community there will also be few doctors who need to lose their own health, that others may recover.

The results of self-sacrifice not unfrequently injure others.

The mother who daily sacrifices time, energy, recreation, and intellectual advantages for her children, even if she does not destroy her own physical health and mental efficiency, may cause the lives of her loved ones to become helpless, narrow, incomplete, and less valuable to others. Self-sacrifice, when carried to an extreme, is likely to be very unfavourable to the personality development of all concerned. This is surely the case when such unselfishness results in physical and mental injury to the sacrificer having an inferiority complex, and a superiority complex and selfish dependency on the part of the one for whom the sacrifice was made.

It is true that self-sacrifice is a very general and useful characteristic when helpless young are in need of care. To continue to sacrifice for them as they grow older is, however, to prolong infantile helplessness and make the next generation of parents less capable and less self-sacrificing. In other words, prolonged self-sacrifice, besides often lowering the health of the sacrificer is likely, if carried too far, to make the next generation less efficient in caring for those who need it, and thus such conduct is self-destroying.

Moderate and temporary self-sacrifice in the sense of giving up present ease or satisfactions in order that future advantages may be realized by self and others, is justified in all nature and especially in civilized life. The animal, and especially the human being, living only for his own momentary satisfaction is not likely to get so many satisfactions nor to live as long or as vigorously as the one acting for his own future and the good of his group. Without acting individually and co-operatively in the way of giving up immediate advantages for more remote ones, it would be impossible for man to construct tools and machines, to make clothing and shelter, to gain knowledge in advance of need. Neither could he organize means of using the powers of nature and the abilities of human beings in caring for the weak and helpless, and reducing the sickness and death-rates.

A certain amount of giving up of advantages to self in order to help others often excites companions to similar action. Whenever this occurs there is mutual helpfulness and better health practices; but if one continues to act thus in an extreme degree without exciting similar acts in companions, the results will be of an opposite nature. The persons ministered to make less provision for their own future and become less co-operative for future ends. Much charity, like unwise parental care, is an injury to its recipients and to society. Where children continue to need parental help and direction all their lives, and charity is necessary to many adults, there is something wrong with the ethical codes of the people.

Religious teachers have generally exalted the self-sacrifice codes, *sometimes* to an extent unfavourable to individual and community health, but often not more than enough to balance the rather natural tendency to act chiefly for self and for the immediate future. In so far as the practice of the code of self-sacrifice has led to giving up immediate satisfactions for future greater ones, has produced reciprocal action on the part of others, and has led to co-operation for future mutual advantages, it has helped to produce better health and to decrease the death-rate in all civilized lands. It may be that without this ideal having been upheld by religion, men would never have acquired and put into use knowledge of how to maintain health and life to the extent that they have. Enlightened self-interest is not in all instances a sufficient stimulus to actions for the good of all in a distant future, hence fostering the self-sacrifice attitude to a reasonable extent has been of value in promoting the health of the civilized world.

It is worthy of note that the golden rule suggests the ideal of mutuality in that it encourages doing to others as you would desire them to do to you. This may involve going " an extra mile " to help another and a reciprocal service on his part, thus serving mutual interests. If all other conditions were equal in three groups of people except the practice of the code of mutual self-sacrifice and mutual co-operation, there can be little doubt that the average health of the moderately self-sacrificing group would be better than that of the one that encouraged extreme self-sacrifice, or the one that practised extreme selfishness.

MENTAL HEALTH AND ETHICS

Closely related to the bodily vigour standard as established by statistics of disease and death-rates, is the standard of mental health. There can be little question that in general, action favourable to physical health is also favourable to mental health ; and still less doubt that a people having a high degree of mental health will be more likely to know and to use means of promoting physical health. At present statistics based on records of admission to mental hospitals are of some value in determining the mental health of different nations, or of the same nation at different times ; but as yet the data is not complete enough to be entirely reliable.

Again, if science can show that certain practices are favourable to mental health and others unfavourable, it will help in deciding which is the more moral as judged by health results.*

One of the most important influences affecting mental health is the character of the adjustments the individuals of a group make to each other, and to common customs and codes. For example, if a code demands continued action contrary to natural human tendencies, a mental tension and conflict will be produced which will be a prominent factor in the production of unhygienic mental states. The codes that remain *continuously* difficult to adjust to by most people, should be revised by science in the interest of mental health and ultimate good morals.

* This and the preceding discussion is, of course, based on the supposition that a code of action for men is of advantage to creatures of his nature, living in this universe. It does not consider the theoretical question of codes for creatures of a different nature, or in a different or future life. It also assumes that truth is obtained by research rather than by supernatural revelation. It recognizes that visions of truth are experienced by great moral and religious teachers, which may be verified in a subjective or in an objective way. If an objective verification is sought, then scientific methods and results are the most exact and reliable. Whether all these assumptions are acceptable or not, it is the purpose of this discussion to show that the help science may render in determining the value of moral codes is similar to that which it may render in other practical affairs, such as building bridges, manufacturing goods, growing crops, combating diseases, educating children, or making laws regulating banking or insurance.

As previously indicated interactions between human beings develop from two types of relationship : (1) that of inferior and superior such as parent and child, an individual and his king or God, and (2) of comparative equality of members of the same class. In the first case there may be much fear and force involved which is clearly not favourable to normal well-balanced health functioning, or there may be the attitudes of helpfulness and gratitude which are more favourable to the maintenance of mental equilibrium if not too long continued. In the case of persons of the same class, there may be much strife with continual thwarting of one by the other, or friendly competition, reciprocal love and co-operation, with satisfying results to all. The latter is, of course, more favourable to mental health. Religion has generally encouraged the relationship of dominance and subordination, sometimes greatly emphasizing fear, and generally placing most stress on being good to the needy and helpless. Many of the followers of Christianity have inconsistently emphasized brotherly love in human relations, while describing God as in the dominant relation of a stern ruler.

Religious excitement and mental disorders often occur together while in other instances peace of mind is gained by religious beliefs and practices. Any religion that increases mental disorders in those professing and practising it is, according to this standard, not as good a guide of moral action as one that decreases them. The same may be said not only of church teaching, but of laws and rules made by the state and by educational and other institutions, some of which have been decidedly unfavourable to mental health, *e.g.* extreme condemnation of unbelief and disobedience.

Any institution, public or private, that exercises a dominating influence over many individuals for a considerable portion of the time is good from the moral point of view in proportion as it increases rather than decreases the mental health of those much under its control, and its rules and traditions are, as a whole, thus justified.

z

CODES AFFECTING RACE BETTERMENT

With the development of scientific knowledge of heredity, birth control, and eugenics, codes that influence the distant future of the race must be evaluated in the light of science. The ethical and legal codes relating to marriage and parenthood certainly need to be revised so that the general average of the mental and physical health of future generations shall be increased rather than lowered. It is an evident truth that only an intelligent people will maintain codes of action favourable to general good health. Codes that perpetuate every sort of marriage, and the birth of all sorts of children must, as knowledge advances, and science is able to state with certainty the laws of heredity, be changed so that there will be less mismating of human beings, a decrease in birth of the inferior, and an increase in birth of those superior in physique and intelligence.

Science is not yet far enough advanced to formulate wisely complete rules for securing human beings superior to those we now have, but it is able to say that laws and attitudes favouring practices that are clearly adding to the proportion of inferior individuals born shall be changed, and that attention shall be directed toward positive means of race betterment.

A SCIENTIFIC VIEW OF HAPPINESS CODES

Many subjective standards for judging moral actions have been proposed. Those using some form of happiness standard have been most frequently favoured. The strongest objective support for such theories is found in the pretty general truth that happiness is favourable to health ; hence, whatever in the long run produces most happiness is likely to be shown in better health of the people who are happy in their mode of life, or in other words, who enjoy living as their codes prescribe. A new code may be disagreeable only at first, but if a supposed duty never comes to give pleasure to the majority of persons who perform it, and if there are signs of decreasing normality of functioning of mind and body of those practising its observance, the presumption is against the requirement being adapted to the people under the conditions in which they are living. Substantial truth-telling to those among whom one continually associates, is undoubtedly, for most persons in most situations, favourable to happiness and to physical and mental health of all concerned ; but *literal exact* truth-telling at all times has disadvantages. With different early training and customs, the amount of frank and exact speaking required in courteous intercourse may be increased. Yet to require literal and exact truths from hostesses, poets, artists, and humorists would detract much from healthful mental activity of the imagination, and the enjoyment of literature and life.

In a large proportion of cases, acts that are admittedly wrong according to almost any generally accepted standards of goodness may bring immediate happiness, but may destroy the possibility of future happiness. Most moral actions sacrifice something present for a greater good in the future. There is little need to dispute whose happiness is to be considered, since generally speaking, the happiness resulting from universal and continued actions of a certain type is not taken from one and given to another, but has the element of mutuality. Indeed this is the best way of judging the ultimate or sum total of happiness. In a lottery, happiness is not mutual, but many are unhappy for the happiness of a few. On the other hand, the happiness that comes from real increase of prosperity in one industry such as farming, extends to those engaged in manufacturing, transportation, education, etc. Æsthetic and intellectual pleasures are not transferred from one to another but are mutually enjoyed in a greater degree because others also are enjoying them.

Attempts to measure happiness directly have not been very successful since it is a subjective state ; nor should it be admitted that happiness is the only desirable end. People continue to strive for ends that neither they nor anyone else can see as being the means of getting the greatest happiness, *e.g.* to solve a puzzle or a mathematical problem, make an invention, climb a mountain, explore a wilderness, conquer a kingdom, build a great fortune. Man's nature and habits cause him to persist in such acts without weighing happiness effects.

Objective evidence of the sort of strivings which give satisfaction may be obtained by determining what ends are most universally and persistently sought. When attempts are made to compare pleasures, time measurements may be employed as objective ends, *e.g.* the pleasure of taste, touch and smell are inferior to sight and hearing, not in intensity, but in the number of hours per day that they can be used without decrease in the enjoyment. Æsthetic, social, and intellectual activities and their accompanying satisfactions are clearly more varied and lasting than those of the senses. They also contribute more to the pleasure of the imagination and to mutual pleasures. In general, the moral plane of a people bears some relation to the dominance of other than purely sensory satisfactions, and hence is in part subject to statistical measurement of evidence of mechanical, artistic, social and intellectual activities.

Another principle more important than all of these must be recognized, *i.e.* that of balance and harmony. Taste sensations, though low in the enduring satisfaction they give, need to be satisfied, or æsthetic and other pleasures become impossible. On the other hand, a meal without æsthetic accompaniments of clean linen, bright silver, flowers, and socially agreeable companionship is less pleasurable and less digestible. Just as a proper balance of physiological processes is necessary to physical life and health, and mental activities to mental health, of economic activities to prosperity, and of individuals, classes, and institutions to social stability, so is harmony of individual and group codes necessary to moral welfare. One of the best ways of judging the value of any moral precept, custom or law is whether its effect after a sufficient length of time is to increase balance or harmony as shown (1) in physical and mental health of individuals; (2) in decrease in number of individuals who violate the regulations; (3) in its effects on economic prosperity; (4) in its decrease of conflict between classes and institutions; and

(5) in increase of co-operative activity of all sorts. Indexes or standards are being developed in all these lines which make it possible to throw light on the comparative value of various regulatory codes.

The final result of a whole set of social and moral codes may be measured more readily than can the value of one alone. A new law has the temporary effect of disturbing the balance unless it is new as a law only, having been a general custom for some time. Some persons change their action in conformity with it, while others are stirred to opposition or to secret violation. It is a long while before its real influence on health, prosperity, happiness, and harmony are shown by statistics, especially if many influences have been modifying the data, *e.g.* laws regulating liquor sales.

SCIENTIFIC CODE MAKING

Has the time come for moral codes to be dictated entirely by scientists ? The teachings of past experience in every field compel a negative answer. A similar answer must be given to the question, " Should moral codes be dictated entirely by religious authorities ? " Religion from the personal and subjective point of view has given varied and wonderful pictures of ideal conduct, while common-sense experience, supplemented by exact science, has shown the objective results of the attempt to order human behaviour in accordance with the various codes. Religion has revealed ideals that science would never have seen, and has inspired more vigorous activity for their realization than science can arouse in most persons. Science, on the other hand, has shown that some religious ideals were inconsistent with the realization of others, and that many of the means prescribed by religion were ineffective and wasteful. Some religious ideals, when not opposed to health practices, were ineffective as the sole means of getting results. No doubt a strong desire for health, wisdom, and goodness is an important help in their attainment, but merely wishing or praying is usually not as sure and efficient a means of obtaining them as the means discovered by science in its studies of nature and human nature. The scientist who attempts to prescribe codes of human conduct without regard to the religious nature of man is perhaps as likely to fail as the religionist who prescribes codes without regard to truths of nature and human nature revealed by scientific research.

Besides, the general truth must be recognized that in every field science must have made very considerable advance in the study of activities of any kind before it can prescribe better methods of getting practical results than exist and have been approved by common-sense experience. Many of the early attempts to direct agricultural operations scientifically were failures. It is now generally understood that a laboratory discovery of probable value must be tested in the field under various conditions before attempting to say with assurance what rules, if followed, will give better crops. Observed verification is necessary to establish a scientific theory as a separate truth ; then another verification to establish its value in a given application.

At the present time science can formulate many general truths or principles of human conduct and of how they work under many conditions. Science can endorse some means of reaching desirable social and moral results with a good deal of assurance, but it is yet far from being in a position to prescribe *all* moral codes and secure their dominance. It may be doubted whether it can ever do so without the help of the subjective and religious point of view. In the meantime, the scientific and the religious attitudes in human affairs are not exclusive of each other, but there may be mutual respect, criticism, and reciprocal use of what each offers. If it were admitted that one must ultimately give way to the other, there would be a serious disturbance of social life if the change were suddenly made.

SELECTED RESEARCHES

"CRIME AND CUSTOM IN SAVAGE SOCIETY."
By Bronislaw Malinowski. *Quoted by Permission.*

. . . One day an outbreak of wailing and a great commotion told me that a death had occurred somewhere in the neighbourhood. I was informed that Kima'i, a young lad of my acquaintance, of sixteen or so, had fallen from a coco-nut palm and killed himself.

I hastened to the next village where this had occurred, only to find the whole mortuary proceedings in progress. This was my first case of death, mourning, and burial, so that in my concern with the ethnographical aspects of the ceremonial, I forgot the circumstances of the tragedy even though one or two singular facts occurred at the same time in the village which should have aroused my suspicions. I found that another youth had been severely wounded by some mysterious coincidence. And at the funeral there was obviously a general feeling of hostility between the village where the boy died and that into which his body was carried for burial.

Only much later was I able to discover the real meaning of these events ; the boy had committed suicide. The truth was that he had broken the rules of exogamy, the partner in his crime being his maternal cousin, the daughter of his mother's sister. This had been known and generally disapproved of, but nothing was done until the girl's discarded lover, who had wanted to marry her and who felt personally injured, took the initiative. This rival threatened first to use black magic against the guilty youth, but this had not much effect. Then one evening he insulted the culprit in public—accusing him in the hearing of the whole community of incest and hurling at him certain expressions intolerable to a native.

For this there was only one remedy ; only one means of escape remained to the unfortunate youth. Next morning he put on festive attire and ornamentation, climbed a coco-nut palm and addressed the community, speaking from among the palm leaves and bidding them farewell. He explained the reasons for his desperate deed and also launched forth a veiled accusation against the man who had driven him to his death, upon which it became the duty of his clansmen to avenge him. Then he wailed aloud, as is the custom, jumped from a palm some sixty feet high and was killed on the spot. There followed a fight within the village in which the rival was wounded ; and the quarrel was repeated during the funeral.

Now this case opened up a number of important lines of inquiry. I was here in the presence of a pronounced crime : the breach of totemic exogamy. The exogamous prohibition is one of the corner-stones of totemism, mother-right, and the classificatory system of kinship. All females of his clan are called sisters by a man and forbidden as such. It is an axiom of Anthropology that nothing arouses a greater horror than the breach of this prohibition, and that besides a strong reaction of public opinion, there are also supernatural punishments, which visit this crime. Nor is this axiom devoid of foundation in fact. If you were to inquire into the matter among the Trobrianders, you would find that all statements confirm the axiom, that the natives show horror at the idea of violating the rules of exogamy and that they believe that sores, disease and even death might follow clan incest. This is the ideal of native law, and in moral matters it is easy and pleasant strictly to adhere to the ideal—when judging the conduct of others or expressing an opinion about conduct in general.

When it comes to the application of morality and ideals to real life, however, things take on a different complexion. In the case described it was obvious that the facts would not tally with the ideal of conduct. Public opinion was neither outraged by the knowledge of the crime to any extent, nor did it react directly —it had to be mobilized by a public statement of the crime, and by insults being hurled at the culprit by an interested party. Even then he had to carry out the punishment himself. The " group-reaction " and the " supernatural sanction " were not, therefore, the active principles. Probing further into the matter and collecting concrete information, I found that the breach of exogamy—as regards intercourse and not marriage—is by no means a rare occurrence, and public opinion is lenient, though decidedly hypocritical. If the affair is carried on *sub rosa* with a certain amount of decorum, and if no one in particular stirs up trouble—" public opinion " will gossip, but not demand any harsh punishment. If, on the contrary, scandal breaks out— everyone turns against the guilty pair and by ostracism and insults one or the other may be driven to suicide. . . .

The two principles Mother-right and Father-love are focused most sharply in the relation of a man to his sister's son and to his own son respectively. His matrilineal nephew is his nearest kinsman and the legal heir to all his dignities and offices. His own son, on the other hand, is not regarded as a kinsman ; legally he is not related to his father, and the only bond is the sociological status of marriage with the mother.

Yet in the reality of actual life the father is much more attracted to his own son than to his nephew. Between father and son there obtains invariably friendship and personal attachment ; between uncle and nephew not infrequently the ideal of perfect solidarity is marred by rivalries and suspicions inherent in any relationship of succession.

Thus the powerful legal system of Mother-right is associated with a rather weak sentiment, while Father-love, much less important in law, is backed by a strong personal feeling. In the case of a chief whose power is considerable, the personal influence outweighs the ruling of the law and the position of the son is as strong as that of the nephew.

That was the case in the capital village of Omarakana, the residence of the principal chief whose power extends over the whole district, whose influence reaches many archipelagoes, and whose fame is spread all over the eastern end of New Guinea. I soon found out that there was a standing feud between his sons and his nephews, a feud which assumed a really acute form in the ever recurrent quarrels between his favourite son Namwana Guya'u and his second eldest nephew Mitakata.

The final outbreak came when the chief's son inflicted serious injury on the nephew in a litigation before the resident government official of the district. Mitakata, the nephew, was in fact convicted and put to prison for a month or so.

When the news of this reached the village, the short exultation among the partisans of Namwana Guya'u was followed by a panic, for everyone felt that things had come to a crisis. The chief shut himself up in his personal hut, full of evil forebodings of the consequences for his favourite, who was felt to have acted rashly and in outrage of tribal law and feeling. The kinsmen of the imprisoned young heir to chieftainship were boiling with suppressed anger and indignation. As night fell, the subdued village settled down to a silent supper, each family over its solitary meal. There was nobody on the central place—Namwana Guya'u was not to be seen, the chief To'uluwa hid in his hut, most of his wives and their families remained indoors. Suddenly a loud voice rang out across the silent village. Bagido'u, the heir-apparent, and eldest brother of the imprisoned man, standing before his hut, spoke out, addressing the offender of his family :—

" Namwana Guya'u, you are a cause of trouble. We the Tabalu of Omarakana, allowed you to stay here, to live among us. You had plenty of food in Omarakana, you ate of our food, you partook of the pigs brought to us as a tribute and of the fish. You sailed in our canoe. You built a hut on our soil. Now you have done us harm. You have told lies. Mitakata is in prison. We do not want you to stay here. This is our village ! You are a stranger here. Go away ! We chase you away ! We chase you out of Omarakana."

These words were uttered in a loud piercing voice, trembling with strong emotion, each short sentence spoken after a pause, each like an individual missile, hurled across the empty space to the hut where Namwana Guya'u sat brooding. After that the younger sister of Mitakata also arose and spoke, and then a young man, one of the maternal nephews. Their words were almost the same as in the first speech, the burden being the formula of chasing away, the *yoba*. The speeches were received in deep silence. Nothing stirred in the village. But before the night was over, Namwana Guya'u had left Omarakana for ever. He had gone over and settled in his own village, in Osapola, the village whence his mother came, a few miles distant. For weeks his mother and sisters wailed for him with the loud lamentations of mourning for the dead. The chief remained for three days in his hut, and when he came out looked older and broken up by grief. All his personal interest and affection were on the side of his favourite son, of course. Yet he could do nothing to help him. His kinsmen had acted in complete accordance with their rights, and, according to tribal law, he could not possibly dissociate himself from them. No power could change the decree of exile. Once the " Go away "—(bukula), " we chase thee away "—(kayabaim) were pronounced the man had to go. These words, very rarely uttered in dead earnest, have binding force and almost ritual power when pronounced by the citizens of a place against a resident outsider. A man who would try to brave the dreadful insult involved in them and remain in spite of them, would be dishonoured for ever. In fact, anything but immediate compliance with a ritual request is unthinkable for a Trobriand Islander.

The chief's resentment against his kinsmen was deep and lasting. At first he would not even speak to them. For a year or so, not one of them dared to ask to be taken on overseas expeditions by him, although they were fully entitled to this privilege. Two years later, in 1917, when I returned to the Trobriands, Namwana Guya'u was still resident in the other village and keeping aloof from his father's kinsmen, although he frequently paid visits to Omarakana in order to be in attendance on his father, especially when To'uluwa went abroad. The mother had died within a year after the expulsion. As the natives described it : " She wailed and wailed, refused to eat, and died." The relations between the two main enemies were completely broken, and Mitakata, the young chieftain who had been imprisoned, had sent away his wife, who belonged to the same sub-clan as Namwana Guya'u. There was a deep rift in the whole social life of Kiriwana.

The incident was one of the most dramatic events which I have ever witnessed in the Trobriands. I have described it at length, as it contains a clear illustration of Mother-right, of the power of tribal law and of the passions which work in spite of it.

The case though exceptionally dramatic and telling is by no means anomalous. . . .

"RECENT IMPROVEMENTS IN DEVICES FOR RATING CHARACTER." By MARK A. MAY and HUGH HARTSHORNE, Yale University. From *The Journal of Social Psychology*, February 1930. *Quoted by Permission.*

Rating scales and rating devices as scientific instruments for the investigation of character and personality have, during the past decade, fallen into considerable disrepute. . . .

. . . This paper is concerned mainly with the description of improvements in technique. . . .

. . . We first went through a thesaurus and selected all the words descriptive of extremes of behaviour tendencies. Samples of the selected pairs are : brutal-humane, stingy-generous, selfish-unselfish, and tolerant-intolerant. From a long list we selected 80 pairs of antonyms (160 words) and printed them on two sheets. Each sheet contains the antonyms of the other. Thus if the word " brutal " appears on sheet A, the word " humane " will appear somewhere on sheet B. Both sheets were checked for each pupil and often by two teachers. Sheet A was checked first and sheet B a week later. . . .

Some of the advantages of this scheme are : (1) It furnishes excellent data for determining reliabilities. By comparing the words checked on sheets A and B, a detailed study may be made of the consistencies or inconsistencies of the rater. If, for example, a teacher checks a pupil as " tolerant " on sheet A and as " intolerant " on sheet B, we have for this pair of words a complete inconsistency. If this happens often enough the coefficient of reliability could actually be negative. That it does not happen will be seen from the coefficient of reliability, which is ·88 for the whole instrument. . . . If a teacher is prejudiced against a pupil, she may check against him all the bad words on the list, or she may show her goodwill towards him by checking all the good words. This technique provides two ways of allowing for such extremes. One is by adopting a scoring plan that will eliminate them ; the other is to leave them all in and correct all subsequent correlations for their effects. . . .

The scoring plan used by the Inquiry is briefly as follows : The words were classified roughly according to certain general behaviour tendencies which we were studying in other ways. For example, all the words referring to co-operative or service tendencies were grouped. For each group of words, the pupil was given a score of plus, minus, or zero for each sheet. If the number of positive words checked exceeded the number of negatives, the score was plus ; if the negatives exceeded the positives, it was minus ; if they balanced, it was zero ; or if no words in that group were checked, it was zero. Since there were four sheets for each pupil, the scores ranged from plus four to minus four. Thus the score or rating is determined not by the total number of words checked but by the sign value of their algebraic sum. . . .

The " Guess Who " Test

This is a device for securing the opinions of pupils concerning each other. It is a modification of the matching device described above, except that here the pupils themselves do the rating. The sketches are much shorter, some of them but a single sentence, but there are many more of them. The sketches are printed on a folder entitled the " Guess Who " test. The reason for calling it a test is to induce the test set or attitude on the part of the pupils and to push to the background the rating set, or the " tattling " attitude. If the pupils feel they are being tested, they are much more likely to be frank and unprejudiced in giving their opinions of their classmates. The directions and some of the sketches are given as follows :

The " Guess Who " Test

Here are some little word-pictures of children you may know. Read each statement carefully and see if you can guess whom it is about. It might be about yourself. There may be more than one picture for the same person. Several boys and girls may fit one picture. Read each statement. Think over your classmates and write after each statement the names of any boys or girls who may fit it. If the picture does not seem to fit anyone in your class, put down no names but go on to the next statement. Work carefully and use your judgment.

4. This is a jolly good fellow—friends with every one, no matter who they are.
5. This one is always picking on others and annoying them.
6. Here is a crabber and knocker. Nothing is right. Always kicking and complaining.

There are 26 sketches. About half are positive (as, for example, number 4 above) and half negative (as number 5 above). A child's score is the number of positive mentions he receives minus the number of times his name appears on the negative items. This crude scoring technique could be refined by scaling the items.

Some of the advantages of this technique are the following. (1) It makes possible the securing of opinions of pupils concerning each other, which could not be accomplished by the use of the usual rating scales. (2) By making it a guessing game, we get away from the rigidity of rating scales without sacrificing anything in the way of accuracy. (3) The fact that the rater does not sign his name and the fact that the word " test " appears on the blank are both favourable to securing unbiased opinions. (4) The instrument has a high reliability. Figured by the split-form technique it has a self-correction of ·90 and a predicted reliability of ·95. But this is probably higher than it would be if we repeated the test using two similar forms. Our guess is that two similar forms of this test would correlate about ·90 provided each form contained 24 traits or items. By increasing the items to cover a wider variety of behaviour tendencies, the repeat reliability could be raised to ·95.

. . . The average intercorrelation of the three sets of teacher ratings is ·80. . . .

. . . The correlations between teachers' opinions as expressed on the check lists, conduct records, and deportment (portraits were not used in this), and the score on the pupils' " Guess Who " test is, for a school population of 800, grades 5 to 8, ·477. This may be taken as a measure of what the teachers and pupils have in common when judging any pupil. This common ground is probably observed conduct.

. . . No one has ever determined the relation between true reputation, which includes prejudice, and true conduct as measured by objective tests.

We have made a beginning at this while developing a battery of objective character tests. We have measured four behaviour tendencies. These tendencies are (1) the tendency to deceive, (2) the tendency to help or to be of service, (3) the tendency to self-control, and (4) the tendency to persistence. . . . The correlations between reputation and test scores are low. They vary from ·10 to ·30.

These low correlations indicate that conduct, as measured by objective tests, and reputation for behaviour tendencies have very little in common. The common elements are probably represented by the degree to which the ratings are based on observations of conduct. . . .

SUGGESTED READINGS

Until recently Ethics has belonged to philosophy, rather than to science. The transition to the scientific approach has been facilitated by the writings of Hobhouse, describing the evolution of ethical practice. One of the best theoretical discussions favourable to an objective study of ethics, is that of :

STAPALDON, W. OLAF, *A Modern Theory of Ethics*, 1929.

The following books are concerned with facts and practices bearing on ethical problems :

FOLSOM, JOSEPH K., *Culture and Social Progress*, 1928.

HEALY, WILLIAM, and BRONNER, AUGUSTA, *Delinquents and Criminals, their Making and Unmaking ; Studies in Two American Cities*, 1926.

HOBSON, J. A., *Economics and Ethics*, 1929.

POUND, ROSCOE, *Law and Morals*, 1924.

TAEUSCH, CARL F., *Policy and Ethics in Business*, 1931.

TUFTS, JAMES, *Our Democracy, its Origin and its Tasks*, 1917.

Special ethical codes proposed and in practice are given in the following :

FREDERICK, J. G., *Book of Business Standards*, 1925.

HERMANCE, EDGAR L., *Codes of Ethics Handbook*, 1924.

LEE, JAMES, *Business Ethics ; a Manual of Modern Morals*, 1926.

LORD, EVERETT W., *Fundamentals of Business Ethics*, 1926.

PAGE, EDWARD D., *Trade Morals ; their Origin, Growth, and Province*, 1913.

TAEUSCH, CARL F., *Professional and Business Ethics*, 1926.

The following books and articles show that an experimental science of ethics is being developed :

ANDERSON, ALICE, and DVORAK, BEATRICE, " Difference between College Students and their Elders in Standards of Conduct," *Journal of Abnormal and Social Psychology*, Oct.-Dec. 1928.

HARTSHORNE, HUGH, and MAY, MARK A., *Studies in Deceit*, 1928.

MAY, MARK A., and HARTSHORNE, HUGH, " First Step toward Measuring Attitudes," *Journal of Educational Psychology*, page 145, 1926.

SHAW, C. R., " Does the Community Determine Character ? " *Religious Education*, pages 24 and 409, 1929.

SHAW, C. R., and others, *Delinquency Areas*, 1929.

WASHBURNE, JOHN N., " An Experiment in Character Measurement," *Journal of Juvenile Research*, January 1929.

CHAPTER XV

MAN, THE MASTER OF LIFE, DEVELOPING
A SCIENCE OF ETHICAL LIVING

I

HIS RELATION TO LIFE IN GENERAL

Life has Increased

Attempts to measure the time the earth has existed and to estimate how long it may be expected to endure in approximately its present state have led to the use of larger and larger figures. At present the statement of time is no longer expressed in millions but in billions of years. Theories as to the meaning of changes in the earth that have, and are likely to take place, are still unproven. We are not sure that " through the ages an increasing purpose runs ". The one thing that all scientists accept is that each new condition of the earth inevitably comes as the result of uniform laws acting upon what has existed. With this as a basis it is possible to discover much and infer more regarding the past history of the universe.

A broad survey of geological facts makes it clear that in remote times there were few if any living organisms on the earth. One-celled organisms of a low type first existed, and these made conditions favourable for the development of other types. Chlorophyl-producing plants which by the aid of the sun change the inorganic substances of air and soil into organic compounds, finally appeared and made possible the development of animal life, which must usually have organized matter for sustenance. After that, countless species of plants and animals appeared and flourished for indefinitely known periods, many of them ceasing to exist, and giving place to others of more complex organization. Then as now, there was a struggle of each species with the others for its continued existence and increase.

Another and more fundamental truth is sometimes ignored : *i.e.* the continuation of each species depends upon the presence of others. The lion must have some vegetable-eating animal upon which to feed, and grass will not grow without bacteria in the soil, earth-worms to loosen it and perhaps insects to fertilize blossoms. Every addition of a new species to plant life makes it possible for new varieties of animals to exist, and these for still others. The much-emphasized conflict between species does not usually exterminate them but kills the weaker individuals and keeps one species from over-running the earth, and then dying out for lack of the others upon which its life depends. Competition limits the number of individuals in each species while increase in number of species makes it possible for vastly more life to exist on the earth then when there were fewer varieties of living creatures. Whether the maximum has as yet been reached we do not know.

Man has Modified and probably Increased Life

When man first appeared there were many forms of life upon which he could feed with no danger of exterminating any of them. With his increased numbers and his great and growing knowledge and use of tools, machines, and nature's forces, he has now become the most important single influence affecting the amount of life the earth shall bring forth. His efforts are naturally directed toward making it support greater numbers of his own species. In doing this he destroys some species, limits the number of others, increases the growth of a few, and changes some of them into varieties almost as distinct as natural species. In this country in spite of the large amount of land covered with houses and roads, food for a hundred times as many human beings as was supplied by the whole land before man interfered with what grew upon it, is now produced. Domesticated plants and animals have largely taken the place of wild ones. By the use of improved seed, fertilizers, and methods of cultivation more human food is produced than was supplied by the many species growing under natural conditions.

It is probable that the total life as measured in metabolic activity of all living things is now much greater in this country than it was before the coming of the white man, but extensive calculations would be necessary to be sure whether man is really adding to the total of life on earth or not. He has destroyed a few species, while greatly increasing varieties and numbers of those useful to him.

Ethics and Increase of Life

There is no question that he is destroying some forms of life and increasing others in such a way that the earth may support an immensely larger number of human beings. In general, sentiment has favoured this attitude of increasing the means of living for man regardless of what species of life is exterminated. The passenger pigeon and other species have been destroyed and depleted, largely for the pleasure of hunting rather than to get food. Far-sighted people are now advocating the preservation of many species for the pleasure of enjoying their beauty, and also for the value of each species in continuing the existence of a large amount of life on the earth. Exceptions to this are made in the case of disease-producing germs, and of plants and animals that injure food crops. Man as the master of life can either increase or decrease the sum total of life existing on the earth in the present and future years. Many injurious microbes, insects and mammals still flourish in spite of man's activities, but if he persistently devoted his efforts to the destruction of any one species, such as typhoid germs, mosquitoes or rats, there is little doubt that he would succeed. With such power in his hands, shall man deem it his duty to act in such a way as to increase the sum total of life on the earth ?

It is clearly the place of science to determine the effects upon other species, especially man, and upon the total of life upon earth, of causing certain species to increase and others to decrease or to cease to exist. If it should be found that a policy which increases the number of human beings and adds to their satisfactions also adds to the total sum of life on earth, it would make little difference which idea con-

2 A

trolled behaviour—that of advantages to the species man, or that of general increase of life on earth. Such questions as experimentation on animals would be settled in the same way, by computing either the effect on total sum of life or on advantages to the human species.

If the advantages to man and the increase of the sum total of life should (as is unlikely) prove to be contradictory to each other, then there is little doubt that man, in accordance with the universal tendency of each species to act for its own advantage, would make increase of life in general a goal subordinate to that of gaining advantages for self. He has always acted thus, and science will simply enable him to do it more effectively.

Notwithstanding this truth, science can greatly modify man's ethical codes by showing hitherto unknown and remote consequences of their observance. Conservation of nature's long-neglected resources is proved by science to be of advantage to man, and as a consequence is being practised much more than formerly. The general effect of scientific advance is to modify the codes of conduct on account of the definite knowledge of consequences that are revealed. It is probable that the more he does this, the more it will be found that what is of advantage to the controller of life on earth is favourable to an increase in the sum total of life that may exist.

Whether or not this proves to be the case, it is only by scientific research that it will be possible to decide on the right policy with regard to various creatures. At present, some states give rewards for destroying animals that in other states are protected by fines. Some of these seeming inconsistencies may have temporary justification in being intelligent attempts to restore a balance in nature that has been disturbed by the action of man. There is no question, however, that both temporary and permanent policy should be guided by scientific researches which show the immediate and remote effects of destroying or protecting crows, foxes, etc.

The most difficult problems for science to solve arise when the several advantages to man seem to be in opposition, e.g. a garden of vegetables to maintain life, or a garden of flowers to make life worth while. Such a question is a small problem of the same type as the big one, as to whether it is better to have large numbers of human species live in a given region or on the earth as a whole, on a basis of mere subsistence, or to have smaller numbers on a luxury basis. If science could measure the total life satisfactions of a thousand persons merely existing, and of five hundred getting the æsthetic and social satisfactions involved in a luxury standard of living, the questions might be settled. This may eventually be possible.

Even now, science may partly solve the problem by objective facts. It can undoubtedly show that a high standard of living tends to increase productiveness, so that a population with such a standard can produce enough to have both necessities and luxuries. There is also evidence that many people who have been living on a luxury standard will not lower it in order to have more children. On the other hand, some will have children even though the chances of keeping them even on a subsistence basis are not favourable. The general effect of increased scientific knowledge is to increase population and raise standards as much as possible, and after that to limit population rather than to lower standards of living.

Economy in Perpetuating Life on the Earth

The numbers of species of animals now inhabiting the earth are greater now than formerly ; also more of them survive and by less wasteful means. The lower animals, such as insects and fishes, appeared earlier than birds and mammals. They survive as species by producing enormous numbers of individuals, the majority of which never reach adult life, while the higher and later appearing animals produce fewer young, a much larger proportion of which survive because the genes are kept from danger within the body of the mother, and the young are cared for after birth until able to live independently. Of all creatures man depends least on fertility, and most on parental care for survival.

The difference between savage and civilized peoples is also very marked as shown by birth-rates and death-rates. In the most enlightened groups the birth-rate is under 20 per thousand, and the death-rate little more than half that ; while in the least enlightened there may be a birth-rate of 50 or more per thousand, a third to a half of whom die in infancy.

Man has modified the birth-rate of many domestic animals and arranged so that most of those born live to maturity. When a people takes steps to keep alive as long as possible all the individuals who are born, and to limit population when necessary by decreasing births instead of allowing many to die of starvation, disease, and warfare, they are following the example of nature as exemplified in the history of the earth.

If it is admitted that abundance of life on the earth, and for man in the fullest sense of the word, is that for which Jesus came, then science offers the best guide to that goal. As various suggestions are made as to what action should be taken to increase any form of life on earth, or any phase of the complex life of man, science is often prepared to show which of various proposals will, on the whole, and in the long run, most effectively achieve the desired results ; it will be able to do this more generally and accurately, and hence will determine what ethical ideals and practices shall survive in so far as abundance of life is accepted as a desirable goal.

Man, like all other creatures, is so organized as to act in ways favourable to his survival individually and as a species, but he, more than any other, makes over his environment so as to live more abundantly. To this end he uses his intelligence and performs most of his acts with reference to future results. Scientific methods have built up knowledge of means many times as reliable as those any one person, however gifted, could acquire in a lifetime, that may be employed in gaining near and remote advantages. This accumulated, well-tested knowledge is now used as a guide in nearly all processes of every industry. When science has accumulated a similar body of knowledge regarding living things, and especially regarding man and his behaviour, it will serve as a guide in all human affairs, including those designated as social and moral, or ethical. While the help science may give to various forms of art and religious beliefs and practices will be considerable, yet it will be less than in material affairs. It is certain, however, to determine in part what artistic and ethical ideals shall survive.

Indications of Amount of Life

The life phenomena of plants is closely correlated with the amount of chlorophyl produced, and this is measurable. The physiological life of animals is closely correlated with basal metabolism, which can be determined for each species. The amount of energy used by animals and men in various typical activities under given conditions may also be measured. If such measurements are made, it will be possible, for example, to compute the comparative amount of life exhibited by a turtle living a hundred years and a squirrel living ten years. On such a basis, the life of a squirrel would probably exceed in quantity by several times that of the turtle. This gives us a starting-point, but not much more, for measuring life.

We shall make some further advance when we study each species of animal to see how well its activities are correlated and integrated, so that they contribute to physiological functioning and cause each movement to aid rather than hinder in making others. For example, the efficiency of a horse as a draught animal, compared with a cow, could be determined by the number of calories of food needed to enable each to draw a ton load a thousand miles. No exact measurements have been made, but observation indicates that dogs are more economical as draught animals than either horses or cows, at least in the Arctics. The comparative efficiency of animal organisms will probably be measured sometime nearly as accurately as that of steam-engines. The objective efficiency of individuals and of races of men as physiological mechanisms may also be measured, and the effects of various hygienic and educational practices on efficiency calculated. These measurements will enable us to determine the potential amount of work that persons of different heredity, regimen, and training may do. Such knowledge may guide eugenic, hygienic, and educational programmes and thus be a basis for many moral practices and laws.

We must recognize, however, that the possession of life power by plant, animal, or human being, however efficiently it may be used in preserving and prolonging its own life, does not necessarily insure that it may not be used in destroying other living things. If increase of the total sum of life on the earth and its perpetuation is supposed to be desirable, then there must be found some way of measuring the effects of behaviour of one creature upon all others. The new science of ecology is bringing to light many unsuspected relations of plants and animals to each other. The sciences of economics and sociology are revealing the significance of competitive and co-operative activity as compared with unorganized individual behaviour. Whatever is learned of how individuals may economize their own energy, and of how energy may be economized in co-operating with others, will aid in forming standards by which to judge conduct as good or bad.

With such standards we would be far on the road to the establishment of a science of ethics. For example: it would not be difficult to show that for a people trying to co-operate efficiently, lying and cheating among individuals of the group are uneconomical means of gaining ends; nor that for one nation to rob another is far less advantageous than it is to establish mutually profitable exchange of products.

Such a scientifically selected code of ethics would not, however, directly help in choosing ends toward which behaviour is to be directed. One group may try to get as much sense pleasure as possible, and science may show them how to do it. Another group may seek æsthetic and intellectual satisfactions and receive some aid from science in doing so. Science may, however, give help by showing that more possibilities of human living may be gained by trying to attain both types of ends in a moderate degree. The gain is probably similar to that of co-operative action over individual action.

The value of the sense satisfactions is to be determined not wholly by measuring them as to intensity and duration, but by their effect upon the attainment of other ends, such as æsthetic and social satisfactions. Too much indulgence in the enjoyment of food may interfere not only with future satisfactions of appetite, but also with social æsthetic and intellectual pleasures. The more we learn of what promotes physical and mental hygiene, the more surely may we decide what ethical codes are the better as indicated by effectiveness in getting many ends that human life is capable of realizing.

II

INTERRELATIONS OF MEN

Tribal Ethics and World Ethics

An isolated group in their adjustments to each other develop forms of conduct which give a certain degree of balance and consistency to their group living. These ways of acting are relatively satisfactory and any marked variations from them by individuals are resented. This approved behaviour is not the same for all, but specialized according to sex, age, and class action and reaction. Men have certain duties and responsibilities, and women others ; age carries with it certain deferences and responsibilities, especially within the family. Also there are usually several classes of persons who behave differently toward each other than toward individuals of their own class. Where a group have lived in intimate association for many generations there is little active opposition to the customs and precepts, though there may be various infractions of the accepted codes which are punished. These ways of acting in every stable society constitute the tribal mores or ethics. An adjoining group of people may have quite a different system of ethics maintained within its group, although members of the two tribes often come in contact with each other.

If, in their earlier meetings, hostility is shown by members of one group, then those of the other will respond by hostility or fear. This tendency to be influenced by what the other does results, after varied actions and reactions, in the development of accepted practices between the groups. For example, whenever one or more members of tribe A are killed by individuals of tribe B, then an equal number of tribe B must be killed. This limits the natural tendency of each to kill and sometimes decreases warfare between the two tribes. Older men try to restrain the hot-headed younger ones, and in order to avoid frequent disturbance of comfort through raids, arrangements are made between leaders of the two tribes when there are killings to make reparations by giving up the proper number to be executed, or by payments of some kind. In other words, tribes, like individuals associating with each other, change their behaviour according to the reaction of others, until they develop types of conduct that are relatively satisfactory. These relations may be either of dominance and subordination, of competitive equality, or sometimes of mutuality and co-operation.

Within the tribe, especially in the family, situations are sure to arise where mutual interests can be gained only by co-operation. Trade involves some elements of mutuality, while joint production and dividing what is produced, is a typical example of co-operation associated with some competition as to who shall get the most for the effort he has put forth. Property, and labour or service codes, inevitably grow out of such situations within the tribe. These are more or less just between individuals and classes, in proportion as needs and supplies are nearly equal. One who has plenty of food may have to be given extra inducements to get him to help build a boat, or to get him to exchange labour or some other article for food of any kind.

When two tribes attempt to get fruits or game in the same region at the same time, conflicts which interfere with either group getting food are likely to arise. If the two tribes are equally strong and there is enough food for both, there usually develops some sort of an agreement as to when, where, or how much each may take. Each is held more or less closely to the agreement by the knowledge that the other will retaliate if the code is not observed. Where one tribe is stronger, or the food supply is inadequate for both, the matter is likely to be settled by force, the weaker being destroyed, enslaved, or driven away.

Conflict between tribes usually stimulates co-operation of members within the tribe. Co-operation and mutuality of group with group may be developed when two weaker tribes are menaced at the same time by a stronger, and are induced to unite to save themselves.

Comparatively few tribes have been so isolated that they did not come in contact with other tribes. The occasional wanderer is likely to be killed, but may be treated kindly or even adopted into the tribe he visits. Where there are frequent meetings of members of the two tribes, either fighting or trading is likely to result. In either case if the two tribes are nearly equal, after a few generations of intercourse they develop well-understood customs of warfare or of trading. The war customs may recognize it as legitimate to kill all ages and sexes, or to kill warriors only, or only those who do not surrender ; or still more surprising, there may be little or no killing because damages will have to be paid for severe injuries. This is analogous to rules of boxing that limit the modes of attack, and to the war rules of civilized nations prohibiting the use of gas, etc.

The trading customs may take the form of " gifts ", of barter, or of buying or selling with some accepted medium of measuring values and exchanging goods. In the " gift " system self-interest and responsibilities are involved just as much as in bargaining, and standards of acceptable conduct are just as well established. Each " gives " what he thinks will bring the most in return " gifts ".

Nations, ancient and modern, act like tribes, in so far as conditions are similar. International customs and laws, such as there are, have developed in accordance with the same principles of human nature as the individual and tribal codes. These are chiefly of two kinds—one of rules governing warfare, and the other governing the treatment of the members of other nations, especially princes or officials. Failure of one nation to show due courtesy to officials of another, has been a frequent cause of war, as has also the mistreatment of visiting citizens.

Not only the person but the property of a traveller is to

be guarded by a nation, if its own citizens are to be free to visit foreign countries. If one nation requires a passport, the other is likely to do so. The customs and codes accepted by all civilized nations represent the most satisfactory adjustments that have been found for the situations that frequently arise. Further development of international and world ethics depends upon the frequency with which situations of various types occur ; and upon intelligent effort to find the most satisfactory adjustment between nations without trying to force compliance with the decision made by one upon another.

Changes Favouring a World Ethics

The changes now occurring in the relations of nations to each other are largely the result of man's inventions and the consequent widening of social influences.

Means of transportation have made travelling to a nation a thousand miles away as easy as it formerly was to visit in the next county. Already the rights of travellers are recognized and guarded by about the same sort of regulations in all civilized countries, and in many not thus classified. Nearly one-half million Americans now travel to other countries each year.

Means of transportation, travel bureaus, and financial institutions are so well developed that travel in, or trading with Brazil is as easily effected as exchange of goods between a farmer and the people of a town a few miles away. The situations arising from travelling and trading in a foreign country are no longer a mere matter of protection of person and property against violence, but of guarding both in a great variety of ways. General practices and even legal procedure are being modified into a common type.

Partly because of increased international travel and trading, and partly for other reasons, world-wide means of communication by mail, telegraph, telephone, and radio have developed. International postal regulations have long existed, and similar ones for telegraph and radio are developing.

For like reasons, the regulations governing the operations

of ships on the high seas, and airplanes are similar. Money
and credit are also being rapidly internationalized.

On account of capital investments in foreign countries and
the relations of industries to each other, every nation is
affected by what is being done, and how it is being done, in
every other country. For example, the hours of labour are
being restricted in all countries with the hope of making them
the same everywhere.

Common interests are being found and common legislation
is being made in such diverse things as protection of migratory
birds and animals, such as ducks, and seals, in the sale of
poisons and drugs, and in the development of power stations.

National governments and large organizations, industrial,
educational, philanthropic, and scientific are concerned in
realizing certain ends by common means. As a result there
are many activities of modern life that will be of as common
interest to the people of all nations as they are to families in
the same town, and will therefore be regulated in the
same way by nations far distant from each other in
space.

With more common action by governments ; more common
practices by international organizations, economic, educational,
etc. ; more uniformity of culture in all parts of the world,
there will develop world ethical codes dominant over those of
nations and tribes, very much as tribal or community codes
dominate family life, or national law dominates that of the
states.

Formerly, distant nations were not closely enough in touch
with each other to compete ; and the nearer ones were just
close enough to bring about conflicts, but not to develop many
fixed customs of behaviour toward each other. There was
much competition for territory and power, and frequent
combinations of weaker to resist stronger.

The present situation, with all nations in close association
and with many common interests, is far more favourable to
the development of international law as well as common
ethical practices. Arbitration and international courts have
inevitably taken the place of war in settling national disputes,

just as referees and courts took the place of individual fighting because they accomplished the results desired more efficiently. The League of Nations council and assembly give opportunity for discussion by representatives from all nations regarding questions of dispute and of mutual interests. Some organization of this sort was the inevitable result of all nations being brought into close relation by modern inventions and organizations. It is doubtful whether there will ever be an attempt to *force* a nation to obey any rule or decree made by the court or assembly, but these organizations are an important medium for promoting and fostering common actions. Nations, like individuals, are influenced by the behaviour of other nations, and in the course of time would be acting much alike even without special effort to get them to agree on common regulations. The League will greatly hasten this natural process.

With the development of many common interests and with the idea of consultation and judicial decisions substituted for force, it is inevitable that the relation between nations will become that of equality rather than of dominance and submission. Competition will continue, but much of it will be of a different type from that formerly most prominent. Competition in a form which causes one to lose what the other gets, and in which each profits in proportion to the losses of the other, as in war and seizure of territory, is giving place to competition for superiority in industrial, artistic, and intellectual lines in which the gains of all are greater because each stimulates the others to higher efficiency.

This change has been brought about partly because of developments which have given all nations common economic and other interests, and partly because science has shown the remote results of actions. To kill another nation industrially or culturally, is to lose an important customer and a stimulating competitor. Figuratively speaking, the enlightened master of the world, instead of killing his neighbour's golden-egg-laying geese, will attempt to rear a better variety of his own which will give him much more gold.

Science and World Ethics

Religions, arts, traditions, industries, and many social customs will probably continue to preserve their local character for many generations, but modern machines will be introduced everywhere and with them some knowledge of science, which will more and more become a guide in dealing first with things, then with people and organizations.   Industries in all parts of the world are succeeding in proportion as science is the guide in dealing with materials, and in forming and conducting industrial organizations.   Humanitarian and other organizations are looking to science for guidance, and ultimately science will be asked to help direct social, moral, and religious activities of all sorts.

There is no such thing as individual and national diversities in science.   In its very nature it is general, impersonal, and verified by the same sort of objective facts.   There may be a national art, literature, or religion, but not a national science.   Whatever degree of certainty and exactness it may attain in any field can be utilized everywhere.   This means that as science is invoked to help solve social and ethical problems it will endorse the same sort of procedure in all parts of the world, in so far as conditions are the same.   As shown above, similarity in cultures is rapidly increasing as scientific knowledge accumulates.

In the meantime the variations in codes temporarily prescribed by science for different countries will be analogous to the individual prescriptions in physical and mental hygiene, but no less in accord with general truths of science.   Everywhere the causes discovered in one country will have the same effects as in another country in so far as conditions are the same.   Science will therefore be able to show each nation how to bring about a better balance of important activities without at once adopting exactly the same codes.

With all nations brought into close relations with all others and guided by common scientific knowledge in controlling their environment and directing their activities, the people of all nations will become more and more alike.   Special adaptations will continue, but economic and ethical behaviour will rapidly become more uniform. Religious practices, arts, and some social customs, will longer retain their national characteristics. New conditions and inventive genius of individuals will continue to produce variations, but science will more and more determine what ones shall survive by showing their immediate and remote effects upon all phases of human living. Scientific selection will determine what cultures shall survive just as nature determines what species shall continue to live. Thus will man, the master of life, order his own life, not merely by his individual intelligence and the experience of his ancestors, but by the accumulated results of scientific research into the truths of nature and human nature.

SELECTED RESEARCHES

"ECOLOGICAL CONDITIONS IN NATIONAL FORESTS AND IN NATIONAL PARKS." By Dr. CHARLES C. ADAMS, N.Y. State College of Forestry, Syracuse, N.Y. From *Scientific Monthly*, June 1925. *Quoted by Permission.*

Conditions in the Grand Canyon National Park : . . . The ecological conditions were already greatly modified from a natural wild park when it became a national park. . . . This excessive overgrazing has made the south rim of the canyon as severely overgrazed, primarily by domestic animals, as is the north rim in the Grand Canyon Game Preserve, with its excessive number of deer and domestic animals, combined. This is a deplorable condition, which influences the wild life, changes the character of the vegetation, favours the erosion of the soil and produces conditions directly the opposite of the intention of a national park. . . .

At the Toronto meeting of the Ecological Society of America on December 28, 1921, it passed the following resolutions :

Whereas one of the primary duties of the National Park Service is to pass on to future generations, unimpaired, the wilderness of the parks, including their native plants and animals ; and

Whereas there are many educational and scientific reasons why the native plants and animals should remain unmixed through importations of other organisms not native to the parks ; therefore be it

Resolved, That the introduction of non-native plants and animals in our National Parks be *strictly forbidden* by the park authorities, it being expressly intended that the planting of non-native trees, shrubs, and other plants, as well as the stocking of waters with fish not native to the region, is strongly opposed. . . .

"SOME STATISTICAL ASPECTS OF LIVINGNESS." By Professor D. FRASER-HARRIS, London, England. From *The Scientific Monthly*, August 1927. *Quoted by Permission.*

Dr. Waller placed a seed of the scarlet runner (Phaseolus) in connection with a sensitive galvanometer, and stimulated the seed by passing through it the discharge from a Leyden jar. As a result of this, the seed made a " response " whose electrical counterpart was seen and measured in the galvanometer. The electro-motive force of these momentary currents can be measured in fractions of a volt.

The following table gives the results at a glance, when seeds ranging from one to five years old were stimulated :

Years Old.						Volts.
1	.	.	.	.	.	0·0170
2	.	.	.	.	.	0·0050
3	.	.	.	.	.	0·0043
4	.	.	.	.	.	0·0036
5	.	.	.	.	.	0·0014

These investigations are particularly interesting both on account of their novelty and their exactitude. We can say, for instance, that the four-year-old seed was 4·72 times less alive than the seed one year old. Or we can state that the one-year-old seed was twelve times more living than the five-year-old. The great accuracy of this method is due to the fact that the measurement of the electro-motive force of currents in the galvanometer is so precise. . . .

Accordingly we find the most striking quantitative differences between the various rates of propagation of nerve-impulses in animals arranged in an ascending scale. The rate is stated in metres per second :

Animal.						Rate of Nerve Impulse, Metres per Second.
Limulus, a crab (nerves of heart)			.	.		0·40
Limax, a slug	.	.	.	.	.	1·25
Cuttle-fish	.	.	.	.	.	2·00
Limulus (nerves of body)			.	.	.	3·25
Hagfish	.	.	.	.	.	4·50
Lobster	.	.	.	.	.	12·00
Snake	.	.	.	.	.	.	14·00
Frog	.	.	.	.	.	.	28·00
Man	.	.	.	.	.	.	120·00

From these results we are permitted to say that the intensity of livingness in a human nerve is ten times that of the nerve of a lobster, thirty times that of a hagfish and sixty times that of a cuttle-fish. . . .

The physiologists can estimate the amount of oxygen in the blood going to a muscle and also the oxygen in the blood coming from the muscle, the difference between these being the quantity of this gas retained by the muscle selected.

In the following table, a muscle in four different physiological conditions was investigated—fully active, gently active, in true physiological repose (that is, not contracting at all), and finally after its nerves had been severed.

State of Muscle (Cat).	Cc. of Oxygen Absorbed per Gram of Muscle per Minute.
Fully active	0·08
Gently active	0·02
In true physiological rest	0·006
After nerves were cut	0·003

Here we have a quantitative chemical method which enables us to say that a muscle in full contraction is thirteen times as active as it is when at rest. . . .

The same chemical method has been successfully applied to the study of the livingness of the heart of the cat. It was found that when that organ was beating normally, it utilized 0·014 cc. of oxygen per gram per minute. When it was artificially stimulated to extreme activity, the figure rose to 0·08 ; but when on the other hand, it had become slow and feeble, the figure sank to 0·007. . . .

The living glands have been investigated in exactly the same way, as the following table shows :

Type of Gland.	Cc. of Oxygen Utilized per Gram per Minute.
Pancreas (acting normally)	0·03
,, (stimulated artificially)	0·10
Kidney (acting normally)	0·03
,, (stimulated)	0·07
Liver (in inanition)	0·005
,, (well nourished)	0·05

. . . The liver in a starving condition is ten times less alive than when thoroughly nourished.

A rather different line of research may be pursued.

The more sluggish a muscle or other organ is, the longer it can survive after the death of the animal of which it was a part. For it must be remembered that an animal can die as a whole (somatic death) and yet its various tissues, for instance its muscles, can live for longer or shorter periods.

Thus, whereas the muscle of the human heart is alive two hours after bodily death, the body muscles are alive five to six hours thereafter. And whereas the muscles of a rabbit will live for eight and a half hours after the death of the animal, those of a sheep will survive for ten and a half, those of a dog for eleven and three-quarters, those of the cat twelve and a half, and those of the frog for from twenty-four to forty hours.

There is still another method open to us, at least as regards a muscle, namely, to calculate the time occupied by the muscle in performing a single act of shortening or the twitch. If we compare two types, the one of extreme sluggishness such as the muscles of the tortoise, and the other of extreme activity, such as the wing-muscle of a wasp, we shall find that, whereas the former takes 1·8 seconds to perform a single shortening, the

2 B

latter takes only 0·009 of a second. In other words, the wasp's muscle " works " two hundred times as rapidly as the tortoise's.

The notion of speed in connection with life is by no means unfamiliar. . . .

This absorption of oxygen is directly proportional to the muscular activity of the animal.

A horse at rest, walking and trotting absorbs per minute 1·6, 4·7 and 8 litres of oxygen, respectively. Therefore, the intensity of its muscular activity is five times greater when trotting than when at rest. . . .

SUGGESTED READINGS

The development of life on earth is described in the following books :

MASON, FRANCIS, ed., *Creation by Evolution*, 1928.
MORGAN, J. DE, *Prehistoric Man*, 1924.
OSBORN, HENRY F., *Origin and Evolution of Life*, 1917.
PERRIER, EDWARD, *The Earth before History*, 1925.

Many researches upon the biological value of various species have been published by the United States Department of Agriculture. Sample studies of the earth's product in relation to ecology and human utilization are summarized in three articles : COHN, ALVIN R., in *Ecology*, July 1929, presents evidence that the introduction of carp into a small lake resulted in the diminution of vegetation in the lake, and the extinction of several native species of fish. BARNES, CARLETON P., " Land Resource Inventory in Michigan," *Economic Geography*, Jan. 1929, reports the work of a committee of the Michigan Academy of Science appointed to investigate cut-over lands, which has developed methods of determining which portions may best be used for reforestation, recreational purposes, water-power, preservation of wild life and agricultural products of various kinds. FABER, HAROLD, *A New Method of Comparing the Productivity of Crops on Arable Land in England, Wales, Scotland and Denmark*, shows the relative productivity of these countries by statistics of dry matter produced per acre, and measurements of the relative food-value for men and animals of the different crops produced. For the years 1923–27 the figures are : England and Wales, 40 ; Scotland, 43·4 ; Denmark, 50·2.

The interrelations of men are presented in three recent books :

GIBBONS, HERBERT A., *Nationalism and Internationalism*, 1930.
RANDALL, JOHN H., *A World Community*, 1930.
STRATTON, G. N., *Social Psychology of International Relations*, 1929.

INDEX